Techniques in Knee Surgery

Techniques in Knee Surgery

■

Editors

Christopher D. Harner, M.D.

Professor
Department of Orthopaedic Surgery
University of Pittsburgh
Pittsburgh, Pennsylvania

Kelly G. Vince, M.D., F.R.C.S. (C)

Associate Professor
Department of Orthopaedic Surgery
University of Southern California
USC University Hospital
Los Angeles, California

Freddie H. Fu, M.D., D. SC. (Hon)

David Silver Professor and Chairman
Department of Orthopaedic Surgery
University of Pittsburgh
Chief
Department of Orthopaedic Surgery
UPMC Presbyterian
Pittsburgh, Pennsylvania

Associate Editor

Patrick E. Greis, M.D.

Assistant Professor
Department of Orthopaedic Surgery
University of Utah
Salt Lake City, Utah

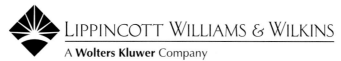

LIPPINCOTT WILLIAMS & WILKINS

A **Wolters Kluwer** Company

Philadelphia • Baltimore • New York • London
Buenos Aires • Hong Kong • Sydney • Tokyo

Acquisitions Editor: James Merritt
Developmental Editor: Sarah Fitz-Hugh
Production Editor: Jodi Borgenicht
Manufacturing Manager: Colin Warnock
Cover Designer: Karen Quigley
Compositor: Maryland Composition

© 2001 by LIPPINCOTT WILLIAMS & WILKINS
530 Walnut Street
Philadelphia, PA 19106 USA
LWW.com

Printed and bound in China

Library of Congress Cataloging-in-Publication Data

Techniques in knee surgery/editors, Christopher D. Harner, Kelly G. Vince, Freddie H. Fu.
   p. ; cm.
   Includes bibliographical references and index.
   ISBN 0-683-18048-7
   1. Knee—Surgery—Atlases. 2. Knee—Wounds and injuries—Atlases. 3.
Knee—Diseases—Atlases. I. Harner, Christopher D. II. Vince, Kelly G. III. Fu, Freddie H.
[DNLM: 1. Knee—surgery—Atlases. 2. Knee Injuries—surgery—Atlases. 3. Knee
Prosthesis—Atlases. 4. Ligaments, Articular—surgery—Atlases. 5. Patellar
Ligament—surgery—Atlases. 6. Surgical Procedures, Operative—methods—Atlases. WE
17 T2555 2000]
RD561.T43 2000
617.5′82—dc21

                                                       00-038431

---

10 9 8 7 6 5 4 3 2 1

To Dr. John Insall who as a surgeon, teacher, and investigator has been an inspiration to so many of us.

■ CONTENTS

Contributing Authors   ix
Preface   xiii

1. Arthroscopic Meniscal Repair   1
   Mark Miller and Christopher G. Palmer

2. Meniscal Allograft Reconstruction: An Arthroscopically Assisted Technique   10
   Darren L. Johnson and Raymond L. Neef

3. Microfracture Procedure for Treatment of Full-thickness Chondral Defects:
   Technique, Clinical Results, and Current Basic Science Status   23
   *J. Richard Steadman, William G. Rodkey, Steven B. Singleton,
   Karen K. Briggs, Juan J. Rodrigo, and C. Wayne McIlwraith*

4. Articular Autologous Chondrocyte Transplant   32
   Ronald A. Navarro and Freddie H. Fu

5. Endoscopic Anterior Cruciate Ligament Reconstruction with Patellar
   Tendon Substitution   41
   Bernard R. Bach, Jr.

6. Endoscopic Anterior Cruciate Ligament Reconstruction Using a Double
   Looped Hamstring Tendon Graft   57
   Todd M. Swenson

7. Two-incision Miniarthrotomy Technique for Anterior Cruciate Ligament
   Reconstruction with Autogenous Patellar Tendon Graft   73
   K. Donald Shelbourne and Thomas E. Klootwyk

8. Arthroscopic-assisted Posterior Cruciate Ligament Reconstruction   83
   Jonathan B. Ticker and Christopher D. Harner

9. Acute and Chronic Injuries to the Lateral Corner: The Popliteus
   and the Lateral Collateral Ligament   95
   Peter T. Simonian and Answorth A. Allen

10. Multiple Ligament Reconstruction   108
    John C. L'Insalata, Paul A. Dowdy, and Christopher D. Harner

11. Technique of Lateral Retinacular Release and Anteromedial Tibial
    Tubercle Transfer   123
    John P. Fulkerson

12. Patellar Instability: Proximal and Distal Realignment   130
    Joseph Abate, Richard D. Parker, and Gary J. Calabrese

13. Surgical Management of Chondral and Osteochondral Lesions of the Knee   140
    Russell S. Petrie, John J. Klimkiewicz, and Christopher D. Harner

14. Arthroscopic Treatment of Degenerative Joint Disease of the Knee   159
    Ashok S. Reddy and Ralph A. Gambardella

15. Subvastus Surgical Approach for Total Knee Arthroplasty   165
    F. Daniel Kharrazi and Kelly G. Vince

16. Surgical Technique for Tibial Tuberosity Elevation   171
    Jeffrey D. Gollish

17. High Tibial Osteotomy: Technique of Plate Fixation   178
     Robert W. Chandler

18. Distal Femoral Osteotomy   186
     Peter J. Evans and Anthony Miniaci

19. Fresh Osteochondral Allografts for Posttraumatic Knee Defects   193
     Allan E. Gross

20. Patellofemoral Replacement   202
     Domenick J. Sisto

21. Surgical Technique for Posterior Cruciate Retaining and Posterior Cruciate
     Substituting Total Knee Arthroplasties   209
     Peter J. Thadani and Kelly G. Vince

22. The Meniscal Bearing Knee   221
     Paolo Aglietti, John N. Insall, Francesco Giron, and Peter S. Walker

23. Soft Tissue Releases for the Valgus Knee   231
     Kelly G. Vince

24. Soft Tissue Releases for the Varus Knee   239
     Kelly G. Vince

25. Reconstruction of Tibial Defects   245
     Sevan G. Ortaaslan and Kelly G. Vince

26. Correction of Fixed Flexion Contracture in Total Knee Replacement   257
     Andrew G. Urquhart and Clifford W. Colwell

27. Supracondylar Fractures Following Total Knee Replacement   264
     Merrill A. Ritter

28. Removal of Metal-backed Patellar Button   268
     Douglas A. Dennis and Anne B. Szymanski

29. Extensor Mechanism Reconstruction with a Semitendinosus Graft   274
     Gerard A. Engh

30. Choices in Coverage for Wound Problems Following Total Knee Replacement   280
     Neil E. Klein

31. Technique of Three-step Revision Total Knee Arthroplasty   291
     Kelly G. Vince

Subject Index   305

■ CONTRIBUTING AUTHORS

Joseph Abate
Orthopaedic Sports Fellow
Section of Sports Medicine
Department of Orthopaedics
The Cleveland Clinic Foundation
9500 Euclid Avenue
Cleveland, Ohio 44195

Paolo Aglietti, M.D.
Professor of Orthopaedic Surgery
First Orthopaedic Clinic
University of Florence
Largo Palagi
Florence
Italy

Answorth A. Allen, M.D.
Assistant Professor
Department of Surgery
Cornell Medical Center
1300 York Avenue
New York, New York 10021
Assistant Attending Physician
Hospital for Special Surgery
535 East 70th Street
New York, New York 10021

Bernard R. Bach, Jr., M.D.
Professor
Department of Orthopedic Surgery
Director
Sports Medicine Section
Rush Medical College
Rush Presbyterian-St. Luke's Medical Center
1725 W. Harrison
Chicago, Illinois 60612

Karen K. Briggs, MBA
Director
Clinical Research
Steadman Hawkins Sports Medicine
    Foundation
181 West Meadow Drive
Vail, Colorado 81645

Gary J. Calabrese, PT
Director
Sports Health Rehabilitation
Department of Orthopaedics
Cleveland Clinic Foundation
9500 Euclid Avenue
Cleveland, Ohio 44195

Robert W. Chandler, M.D.
Orthopaedic Surgeon
10666 North Torrey Pines Road
La Jolla, California 92037

Clifford W. Colwell, M.D.
Orthopaedic Surgeon
Kerlan-Jobe Orthopaedic Clinic
6801 Park Terrace Drive
Los Angeles, California 90045

Douglas A. Dennis, M.D.
Clinical Professor
Department of Mechanical Engineering
Colorado School of Engineering
1600 Illinois
Golden, Colorado 80401
Clinical Director
Rose Institute for Joint Replacement
Rose Medical Center
4567 East 9th Avenue
Denver, Colorado 80220

Paul A. Dowdy, M.D.
Orthopaedic Surgeon
Sports Medicine Institute
Chief
Department of Surgery
Heart of Florida Regional Medical Center
1705 US Highway 27 North
Davenport, Florida 33837

Gerard A. Engh, M.D.
Associate Clinical Professor
Department of Orthopedic Surgery
University of Maryland
22 South Greene Street
Baltimore, Maryland 21201
Active Staff
Department of Orthopedic Surgery
Inova-Mount Vernon
2501 Parkers Lane
Alexandria, Virginia 22306

Peter J. Evans, Ph.D., F.R.C.S. (C)
Assistant Professor
Department of Orthopaedic Surgery
Johns Hopkins University School of Medicine
Baltimore, Maryland

Freddie H. Fu, M.D., D.Sc. (Hon)
David Silver Professor and Chairman
Department of Orthopaedic Surgery
University of Pittsburgh
3471 5th Avenue
Pittsburgh, Pennsylvania 15213
Chief
Department of Orthopaedic Surgery
UPMC Presbyterian
200 Lothrop Street
Pittsburgh, Pennsylvania 15213

John P. Fulkerson, M.D.
Clinical Professor
Department of Orthopedic Surgery
University of Connecticut Medical School
270 Farmington Avenue
Farmington, Connecticut 06032

Ralph A. Gambardella, M.D.
Orthopaedic Surgeon
Kerlan-Jobe Orthopaedic Clinic
6801 Park Terrace Drive
Los Angeles, California 90045
Orthopaedic Consultant
Los Angeles Dodgers
Associate Clinical Professor
Department of Orthopaedics
University of Southern California

Francesco Giron, M.D.
Assistant in Orthopaedics
First Orthopaedic Clinic
University of Florence
Largo P. Palagi 1
Florence 50134
Italy

Jeffrey D. Gollish, M.D., F.R.C.S.C.
Lecturer
Department of Surgery
University of Toronto
Director
Arthroplasty Service
Orthopaedic and Arthritic Institute
Sunnybrook and Womens College Health
   Sciences Center
43 Wellesley Street East
Toronto, Ontario
Canada M4Y 1H1

Allan E. Gross, M.D., F.R.C.S.C.
Professor
Department of Surgery
University of Toronto
Division Head
Orthopaedic Surgery
Mount Sinai Hospital
600 University Avenue
Toronto, Ontario
Canada M5G 1X5

Christopher D. Harner, M.D.
Professor
Department of Orthopaedic Surgery
University of Pittsburgh
4601 Baum Boulevard
Pittsburgh, Pennsylvania 15213

John N. Insall, M.D.
Professor
Department of Orthopedic Surgery
Albert Einstein College of Medicine
Bronx, New York
Chief
Adult Knee Reconstruction
Department of Orthopedic Surgery
Beth Israel Medical Center
New York, New York

Darren L. Johnson, M.D.
Chairman of Orthopaedic Surgery
Department of Surgery
University of Kentucky School of Medicine
Kentucky Clinic, K415
Associate Professor of Surgery
Department of Surgery
Albert B. Chandler Medical Center
800 Rose Street
Lexington, Kentucky 40536

F. Daniel Kharrazi, M.D.
Kerlan-Jobe Orthopaedic Clinic
6801 Park Terrace Drive
Los Angeles, California 90045

Neil E. Klein, M.D.
Attending Physician
Department of Surgery
Downey Regional Medical Center
11500 Brookshire Avenue
Downey, California 90241

John J. Klimkiewicz, M.D.
Clinical Instructor
Department of Orthopaedic Surgery
Georgetown University Medical Center
3800 Reservoir Road NW
Washington, DC 20007

Thomas E. Klootwyk, M.D.
Clinical Instructor
Department of Orthopaedic Surgery
Indiana University School of Medicine
1120 South Drive
Orthopaedic Surgeon
Methodist Sports Medicine Center
1815 North Capitol Avenue
Indianapolis, Indiana 46202

John C. L'Insalata, M.D.
Orthopaedic Surgeon
Orthopaedic Surgical Consultants
9921 4th Avenue
Brooklyn, New York 11209

C. Wayne McIlwraith, D.V.M., Ph.D.
Professor and Director
Equine Sciences and Orthopaedic Research
Colorado State University
Fort Collins, Colorado 80521

Mark D. Miller, M.D.
Orthopaedic Surgeon
W.B. Carroll Memorial Clinic
2909 Lemmon Avenue
Dallas, Texas 75204

Anthony Miniaci, M.D., F.R.C.S.(C)
Head
Sports Medicine Program
Division of Orthopaedic Surgery
University of Toronto
Toronto Hospital
Western Division, ECW 1-036
399 Bathurst Street
Toronto, Ontario
Canada M5T 1S8

Ronald A. Navarro, M.D.
Orthopaedic Surgeon
Kaiser Orthopaedics
25825 South Vermont Avenue
Harbor City, California 90710

Raymond L. Neef, M.D.
Sports Medicine Fellow
Division of Orthopaedics
Section of Sports Medicine
University of Kentucky
Lexington, Kentucky 40536

Sevan G. Ortaaslan, M.D.
Jan W. Duncan Orthopedics
1700 Caesar Chavez Avenue
Los Angeles, California 90033

Christopher G. Palmer, M.D.
Staff Orthopaedic Surgeon
Major, USAFA, MC
4102 Pinion Drive
USAFA, Colorado 80840–1000

Richard D. Parker, M.D.
Head
Section of Sports Medicine
Department of Orthopaedics
The Cleveland Clinic Foundation
9500 Euclid Avenue
Cleveland, Ohio 44195

Russell S. Petrie, M.D.
Staff Surgeon
Department of Orthopaedic Surgery
Hoag Memorial Presbyterian Hospital
1 Hoag Drive
Newport Beach, California 92663

Ashok S. Reddy, M.D.
Peachtree Orthopedic Clinic
2001 Peachtree Road NE
Atlanta, Georgia 30309

Merrill A. Ritter, M.D.
Professor
Department of Orthopaedics
Indiana University School of Medicine
1120 South Drive
Indianapolis, Indiana 46202

William G. Rodkey, DVM
Director, Basic Science Research
Steadman Hawkins Sports Medicine
    Foundation
181 West Meadow Drive
Suite 1000
Vail, Colorado 81657

Juan J. Rodrigo, M.D.
Professor and Surgeon
Department of Orthopaedics
University of California
Davis Medical Center
4860 Y Street
Sacramento, California 95817

K. Donald Shelbourne, M.D.
Assistant Professor
Department of Orthopaedics
Indiana University School of Medicine
1120 South Drive
Orthopaedic Surgeon
Methodist Sports Medicine Center
1815 North Capitol Avenue
Indianapolis, Indiana 46202

Peter T. Simonian, M.D.
Chief, Sports Medicine
Associate Professor
Department of Orthopaedic Surgery
University of Washington
Box 356500
Seattle, Washington 98195

Steven B. Singleton, M.D.
Clinical Associate
Steadman Hawkins Clinic
181 West Meadow Drive
Suite 1000
Vail, Colorado 81657

Domenick J. Sisto, M.D.
Fellowship Director
Sports Medicine
Los Angeles Orthopaedic Institute
4955 Van Nuys Boulevard
Sherman Oaks, California 91403

J. Richard Steadman, M.D.
Orthopaedic Surgeon and Principal
Steadman Hawkins Clinic
Steadman Hawkins Sports Medicine
    Foundation
181 West Meadow Drive
Vail, Colorado 81657

Todd M. Swenson, M.D.
Department of Orthopedic Surgery
Riverview Clinic
Dean Medical Center
580 North Washington Street
Janesville, Wisconsin 53547

Anne B. Szymanski, B.A.
Director of Clinical Research
Denver Orthopedic Specialists, PC
1601 East 19th Avenue
Denver, Colorado 80218

Jonathan B. Ticker, M.D.
Assistant Clinical Professor of Orthopaedic
    Surgery
Columbia University College of Physicians &
    Surgeons
630 West 168th Street
New York, New York 10032
Island Orthopaedics & Sports Medicine, PC
660 Broadway
Massapequa, New York 11758

Peter J. Thadani, M.D.
Attending Physician
Kerlan-Jobe Orthopaedic Clinic
2400 East Katella
Anaheim, California 82806

Andrew G. Urquhart, M.D.
Maumee Bay Orthopedics, Inc.
2702 Navarre
Oregon, Ohio 43616

Kelly G. Vince, M.D., F.R.C.S. (C)
Associate Professor
Department of Orthopaedic Surgery
University of Southern California
USC University Hospital
1450 San Pablo Street
Los Angeles, California 90033

Peter S. Walker, Ph.D.
Professor
Biomedical Engineering
Cooper Union
51 Astor Place
New York, New York 10003
Honorary Professor
Biomedical Engineering
Royal National Orthopaedic Hospital
Stanmore, London
England HA7 4LP

■ *PREFACE*

We had the many thousands of words in the original edition of *Knee Surgery*. Now we have the pictures. Virtually every expert in the field of knee surgery in the United States and several experts from abroad contributed to the original text that described the history, science, decision making, and techniques that enable surgeons to fix the many things that can go wrong with the human knee. Clearly, if surgeons need and want amplification of any aspect of their craft, it is in the actual, hands-on surgical technique, the translation of words into action. Nothing can accomplish this better than an illustrated atlas.

This atlas demonstrates the innuendo of surgical procedures that are performed every day by thousands of surgeons worldwide, in the words and images of surgeons who themselves have performed many thousands of procedures. Surgical solutions to unusual problems that may only be encountered unexpectedly several times in a career have been included. The atlas covers small facets of larger procedures—the tips and tricks that make the long procedure safer, shorter, and more effective. The visual approach is essential, etching itself in the memory perhaps more reliably than words can, ready for retrieval when the moment arrives.

Surgeons live in a visual universe and our patients thrive on our ability to interpret and assimilate what we see and touch. Just as the student initially compiles conceptual, written information and then moves on to visualization of the surgical procedure before participating in real surgical procedures, all surgeons must incorporate, conceptualize, and then visualize information. What better way to see ourselves doing the procedure than to have an image to study? In this regard *Techniques in Knee Surgery* is the inevitable and necessary picture that is worth a thousand words.

Kelly G. Vince, M.D., F.R.C.S.C.

Techniques in Knee Surgery

MARK MILLER
CHRISTOPHER G.
PALMER

1

Arthroscopic Meniscal Repair

Although the first open meniscal repair is thought to have been performed by Annandale in 1885 (1), it has taken a century for the procedure to become popular. In 1936 King (2) first reported meniscal healing in a series of canine experiments. It also was King who first described postmeniscectomy degenerative arthritis. In 1948 Fairbank (3) published the classic description of postmeniscectomy degenerative changes seen on radiographs. Nevertheless, it would be several years before partial meniscectomy replaced total meniscectomy as standard of care in the treatment of meniscal injury.

Pioneers of open meniscal repair include Dehaven (3a), Henning (4), and others who did clinical studies which helped to popularize this technique. It was not until the mid-1970s that arthroscopic meniscal repair first was described in a small series of patients by Ikeuchi (5). More recent proponents of arthroscopic meniscal repair including Henning (4), Cannon and Vittori (6), and others have encouraged surgeons to "save the meniscus" whenever possible.

Open meniscal repair generally is limited to peripheral tears within several millimeters of the meniscosynovial junction of the posterior one third of the lateral or medial meniscus. Although there are advantages and disadvantages to the arthroscopic inside-out and outside-in meniscal repair techniques, the indications are similar and the choice is largely a function of surgeon's preference. Indications for meniscal repair are based on a firm understanding of meniscal function and the literature. Other important considerations include patient age; chronicity, type, size, and location of the tear; and associated ligamentous injuries.

Menisci have been shown in biomechanical studies to play an important role in load transmission, transmitting approximately 50% of the weight-bearing forces in extension, and 85% in flexion. Meniscectomy reduces this function by 50 to 70% (7). The menisci also have been shown to be important in joint stability and congruity (8), joint lubrication and nutrition (9), and shock absorption during the gait cycle.

Successful meniscal repair is linked intimately to an adequate peripheral blood supply. Arnoczky and Warren (10) described the microvascular anatomy of the meniscus in 1982. They demonstrated a perimeniscal plexus that supplied the peripheral 10 to 25% of the meniscus. This landmark work resulted in a classification of meniscal tear zones based on location and corresponding vascular supply: zone 1, or red–red zone, at the periphery of the meniscus completely within the vascular plexus with excellent healing potential; zone 2, the red–white zone, at the border of the vascular zone with good healing potential; and zone 3, the white–white zone, within the avascular region of the meniscus with poor healing potential (Fig. 1-1).

Preoperative information obviously plays a role in treatment of meniscal injuries. There are well-described physical findings and imaging studies to identify meniscal tears, but our review of the literature revealed no consistent findings to predict whether a meniscal tear likely is suitable for repair. Diagnostic studies such as double-contrast arthrography still are useful tools in evaluating meniscal lesions. A vertical tear near the meniscosynovial

■ HISTORY OF THE
TECHNIQUE

■ INDICATIONS AND
CONTRAINDICATIONS

1

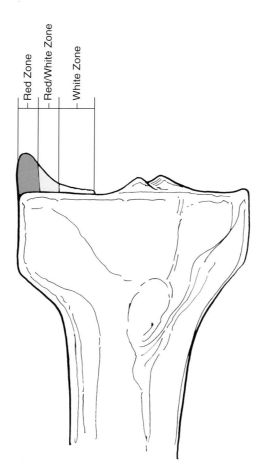

Red Zone

Red/White Zone

White Zone

FIGURE 1-1

Meniscal zones are based on healing potential. The red–red zone has the best healing potential.

junction with minimum staining of the meniscus indicates a high probability of a successful repair. More recently, with improved understanding and resolution of magnetic resonance imaging, arthrography largely has been replaced for the evaluation of meniscal tears. Accuracy of magnetic resonance imaging reportedly is 93 to 98% in detecting medial meniscal tears, and 90 to 96% for lateral meniscal tears (11).

The ideal candidate for meniscal repair is a relatively young individual with an acute, longitudinal tear of the meniscus that is 1 to 2 cm in length in the vascular peripheral zone, with an intact or reconstructed anterior cruciate ligament (ACL) (6). There seems to be little consensus on the indications outside these ideal parameters. Several studies have disputed the notion that the ability of a meniscal lesion to heal is dependent on the patient's age (12,13). Other basic science research, however, has confirmed that the healing stages of the meniscus mirror those of other connective tissues, suggesting that age and general condition do affect the outcome of attempted repairs (14). There has been some controversy concerning the ideal length of time between injury and repair. A recent study suggested that meniscus repair within 8 weeks of injury has better results. This study, however, made the observation that tears repaired after 8 weeks tended to be more complex (13).

One of the most important clinical factors is the functional status of the ACL. Several investigators have reported markedly decreased healing rates in ACL-deficient knees (6,15). Lynch et al. (16) reported better success in ACL reconstructions that included meniscal repair for associated meniscal tears rather than partial or total meniscectomy (16). The rate of successful meniscal repair is reportedly higher with simultaneous ACL reconstruction because of increased biomechanical stability and hemarthrosis, which may stimulate meniscal healing.

Relative contraindications to repair include tears that are considered stable, such as partial-thickness tears, or those that cannot be displaced more than several millimeters from the peripheral rim. These tears are best left alone. Other contraindications are complex tears in which an anatomic reduction of the torn meniscal edges is not feasible, such as degenerative tears with multiple cleavage planes or multiple levels of longitudinal tearing. These tears are treated best with partial meniscectomy. Tears in the relatively avascular zones of the meniscus are also relative contraindications for repair.

Anesthesia Anesthesia is largely a matter of surgeon's preference. Traditionally, arthroscopy has been carried out under general anesthesia or regional block. Local anesthesia using either a single preoperative injection or continuous infusion has been described as a reasonable alternative to general or regional anesthetics. Martin et al. (17) detailed a technique using 20 to 25 mL of 1% lidocaine with 1:200,000 units of epinephrine to infiltrate portal sites and 20 mL of 0.25% marcaine with epinephrine mixed with 10 mL of 1% lidocaine with epinephrine for intraarticular injection. There are several potential problems associated with the use of local anesthetic in knee arthroscopy. Although the addition of epinephrine theoretically makes the use of a tourniquet unnecessary, this is often not the case. Patients often become intolerant of a tourniquet placed on an unnanesthetized thigh after 20 to 30 minutes. Also, patients with relatively tight knees requiring moderate valgus and varus stress for joint visualization may experience undue discomfort with only a local anesthetic. Finally, patients may move their legs spontaneously at inopportune times. It is for these reasons our preference is for general or regional anesthetic.

Surface Anatomy Before beginning any arthroscopy with or without anticipated meniscal repair, it is important to understand relationships of surface anatomic landmarks and to be able to mark them accurately. The patella, the medial and lateral femoral condyles, the tibial plateau, the tibial tuburcle, both edges of the patellar tendon, and the fibular head all should be palpated and outlined with a marking pen. The posterior edge of the iliotibial band, the biceps femoris tendon, the lateral collateral and medial collateral ligaments, and the medial hamstring complex also should be palpated. Marking these structures before insufflation of the knee may facilitate later placement of portals and incisions.

Skin Incisions Several considerations need to be made before creating arthroscopy portals or surgical incisions. Regardless of the use of epinephrine in the arthroscopic saline, it is wise to place a tourniquet preoperatively as proximally as possible on the thigh, as a backup. Meniscal repair may be accomplished with a lateral post and the foot of the operating table extended, or with a circumferential thigh holder with the table flexed. Some surgeons prefer a lateral post, because they feel a thigh holder may limit knee flexion or exposure. We routinely use a thigh holder in conjunction with a tourniquet and have not found this to be a problem. Placing the tourniquet or thigh holder too distally, however, or placing the knee too close to the flex point in the operating room table may limit necessary exposure to the knee. It is also important to recognize that a tight thigh holder may have a tourniquet-like effect during extended procedures.

Standard diagnostic arthroscopy portals are used to identify a potentially repairable meniscal tear. Correct portal placement is crucial to allow complete visualization of both medial and lateral menisci. The use of a 70-degree arthroscope with a modification of the technique of Gillquist et al. (18) may be necessary for adequate inspection of the posteromedial joint. This is accomplished most easily with the knee in flexion as a blunt obturator is passed through it between the medial femoral condyle and the posterior cruciate ligament through the inferolateral portal. The edges of the torn meniscus and adjacent synovium are abraded with a motorized shaver or rasp prior to repair to stimulate blood flow and to remove any fibrinous debris that would hinder repair.

Outside-in Technique There are at least four techniques for meniscal repair: open, "outside-in," "inside-out," and the most recently developed, "all-inside." We describe what we believe to be the most popular methods. The outside-in technique of meniscal repair offers several advantages over open repair. It is more versatile, because it allows access to the an-

■ SURGICAL TECHNIQUES

terior and middle thirds of the meniscus. It also requires little in the way of expensive instrumentation. By using separate 1- to 2-cm incisions for each pair of sutures, there is also
less soft-tissue dissection around the neurovascular structures. These incisions are made
perpendicular to the joint line on the posteromedial or posterolateral corners of the knee.

For medial meniscal repair, positioning the knee in flexion has been recommended for
easier placement of sutures away from the saphenous nerve. The anatomic course of this
nerve must be understood before attempting dissection on the medial aspect of the knee.
Proximal to the joint line, the nerve lies deep to the investing fascia of the knee and the sartorius muscle as it runs along the muscle's posterior edge. The nerve may not emerge from
this subbfascial location until a point well distal to the joint, as it pierces the inferior portion of the sartorius. It is at this level that the nerve gives off its infrapatellar branch, with
the main branch continuing distally down the medial aspect of the leg with the greater
saphenous vein. The nerve often can be located by arthroscopic transillumination of the
skin on the posteromedial corner of the knee. Laterally, the peroneal nerve is at risk but
should be safe as long as the knee is flexed and there is proper identification of the biceps
femoris tendon. Dissection and needle passage must be kept anterior to the biceps.

After making the small skin incision, blunt dissection is utilized to spread subcutaneous
tissue carefully in a safe plane. A retractor is used to retract neurovascular structures posteriorly during the remainder of the repair. A prebent 18-gauge spinal needle then is
passed under direct arthroscopic visualization from outside the capsule and through the
meniscal tear. Repair generally is initiated in the most posterior portion of the tear. This
sometimes must be altered if visualization of the tear is obscured. The traditional approach

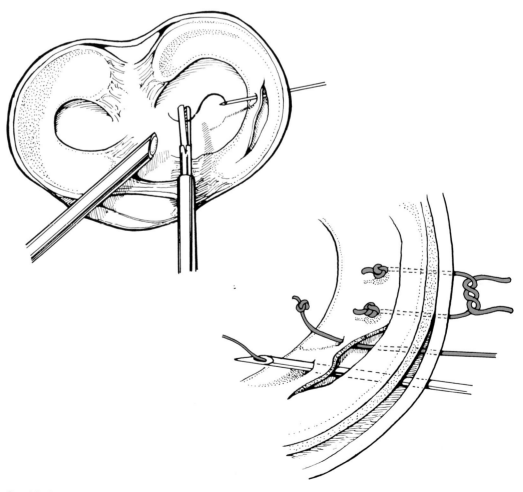

■ FIGURE 1-2   Outside-in technique for meniscal repair. Note that the knot captures the meniscus being repaired.

is to pass the suture through the femoral side of the meniscus, but this too may be altered based on tear configuration and the adequacy of reduction of the torn meniscal edges. With the needle passed across the tear into the joint, an arthroscopic probe or other instrument may be used to push the meniscus onto the needle, and the stylet is removed from the needle. A number 0 polydioxanone suture (PDS) then is passed through the needle into the joint, grasped, and pulled out through the ipsilateral anterior portal. A large "mulberry" knot is tied in the end of the suture before being pulled back into the joint until it abuts snugly against the meniscus (Fig. 1-2). Confirmation of an anatomic reduction of the torn meniscal edges then should be accomplished. A second suture is placed in the same manner 3 to 4 mm anterior to the previous suture.

There are several alternatives to this method of suture placement. One is to tie the loose ends of the two adjacent sutures together before pulling them back into the knee through the anterior portal instead of the individual knots. This creates a horizontal mattress suture and somewhat decreases the mass of a potentially abrasive knot. Another option is to place sutures in a divergent fashion with inferior and superior limbs to achieve a vertical orientation of the sutures, as described by Henning (19). Still another variant of the outside-in technique utilizes a horizontal mattress suture without a knot remaining in the joint. This technique uses a wire loop passed through a second needle to capture the free end of the suture and pull it back through the meniscus. The free ends then are tied snugly to the outside of the capsule.

It generally is recommended that the sutures be spaced every 3 to 4 mm. Sutures should be placed to within a few millimeters of the apices of the tear. Care must be taken to avoid eversion of the torn edges or "puckering" of the meniscus. Any malreduction must be dealt with by suture removal and placement of sutures in another orientation. After suture placement the incisions are irrigated and closed in layers, according to surgeon's preference. We routinely use absorbable fascial and subcutaneous sutures followed by a running, nonabsorbable suture to be removed after 10 to 14 days. A standard knee dressing and brace then are applied.

Inside-out Technique   The inside-out technique of meniscal repair was popularized by Henning in the early 1980s (19). It is perhaps the most popular technique currently used for meniscal repair. In this technique, a similar setup, with a tourniquet and proximal thigh holder or lateral post, is utilized. Again standard diagnostic arthroscopy is carried out, using carefully positioned portals. The edges of the tear and adjacent synovium are rasped.

For medial meniscal tears, a 3- to 4-cm vertical incision is made centered on the joint at the posteromedial aspect of the knee. The placement of the incision may be facilitated by probing the posteromedial capsule just superior the the torn meniscus. The probe often can be palpated from the outside of the knee. The incision usually is located behind the medial collateral ligament. After the skin incision, blunt dissection is carried through the subcutaneous fat layer down to the sartorious fascia. Superior to the sartorius, the fascia is split proximally and distally for several centimeters with the knee kept in flexion. The underlying saphenous nerve and hamstring tendons are retracted medially and posteriorly, exposing the capsule. A popliteal, army–navy, spoon, or other retractor is used to protect these structures throughout the remainder of the repair.

During suture placement, a qualified asistant is crucial. The assistant is responsible not only for needle and suture retrieval but also for retraction of neurovascular structures. Sutures may be placed with the use of a single- or double-lumen cannula system. Specially designed curved Keith needles armed with absorbable 2-0 PDS or nonabsorbable ethibond suture are available commercially. Beginning 2 to 3 mm from the most posterior aspect of the tear, the cannula is placed through the contralateral portal and viewed from the ipsilateral portal. The needle is advanced slowly under strict control of the depth of passage, as the assistant carefully watches for the exiting needle. A thimble may be used by the assistant to palpate the exiting needle. A needle driver is used to retrieve the needle and pull the suture through the meniscus. The needle is cut from the suture, and a second suture is placed in a similar manner 3 to 4 mm anterior to the previous one in a horizontal fashion

(Fig. 1-3). For better coaptation of meniscal edges, some surgeons prefer sutures placed with a vertical orientation using superior and inferior limbs. Regardless of the suture orientation, it is necessary to confirm anatomic coaptation of the torn meniscal edges at this time. Repair then proceeds in a posterior to anterior direction at 3- to 4-mm intervals to within several millimeters of the anterior apex of the tear. It may be necessary to place the knee in more flexion for easier needle retrieval, but this may result in more difficult visualization of the posterior horn of the meniscus.

For lateral meniscal repair, the skin incision is centered on the posterolateral joint line, with the knee in 60 to 90 degrees of flexion. The incision is extended several centimeters proximally and distally in the interval between the posterior aspect of the iliotibial band and anterior aspect of the biceps femoris. As described for medial meniscal repair, the placement of the skin incision may be facilitated by palpation of a probe against the capsule on the outside of the knee. The interval between the iliotibial band and biceps should be identified easily. Care must be taken in avoiding injury to the peroneal nerve by maintaining knee flexion and constant posterior retraction of the biceps femoris tendon.

After the skin incision, the next layer to be encountered is the lateral edge of the gastrocnemius tendon and the posterolateral capsule. These structures are separated by blunt dissection anterior to the gastrocnemius. This allows placement of a retractor and exposure of the capsule. The meniscal repair then may proceed in the manner described for the medial meniscus, using a single- or double-lumen cannula system. Although the double-lumen system may be somewhat faster, it allows less flexibility in placement of sutures. It must be remembered that the popliteal artery is just posterior to the posterior horn of the lateral meniscus. Careful passage of needles in proper orientation under direct vision to a competent and capable assistant is critical to avoid injury to neurovascular structures. After

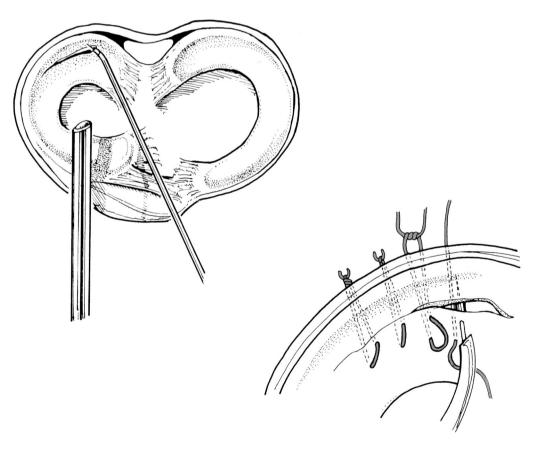

■ FIGURE 1-3

Inside-out technique for meniscal repair. Note that vertical structures provide the strongest repair.

completion of the repair, the wound is irrigated and closed in layers according to the surgeon's preference. A sterile dressing and knee brace then are applied.

Meniscal repair also may be accomplished using an open or all-inside technique. Open repair, as mentioned previously, generally is limited to peripheral tears within several millimeters of the meniscosynovial junction. In this location it may be possible to achieve a more anatomic reduction. The all-inside technique recently described by Morgan (20) may offer a cosmetic advantage and be somewhat faster for those well versed in the procedure, but long-term results are not yet available. Other newer techniques and devices using suture anchors or "arrows" have not been evaluated adequately in controlled clinical trials.

One of the considerations in meniscal repair is whether to use repair-augmentation procedures to optimize healing in a relatively avascular region of the meniscus. Arnoczky et al. (21) have reported successful use of exogenous fibrin clot in a canine model. The fibrin clot is felt to deliver a concentration of mitogenic and chemotactic factors to stimulate cells important in meniscal healing. This clot is made easily using 50 to 60 mL of the patient's blood mixed for several minutes in a glass beaker with a glass rod. The clot then is inserted through an arthroscopic cannula into the repair site just prior to the placement of sutures. The clot also may serve as a scaffolding for further vascular or fibrocartilaginous ingrowth.

Other investigators have reported the use of full-thickness vascular access channels from the periphery of the meniscus to a tear in a relatively avascular zone (14). Blood vessels critical for meniscal healing from the periphery then may grow through the channels. These vascular channels, however, may change the mechanical characteristics and stability of the meniscal rim by disrupting circumferential collagen bundles.

Complications associated with meniscal repair techniques include the general complications related to arthroscopy and those related specifically to meniscal repair. The overall complication rate of knee arthroscopy has been reported to be between 0.8 and 8.2% (22). Excluding failure to heal the repair and retearing, the most common complication of meniscal repair is neurovascular injury. In dissection of the posteromedial knee, the saphenous nerve and its infrapatellar branch are most at risk. Transection, or entrapment of this nerve with suture, may result in a painful neuroma. It cannot be overemphasized that careful dissection and retractor placement are critical to avoid these structures. Needles must be passed and tied under direct vision. The incidence of saphenous nerve injury has been reported between 1.2 and 2.5% (23). On the lateral side of the knee, care must be taken to avoid the popliteal artery and peroneal nerve. These structures are avoided by careful attention to dissection and retractor placement anterior to the biceps femoris with the knee in 60 to 90 degrees of flexion.

There is no consensus concerning the most effective rehabilitation following meniscal repair. There is debate concerning when to allow motion and when to allow weight bearing.

Traditional rehabilitation has allowed early motion but has not allowed weight bearing for 6 to 8 weeks. Some still advocate complete immobilization for 6 weeks following repair of a torn meniscus (24). Others have allowed full weight bearing in the early postoperative period with the knee locked in extension, believing tht the meniscus undergoes little translation with the screw-home mechanism in effect. Our preliminary research in goats (25) and the clinical work of others suggest that immobilization may be unnecessary. The trend is toward more accelerated rehabilitation, and early motion with partial weight bearing seems to cause no change in early clinical outcome. It is important to avoid hyperflexion and squatting activities for several months following repair. After 2 to 3 months, leg-strengthening exercises should be instituted. Paients usually return to activity as tolerated within 3 to 4 months postoperatively.

Most reports of arthroscopic meniscal repair are based on clinical rather than arthroscopic results and probably overestimate the successful healing rate. Morgan and Cascells

■ TECHNICAL ALTERNATIVES AND PITFALLS

■ REHABILITATION

■ OUTCOMES AND FUTURE DIRECTIONS

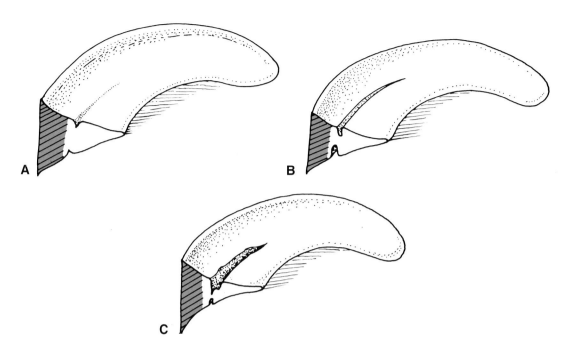

Assessment of healing. **A:** Healed (<10% cleft). **B:** Partially healed (≤50% cleft). **C:** Not healed (>50% cleft).

reported excellent clinical results in 98.6% of their outside-in repairs. Ryu and Dunbar (26) similarly reported clinical healing in 87% of their patients in a 2 year follow-up study.

Routine arthroscopic follow-up of meniscal repairs first was reported by Rosenberg et al. (27) in 1986. They found that at 3 months, 24 of 29 repaired menisci had healed completely. Four of the five that had not healed were in ACL-deficient knees (27). The assessment of healing generally is based on the amount of "residual cleft" at the original repair site (Fig. 1-4). A healed lesion has a cleft less than 10% of the meniscal thickness. A partially healed lesion has a cleft less than 50% of the thickness of the meniscus at any point along the repair. Using these criteria, the literature suggests a complete healing rate of 75 to 90%, partial or incomplete healing in 10 to 15%, and a failure of clinically significant meniscal healing in 5 to 10% (15,27,28).

Although meniscal repair, with proper patient selection, indications, and technique, has enjoyed good initial success, more long-term studies are needed. More research also is needed to document the effectiveness of augmentation procedures. Nonetheless, it is apparent that attempts to repair the meniscus are a much improved form of treatment for meniscal injury than meniscectomy.

References

1. Annandale T. An operation for displaced semilunar cartilage. *Br Med J* 1885; 1:779.
2. King D. The healing of the semilunar cartilages. *J Bone Joint Surg Am* 1936; 18:333–342.
3. Fairbank TJ. Knee joint changes after meniscectomy. *J Bone Joint Surg* 1948; 30B:664–670.
3a. Dehaven KE. Peripheral meniscus repair, an alternative to menisectory. *Ortho Trans* 1981; 5:399–400.
4. Henning CE. Arthroscopic repair of meniscus tears. *Orthopedics* 1983; 6:1130–1132.
5. Ikeuchi H. Surgery under arthroscopic control. *Rheumatology* 1976; 3(special issue):57–62.
6. Cannon WD, Vittori JM. The incidence of healing in arthroscopic meniscal repairs in anterior cruciate ligament reconstructed knees versus stable knees. *Am J Sports Med* 1992; 20:176–181.
7. Fukubayashi T, Kurasawa H. The contact area and pressure distribution pattern of the knee: A study of normal and osteoarthritic knee joints. *Acta Orthop Scand* 1980; 51:871–880.
8. Walker PS, Erkman MJ. The role of the menisci in force transmission across the knee. *Clin Orthop* 1975; 109:184–192.

9. MacConaill MA. The functions of intra-articular fibrocartilages with special reference to the knee and inferior radioulnar joints. *J Anat* 1932; 66:210–227.
10. Arnoczky SP, Warren RF. Microvasculature of the human meniscus. *Am J Sports Med* 1982; 10:90–95.
11. Jackson DW, Jennings LD, Maywood RM, et al. Magnetic resonance imaging of the knee. *Am J Sports Med* 1988; 16:29–47.
12. Hamberg P, Gillquist J, Lysholm J. Suture of new and old peripheral meniscus tears. *J Bone Joint Surg Am* 1983; 65:193–197.
13. Henning CE, Lynch MA, Yearout KM, et al. Arthroscopic meniscal reapir using an exogenous fibrin clot. *Clin Orthop* 1990; 252:64–72.
14. Cabaud HE, Rodkey WG, Fitzwater JE. Medial meniscus repairs: An experimental and morphological study. *Am J Sports Med* 1981; 9:129–134.
15. Morgan CK, Wojtys EM, Cassells CK. Arthroscopic meniscal repair evaluated by second look arthroscopy. *Am J Sports Med* 1991; 19:632–638.
16. Lynch MA, Henning CE, Glick KR. Knee joint surface changes: Long-term follow-up meniscus tear treatment in stable anterior cruciate ligament reconstruction. *Clin Orthop* 1983; 172:148–153.
17. Martin RC, Brown DE, Zell BK, et al. Diagnostic and operative arthroscopy of the knee under local anesthesia with parenteral medication. *Am J Sports Med* 1989; 17:436–439.
18. Gillquist J, Hagberg G, Oretorp N. Arthroscopic examination of the posteromedial compartment of the knee joint. *Int Orthop* 1979; 3:313.
19. Henning CE. Arthroscopic repair of meniscus tears. *Orthopedics* 1983; 6:1130–1132.
20. Morgan C. "All-inside" arthroscopic meniscus repair. *Sports Med Arthroscopy Rev* 1993; 1:152–158.
21. Arnoczky SP, Warren RF, Spivak JM. Meniscal repair using an exogenous fibrin clot: An experimental study in dogs. *J Bone Joint Surg Am* 1988; 70:1209–1220.
22. Delee JC. Complications of arthroscopy and arthoscopic surgery results of a national survey. *Arthroscopy* 1985; 1:214–220.
23. Small NC. Complications in arthroscopy: The knee and other joints. *Arthroscopy* 1986; 2:253–258.
24. DeHaven KE, Stone RC. Meniscal repair. In: Sahriaree H, ed. *O'Connor's textbook of arthroscopic surgery*. Philadelphia: JB Lippincott, 1992:327–338.
25. Miller MD, Ritchie JR, Gomez BA, et al. Meniscal repair: An experimental study in the goat. *Am J Sports Med* 1995:23:124–128.
26. Ryu RKN, Dunbar WH. Arthroscopic meniscal repair with two-year follow-up: A clinical review. *Arthroscopy* 1988; 4:168–173.
27. Rosenberg TD, Scott SM, Coward DB, et al. Arthroscopic meniscal repair evaluated by repeat arthroscopy. *Arthroscopy* 1986; 2:20.
28. Stone RG, Van Winkle GN. Arthroscopic review of meniscal repair: Assessment of healing parameters. *Arthroscopy* 1986; 2:77–81.

DARREN L. JOHNSON
RAYMOND L. NEEF

2

Meniscal Allograft Reconstruction: An Arthoscopically Assisted Technique

■ HISTORY OF THE
TECHNIQUE

Our increasing knowledge of the functions of the human meniscus has led to dramatic changes in the treatment of meniscal pathology. What began with complete meniscal resection has evolved into techniques for meniscal repair and replacement. Meniscal reconstruction is an attempt to preserve the important functions of the human meniscus; it is designed to increase contact area, improve force transmission, decrease contact stress, and support shock absorption, secondary mechanical stability, joint lubrication, and nutrition of chondrocytes (1,2). In performing a meniscal transplantation, the goal is to delay the progressive joint deterioration in those situations in which a total meniscectomy previously has been performed or the magnitude of meniscal injury is so severe so as to prohibit its preservation of structure and function (3,4).

■ INDICATIONS AND
CONTRAINDICATIONS

The indications for meniscal reconstruction currently are being defined. Because there is a lack of uniformity in patient selection, operative technique, follow-up criteria, and successful outcome, determining which patients may benefit most from isolated meniscal reconstruction is difficult. Preoperative variables to consider in deciding if a meniscal reconstruction is indicated include the patient's age, knee stability and alignment, and the degree of compartment wear. At present, it is believed that the patient must be experiencing symptoms of postmeniscectomy syndrome to be a candidate for reconstruction. In the future, prophylactic meniscal reconstruction (in asymptomatic patients) may be indicated in select cases.

The ideal candidate may be a young individual who has undergone complete meniscectomy and is predicted to develop significant degenerative changes. This is especially true of individuals who have undergone removal of the lateral meniscus. Because of the increased load-bearing function of the lateral meniscus, partial or complete removal results in accelerated degenerative changes in the lateral compartment. A second group of patients include those with ligamentous instability and with unrepairable or previously removed menisci. To improve stability within the anterior cruciate ligament (ACL) and medial meniscus–deficient knee, ACL reconstruction may be combined with medial meniscal reconstruction (2,5). By adding a medial meniscal allograft to a ligament reconstruction, improved stability may be achieved. Whether the allograft has any influence on the degenerative process on the joint surfaces has yet to be determined. Additionally, in the individual with posterolateral instability and absence of the lateral meniscus, a combined posterolateral reconstruction and lateral meniscal allograft may be warranted (6). Because of the convex geometry of the lateral compartment, a lateral meniscal allograft may help to control rotation and translation in the knee joint.

In two recent series reported by Garrett (7) and Noyes (8), it appears that meniscal transplantation has a much more predictable outcome in those patients who have only Outerbridge grade I or II articular disease (7,8). Inferior results were seen in those individuals with advanced compartment wear with Outerbridge grade III or IV articular disease or those individuals with incongruent articular services. Currently it is unknown whether meniscal reconstruction would benefit the middle-aged individual with full-thickness articular lesions who is a candidate for an osteotomy. Whether the osteotomy should be combined with the meniscal reconstruction is unclear; however, the reconstruction may improve the load-bearing characteristics of the compartment, decelerate the degenerative changes, and enhance the effect of the osteotomy. The potential of this treatment in this "patient" remains clearly investigational at this time.

Based on the available literature and reports to date, the ideal candidate for a meniscal reconstruction is one who meets the following criteria: 1) young (20–40 years of age) and symptomatic, with documented evidence of a near complete previous meniscectomy or the biomechanical equivalent of a total meniscectomy; 2) ligamentously stable, or ligamentous stability being achieved concurrently with the meniscal reconstruction; 3) Outerbridge grade I or II articular cartilage changes, as determined by the use of a 45-degree posteroanterior flexion weight-bearing radiograph as described by Rosenberg et al. (9); 4) no evidence of malalignment on standing long-cassette radiographs; and 5) failure of diagnostic arthroscopy at the time of reconstruction to reveal any Outerbridge grade IV articular changes or articular incongruity. It is extremely important during the preoperative counseling session to inform the patient that the final decision to perform the reconstruction is made in the operating suite. The authors have found only a small, select number of patients who fit this strict inclusion criteria; however, the results to date, although preliminary, have been encouraging.

■ SURGICAL TECHNIQUES

An arthroscopically assisted technique for meniscal reconstruction using fresh-frozen allograft tissue without disruption of the collateral ligaments or extensor mechanism is described. This technique, utilizing an allograft with preserved anterior and posterior meniscal-horn attachments to cylindrical bone plugs, emphasizes visualization of arthroscopic landmarks for each bony meniscal-horn insertion site, with creation of osseous tunnels at these corresponding sites to allow for anatomic seating of the meniscal allograft (Fig. 2-1).

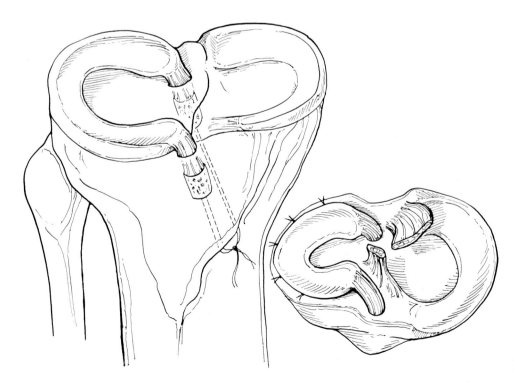

■ FIGURE 2-1

Schematic drawing showing our technique of lateral meniscal reconstruction, with meniscal horns preserved as bone plugs placed into osseous tunnels.

Anesthesia and Patient Positioning   Once satisfactory general or regional anesthesia has been completed, a detailed examination under anesthesia is performed. Integrity of the primary and secondary restraints for each of the six degrees of freedom must be documented. Failure to correct preexisting instability at the time of meniscal reconstruction often leads to surgical failure. The nonoperative leg is placed into a well-leg support that flexes, externally rotates, and abducts the hip and also flexes the knee, thereby moving the unaffected extremity out of the operative field. A well-padded tourniquet is placed proximally on the operative extremity, which then is placed in an arthroscopic leg holder. The foot of the table is flexed to allow for 120 degrees of unrestricted knee flexion.

Diagnostic Arthroscopy and Bed Preparation   Standard anteromedial and anterolateral portals are used for diagnostic arthroscopy to confirm that the patient is a candidate for meniscal reconstruction. Those patients who have higher degrees of articular cartilage damage or articular incongruity are excluded from transplantation. Once a decision has been made to perform the transplant, meticulous preparation of the host bed is done to ensure anatomic positioning and maximal healing potential.

Using a meniscal resector, remaining meniscal tissue is debrided back to the meniscal–capsular junction to ensure peripheral vascular supply to the allograft menisci. Working on the posterior horns of the medial and lateral menisci requires the use of a 70-degree arthroscope and creation of accessory posteromedial and posterolateral portals. Debridement is continued until a meniscal remnant of 1 to 2 mm remains; this acts as a scaffold to help keep the meniscal substitute from translocating inferiorly on the tibia. A rasp is used to abrade the synovium on the superior and inferior surfaces of the meniscal remnant throughout its entirety, to stimulate the perimeniscal capillary plexus, as is done for meniscal repair.

Graft Selection, Sizing, and Preparation   Although autogenous tendons, fat pad, fresh meniscal allograft, and collagen scaffold all have been described as meniscal substitutes, the technique being described here involves the use of fresh-frozen meniscal allograft tissue that has been harvested and procured according to the standards set by the American Association of Tissue Banks.

Precise sizing of the meniscal allograft is required if the meniscus is to regain its stabilizing, load-bearing, and energy-absorptive functions. The current technique for preoperative sizing is a modification of that proposed by Garrett (5). Preoperatively, a true lateral radiograph of the patient's involved knee is obtained. The anteroposterior diameter of the appropriate tibial plateau is measured, taking into account any magnification error. This information (i.e., right, medial, 50-mm anteroposterior diameter) is matched to a specimen that has been measured at the time of harvesting and procurement by the tissue bank. The matched specimen then is delivered as an entire hemisection tibial plateau with preserved bony meniscal attachments.

Intraoperatively, the fresh-frozen meniscal allograft is thawed at temperatures below 40°C to prevent denaturing of the collagen fibers. Using a variety of handheld instruments, each meniscal-horn bony insertion site is prepared to cylindric 8 × 20-mm bone plugs, as is done for a typical bone–patellar tendon–bone ACL reconstruction. Number 2-0 nonabsorbable braided sutures are placed through the root of each meniscal horn and respective bone plug to assist in meniscal insertion, passage, and fixation. The meniscus–bone interface is demarcated carefully with a sterile marking pen to allow for accurate assessment of complete graft seating to the level of the bone–meniscal tunnel junction.

Osseous Tunnel Placement   This technique of meniscal reconstruction involves obtaining fixation of the meniscal allograft through a combination of peripheral meniscal suturing and anchoring of the bone plugs in osseous tunnels located at anatomic locations corresponding to the normal insertion sites of the respective meniscal horns. In a patient who underwent previous complete meniscectomy, there may be no remaining tissue to serve as a "footprint" for tunnel placement. This stimulated work in the laboratory which has defined the true three-dimensional shapes and sizes for each meniscal-horn bony insertion site, along with their respective topographic relationships to one another, the ACL and posterior cruciate ligament tibial "footprints," and the articular surface of the medial and lateral tibial plateaus. In addition, consistently identifiable arthroscopic and radiographic landmarks of the meniscal-horn insertion sites may be utilized for anatomic placement of a meniscal substitute (Fig. 2-2).

The anterior and posterior horn bony root insertion sites of the medial meniscus are best visualized with the arthroscope in the anteromedial and posteromedial portals, respectively. Placement of the tibial guide in the contralateral anterior portal is optimal for each medial meniscal insertion site. Placement of the arthroscope and tibial guide in the anterolateral and anteromedial portals, respectively, allows for optimal visualization and tunnel placement for both lateral meniscal-root bony insertion sites.

Once the anatomic intraarticular tibial attachment site is located for each bony root insertion site, the extraarticular exit is placed over the contralateral portion of the tibial metaphysis at the level of the fibular head, midway between the tibial tubercle and the posteromedial or posterolateral border of the tibia. The advantage of drilling tunnels from the contralateral metaphysis is twofold: Tunnel divergence is greater, providing a larger bony bridge between the two tunnels (i.e., less chance of tunnel "blowout"); and there is a decrease in the bending angle at the meniscal root–bone plug tunnel interface. A longitudinal incision is made in the skin, and periosteal flaps are created. The tibial tunnels are drilled under direct arthroscopic visualization. After insertion of the arthroscopic drill guide in the appropriate anterior portal, a guide wire is drilled through the tibial jig. The tibial guide pin then is overdrilled with an 8-mm cannulated reamer. Using a meniscal resector and arthroscopic rasp, the tibial tunnel is cleared of all soft tissue to facilitate bone plug insertion and prevent graft abrasion at the plateau–tunnel interface.

The anatomic locations of the meniscal bony insertion sites has direct surgical implications. The meniscal posterior horn insertions are directly adjacent to one another, with that of the lateral meniscus being slightly more anterior. Care must be exercised in drilling the posterior osseous tunnels so as to not injure the adjacent structures. If concomitant ligament and meniscal reconstruction is being considered, the insertions of the anterior and

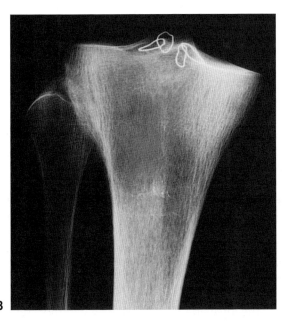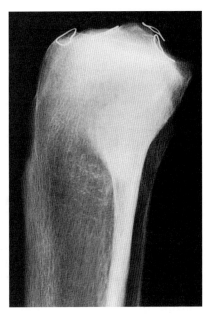

A, B

■ FIGURE 2-2

A,B: Anteroposterior lateral radiographs showing the insertion sites of the meniscal horns. The lateral radiograph also demonstrates the order of the meniscal roots from anterior to posterior: anterior horn medial meniscus, anterior horn lateral meniscus, posterior horn lateral meniscus, posterior horn medial meniscus.

posterior horn of the lateral meniscus need special consideration; each is intimately associated with the other (separated by the lateral tibial spine) and also with the ACL tibial footprint. The anterior horn inserts directly adjacent and parallel to the anterior half of the ACL footprint; the posterior horn inserts directly posterior to the footprint. Thus, a staged procedure is recommended in order to allow for anatomic placement of each bone tunnel without potential blowout of these tunnels into one another. Ligament reconstruction should be performed first to restore normal kinematics, followed by meniscal reconstruction.

Graft Insertion   In an arthroscopically assisted technique, inserting the meniscal allograft into the knee joint is the most technically demanding portion of the procedure. Although some authors have recommended passage of the meniscal allograft from anterior to posterior, this technique advocates posterior to anterior passage to avoid bone-plug fracture. The technique of graft insertion for a lateral meniscal transplant is outlined in Figure 2-3 (10).

Exposure of the posterior border of the lateral collateral ligament laterally or the junction of the posterior border of the medial collateral ligament and the posterior oblique ligament medially is done through an accessory incision, as if performing an "inside-out" meniscal repair (11). A 1.5-cm arthrotomy is made at this junction. With arthroscopic assistance, a suture passer is passed retrograde through the posterior horn tunnel to outside the knee through the posterior arthrotomy. Sutures placed in the posterior horn root and bone plug of the meniscal allograft then are pulled out through the tunnel via the suture passer. Traction is applied only to the suture through the meniscal root; the suture that passes through the bone plug is used for guidance only. Excessive tension on the guide suture may cut through the cancellous bone plug.

After seating of the posterior horn bone plug, a two-step process is used for anterior horn insertion and seating. The suture passer is introduced through the ipsilateral anterior arthroscopic portal and brought out through the posterior capsular incision. The sutures anchoring the anterior portion of the allograft are pulled out the ipsilateral anterior portal, guiding the anterior bone plug along the medial or lateral gutter to the anterior intraarticular portion of the knee joint. The suture passer then is passed retrograde through the anterior horn tunnel into the knee and out through the ipsilateral anterior portal, to accompany the sutures anchored to the anterior bone plug. The sutures are pulled through the anterior tunnel, followed by seating of the anterior bone plug. The meniscal allograft then is seated in its anatomic position, with the anterior and posterior bone plugs in their respective osseous tunnels.

Graft Fixation   Peripheral fixation of the meniscal allograft may be performed using an "outside-in" technique. No tension should be applied to the bone-plug sutures during peripheral fixation. The medial meniscus is sutured with the knee in 10 degrees of flexion to approximate the posteromedial capsular tissue and the meniscus. This also helps avoid posterior capsular plication, which may limit motion postoperatively. The lateral meniscus is sutured with the knee in 50 to 70 degrees of flexion, which allows the peroneal nerve to drop posteriorly behind the biceps. Number 2-0 nonabsorbable braided sutures are placed in a vertical or horizontal fashion. Placement of the sutures on the femoral and tibial surface of the meniscus ensures complete approximation of the meniscal body and capsule. Suture placement should be in 2- to 4-mm intervals, working posterior to anterior to avoid meniscal buckling. After peripheral fixation, tension is applied to the meniscal horn sutures as the knee is moved through a complete range of motion. Meniscal kinematics should be observed as the knee is probed to assess stability and reduction. Finally, the sutures anchoring the tibial bone plugs are tied over the bony bridge separating the tunnels.

Closure and Dressing   Subsequently, the knee and portals are irrigated thoroughly and debrided, and wounds are closed with subcutaneous absorbable sutures. Light sterile dressings are applied, followed by cryotherapy and a hinged knee brace. Patients are placed in a continuous passive motion (CPM) device (0–45 degrees) immediately after the operation and asked to utilize the device 6 to 8 hours per day until 90 degrees of flexion is obtained.

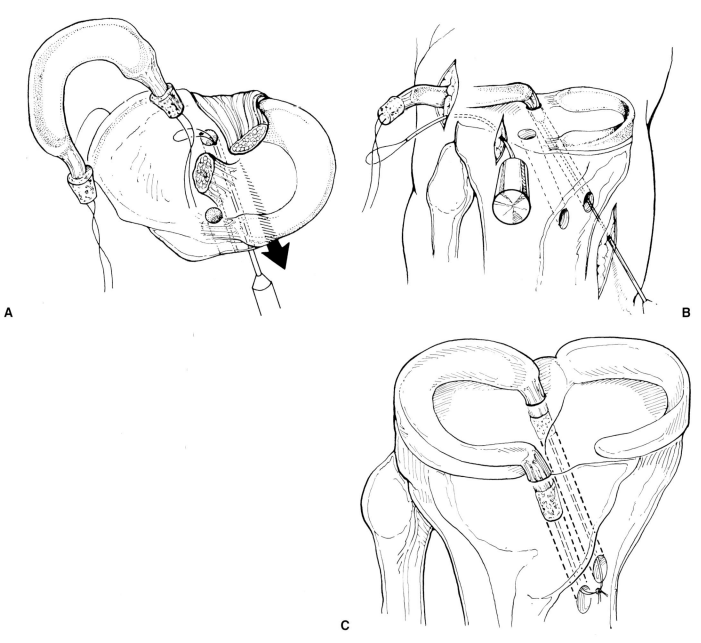

A

B

C

Schematic drawings showing insertion, passage, and seating of a lateral meniscal allograft. **A,B:** Insertion and seating of the posterior horn–bone plug complex. **C:** Insertion and seating of the anterior horn–bone plug complex. (From Johnson DL, Swenson TM, Harner CD. Meniscal reconstruction using allograft tissue: an arthroscopic technique. *Operative Techniques in Sports Medicine* 1994;2(3):223–231, with permission.)   ■ F I G U R E   2 - 3

■ TECHNICAL
ALTERNATIVES AND
PITFALLS

The technique of meniscal allograft preparation and preservation has received consider-able attention in the recent orthopedic literature. Because of difficulty in locating, harvest-ing, and distributing fresh donor allografts to size-matched recipients, as well as the con-siderable risk of disease transmission, fresh grafts seldom are utilized, in favor of banked preserved specimens. Presently, preservation of meniscal allografts involves deep freez-ing, lyophilization, or cryopreservation. Of these three processes, only cryopreservation has been shown to reproducibly maintain a substantial portion (20%) of viable chondro-cytes. Although there is literature to support each of these preservation techniques, there is a trend towards more shrinking, inappropriate remodeling, and greater failure rates in series using freeze-dried and deep-frozen grafts. It also cannot be overlooked that use of gamma irradiation in both the lyophilization and deep-frozen processes may contribute to the relatively less successful results. Finally, cryopreservation is not considered a process through which sterilization can be assured, and the remote risk of disease transmission through the use of cryopreserved tissue continues to be of concern. Therefore, the pro-cesses of freeze drying and gamma irradiation, which are more likely to effectively elimi-nate viral transmission, will continue to have roles in allograft meniscal transplantation.

The most common meniscal replacements used to date include fresh, frozen, and cryop-reserved meniscal allografts (7,8,12). There is a considerable amount of debate about whether the meniscus must contain viable cells at the time of reconstruction or whether it can be nonviable and act merely as a scaffold for migrating cells from the host tissue. A vi-able cell population at the time of reconstruction may be beneficial to the maintenance of the material properties of the meniscal allograft during biologic incorporation. The ratio-nale from maintaining cell viability in meniscus tissue is based on previous studies per-formed on articular cartilage. In recent studies of patellar, meniscal, and ACL allografts by Jackson et al. (13), however, fresh allograft cell DNA was replaced entirely by host DNA by 4 weeks after implantation in goats, suggesting that fresh allograft cells did not remain in the substitute. This evidence raises questions concerning the advantages of using allograft tissue with living cells, which is more expensive and has more complicated surgical logis-tics and a higher potential risk of disease transmission. The majority of scientific investi-gators have transplanted nonirradiated cryopreserved meniscal allograft into the human knee (12).

If the transplanted meniscus is to regain its load-bearing, stabilizing, and energy absorptive functions, it must confirm strictly to the contour of the compartment. To re-produce optimum joint mechanics and meniscal kinematics, isotopic allograft recon-struction is required (i.e., transplantation of the right medial meniscus for right medial meniscal deficiency). Ideally, meniscal size should be matched within 5% (14). Reported techniques of meniscal sizing include magnetic resonance (MR) imaging, computed to-mographic arthrograms, and plain radiographs (5,6). Currently MR imaging and com-puted tomography consistently underestimate the size of the true meniscus; however, this is likely to improve with advancing technology. Preoperative sizing may be per-formed using a plain radiographic technique, as described by Garrett (5) and Johnson (10). It is critically important to maintain close communication with one's local tissue bank to ensure that matched specimens that meet all preoperative requirements are ob-tained at the time of surgery.

The menisci are believed to be "immunologically privileged." This is because the surface of the fibrochondrocytes that express class I histocompatability antigens are isolated from the host immune system by a dense extracellular matrix. No study in the literature to date has reported gross or histologic evidence of an adverse immunologic response to a menis-cal allograft in a patient. Recent studies, however, have shown that normal fresh and frozen human menisci continue to express HLA/ABC and HLA/DR antigens. In transplanting menisci with attached bone there are additional immunologic considerations. There is clear evidence of an immunogenic response against bone. Given the importance of histocom-patibility antigens in transplantation phenomenon, knowledge of the HLA antigen ex-pression is fundamental to understanding the inflammatory, immune, and wound-healing response of the host to the transplanted meniscus, and possible interplay between the graft tissue and the host response. If histocompatibility antigens are present at the time of transplantation, will "tissue matching" enhance meniscal allograft results?

Described surgical techniques for meniscus reconstruction have included both open techniques through an arthrotomy and arthroscopically assisted insertion techniques (5,14). Garrett (5) has described a surgical technique that employs a median parapatellar incision for a medial meniscal transplantation and a lateral parapatellar incision with a tibial tubercle osteotomy for lateral meniscal transplantation. The ipsilateral collateral ligament is removed from its femoral origin and reattached at the conclusion of the meniscal reconstruction. Although technically more demanding, advantages of an arthroscopic insertion technique include decreased morbidity relative to an arthrotomy, avoidance of collateral ligament disruption, and facilitation of early rehabilitation. Ultimately, the technique used is determined by the additional surgery being performed (i.e., ligament reconstruction or osteochondral allograft transplantation).

Once a surgical technique has been selected, the factors most critical to the potential success of the reconstruction are the anatomic placement of the allograft, secure fixation to the periphery, and meniscal-horn attachment to the tibia. Loss of fixation at either the meniscal roots or the periphery leads to failure (4). Peripheral capsular fixation is a prerequisite for biologic incorporation of the graft that occurs from the periphery. Fixation of the meniscal horns on the tibia is a prerequisite for restoration of "hoop stress" within the periphery of the meniscus and prevention of meniscal extrusion (5). The recreation of meniscal hoop stress is believed to be a required stimulus for remodeling of the collagenous network to meet the individual anatomy of the recipient's joint.

Knowledge of meniscal-horn bony insertion site anatomy is imperative in planning meniscal reconstruction. For meniscal cartilage replacement to be potentially successful, the attachment sites of the meniscal horns must be placed similarly, anatomically, to the principals learned with cruciate ligament reconstruction. Recent studies by Johnson et al. (15) and Kohn (21) have defined the bony insertion site anatomy of the human menisci. In addition, arthroscopic landmarks have been described to locate the footprint of the meniscal-horn attachment in those situations in which chronic absence of the meniscus has left no remaining meniscal tissue to serve as a landmark for meniscal allograft placement.

Anchoring of the meniscal horns has been described using soft tissue (4), bone plugs or blocks (14), or a bony bridge connecting the anterior and posterior horns (5). At present, there has been no report of a loss of peripheral capsular fixation. Failure of fixation of the anterior and posterior horn, however, has been reported in experimental and clinical cases (4). It appears that soft-tissue techniques of anchoring the meniscal horns probably do not secure the graft well enough to withstand extrusion forces during weight bearing. Advantages of using menisci with horn attachments preserved to bone plugs or a bony bridge connecting the meniscal horns include increased stability and fixation through bone to bone healing while attempting to preserve hoop stress transfer to the meniscal body (14). In addition, securing bone plugs into osseous tunnels may allow the reestablishment of more normal meniscus mobility and prevent extrusion and changes in meniscal length seen in transplanted allograft menisci with only peripheral fixation. Advantages of using bone plugs over a bone block connecting the meniscal horns include the ability to insert a meniscus with attached bone plugs into the knee using an arthroscopically assisted technique, and the ability to anchor the meniscal roots at their correct anatomic locations. In using an allograft with a bone bridge connecting the meniscal horns, preoperative graft sizing is of extreme importance. Also, the bony bridge graft may be the most difficult one for which to get an exact individual fit, because the size and shape of the meniscus itself. The bone block presents a separate problem. It seems difficult to reproduce the individual bony insertion site anatomy of the meniscal roots with the bone bridge technique. Exact placement of the attachment site is difficult to verify.

The problem of fixation of the anterior and posterior horn of the meniscus allograft using soft tissue or a bony technique has yet to be solved definitively. Although soft-tissue fixation avoids the risk of an immunologic response to allograft bone, anchoring of the anterior and posterior horns with the soft-tissue technique seems to have an increased rate of failure, particularly with extrusion of the meniscus. At present there is no basic science study that documents the recreation of hoop-stress transfer from the meniscal root to the meniscal body with a bony or soft-tissue anchoring technique of the meniscal roots. Fixation of the meniscus to the peripheral capsular rim has not been reported to date to be a problem. It is recommended that the meniscus be fixed to the periphery using a technique similar to that which has been described for meniscal repair. Sutures should be inserted from both the upper and lower meniscal surfaces to approximate the meniscus and capsule completely. Suture placement should proceed from posterior to anterior to avoid meniscal buckling. Once the meniscus has been secured peripherally and at the meniscal-root attachment, meniscal kinematics should be observed closely during probing to assess stability and reduction.

Aside from the issue of graft preservation and sterilization, the most critical factor in the successful outcome of a meniscal allograft transplantation is the ability of the surgeon to carry out the procedure in such a way as to assure that a well-sized graft is securely and evenly affixed at its periphery without damaging the meniscus. It is apparent that the meniscal allograft is a relatively delicate structure and can be lacerated or damaged easily by careless technique. Iatrogenic defects and lacerations can lead to less than desirable long term success rates for meniscal transplantation (16).

■ REHABILITATION

A standard rehabilitation protocol for a patient after meniscal allograft reconstruction has not been determined. Most rehabilitation protocols described have incorporated the knowledge of meniscal repair in the basic science and clinical literature. There have been no data specifically on the stress that is seen at the meniscal tibial attachment of the meniscal horns if the joint is loaded. This information would be critically important in determining a rehabilitation protocol that does not threaten the attachment of the meniscal horns. Most studies employ early passive and active motion to facilitate nutrition of the transplanted meniscus. It is a matter of debate when weight bearing should be initiated and how much weight should be used at certain specific times. Often the protocol used is dictated by the concomitant surgery performed at the time of meniscal allograft reconstruction. Further information is needed to determine the effect of different rehabilitation protocols on incorporation of the meniscal allograft. Postoperative protocols ought to reflect the considerations of postoperative meniscus repair protocols. This involves, in general, limited weight bearing for approximately 6 weeks postsurgery, with progressive advancement. Closed-chain exercises are emphasized. Deep flexion is avoided for the first 6 months. Bicycling, swimming, and straightahead jogging are allowed between 3 and 6 months. Hard running, agility maneuvers, full squats, and return to collision sports are prohibited until after 6 months.

■ OUTCOMES AND FUTURE DIRECTIONS

Meniscal replacement using allograft tissue is currently in its investigational stage. Although reported clinical and basic science studies are limited (4,7,17), they have shown that meniscal allografts heal to the periphery in a manner similar to meniscal tears. Morphologic alterations in collagen architecture as well biochemical differences, however, raise questions concerning long-term viability and function. Unfortunately, most human studies involving meniscal reconstruction have been performed on patients who have either complex problems of joint deterioration with meniscectomy, ligamentous instabilities, or combinations requiring ligamentous, osteochondral, and meniscal reconstruction. "Isolating" the outcome of the meniscus reconstruction in these combined cases is exceedingly difficult. This lack of uniformity in patient selection, operative technique, and follow-up criteria make clinical results in different groups difficult to interpret. At the current time there is no universally accepted method for evaluating the results of meniscus reconstruction surgery. Rating scales may be used that include subjective variables such as pain and swelling. Subjective results of all authors have involved extremely short-term follow-up considering proposed function of the human meniscus. Furthermore, a patient cannot tell if a meniscus is working. Patients often feel that the operation is a success if they do not have postoperative complications.

Currently, there is little correlation between patient symptoms and objective findings. Current methods of objectively evaluating the result of meniscal transplantation include second-look arthroscopy and MR imaging (6,18). Similar to what has been described with the use of MR imaging in the assessment of healing after a meniscal repair, MR imaging is even more difficult to interpret after meniscal reconstruction. Changes in signal characteristic within the meniscal allograft have been seen 6 to 12 months after meniscal allograft surgery. The significance of this remains to be determined. It may be helpful in those clinical situations in which it is felt that the meniscus has detached from its meniscal-horn attachment and displaced into the gutter. Perhaps further enhancement in MR imaging technology and a better understanding of the correlation between MR findings and biologic incorporation will make this a tool for evaluation in the future. At present, it remains clearly investigational. Second-look arthroscopy may be the best way of objectively evaluating the results of meniscal reconstruction at this time (6). Garrett has defined "success" at second-look arthroscopy as incorporation of the allograft, firm attachment throughout its entirety, and absence of allograft shrinkage or degeneration (7). It has been recommended by some authors that all patients have second-look arthroscopies to evaluate the integrity of the meniscal substitute (6). It is important to note on second-look arthroscopy whether the meniscus is healed to the periphery throughout its entirety and is anchored firmly at its meniscal-horn attachments. Shrinkage of the meniscus has been seen in those situations in which the meniscus has become detached from its meniscal-horn attachment or with the use of lyophilized meniscal allografts (4).

The ultimate success or failure of a meniscal reconstruction should not be judged solely on demonstration of allograft incorporation, absence of a decrease in meniscal size, or vascularization of the allograft; rather it should be measured by the ability to prevent or decelerate the progression of degenerative changes of the postmeniscectomy knee or provide additional stability in those knees with ligamentous insufficiency. Allografts must be analyzed not only from a macroscopic and histologic standpoint but also from a functional standpoint. A functional meniscus substitute must demonstrate during mechanical testing the load-bearing characteristics of the femur on the tibia similar to that of the knee without a meniscectomy. At present, there are no noninvasive methods for quantifying and evaluating *in vivo* a meniscal substitute's functional level. In the future, these may include dynamic MR imaging, weight-bearing MR imaging, and the use of sequential technetium scanning as a means of monitoring the restoration of osseous homeostasis after meniscal reconstruction, as has been reported with ACL reconstruction (19).

Zukor et al. (20) were the first to publish clinical results of meniscal allograft reconstruction. They began with the use of fresh meniscal allograft as composite grafts with osteochondral joint segments in patients with posttraumatic joint damage. They performed second-look arthroscopy in eight patients (10 menisci) and subsequent arthrotomy in four patients with five meniscus allografts out of a series of 28 meniscus transplants in 26 patients. Menisci were noted to be stable and have no significant degenerative changes. They noted that the articular cartilage underlying the meniscus always had a "more normal appearance than the rest of the cartilage of the tibial plateau." Milachowski et al. (4) described meniscus allograft transplantation in conjunction with ACL reconstruction in 22 patients. These meniscal reconstructions were performed via an arthrotomy, with peripheral fixation of the meniscus with sutures and anchoring of the meniscus at the anterior and posterior horns with a soft-tissue technique. Frozen menisci were used in six cases and lyophilized gamma-sterilized menisci in 16 cases. Second-look arthroscopy was performed in two thirds of the patients, and at the time of repeat arthroscopy shrinkage of the meniscal implant was seen in both lyophilized and deep-frozen menisci. This was a more frequent finding in the lyophilized gamma-sterilized implants. The authors found no adverse immunologic reactions in either group.

Kohn and Wirth (21) reported their results of 23 patients receiving transplant of lyophilized and deep-frozen meniscal grafts who had concomitant ACL bone–patella–bone reconstruction, with follow-up between 24 and 50 months. Eighteen of 23 patients had follow-up arthroscopy to evaluate the graft. Nearly all grafts had been destroyed or had been reduced significantly in size, with only one graft showing a normal appearance more than 1 year after transplantation.

Garrett (7) reported his results of transplanted fresh and cryopreserved meniscal allografts in 43 patients with 2 to 7 years of follow-up. All cases were performed through an arthrotomy with detachment of the ipsilateral collateral ligament. These reconstructions were very complex; only seven patients of the entire series underwent "isolated" meniscal reconstruction. The menisci were implanted with a bone bridge connecting the anterior and posterior horns. Of the 28 patients who underwent second-look arthroscopy, 20 patients were labeled "successes," because they showed healing of the allograft meniscus to the peripheral rim in the absence of the shrinkage or degeneration. In general, better results were seen in patients who had Outerbridge grade I or II articular cartilage degeneration than in those with grade III or IV.

Noyes (8) reported his results of transplanted irradiated meniscal allograft using an arthroscopically assisted technique in 82 patients followed prospectively over a 2- to 4-year period. Menisci were implanted using a bone-plug technique of the posterior horn and soft-tissue suturing of the anterior horn. Eighty-one percent of the patients had concomitant ACL reconstruction. Using MR imaging and arthroscopic data, it was determined that, of 96 menisci, 22% healed, 34% partially healed, and 44% failed. A significant relationship was found between advanced arthritic changes (grade III or IV) and decreased meniscal healing. Although the meniscal allograft appeared to function and diminish medial joint-line pain in the initial postoperative period, the failure rate increased over the time of the study. This increase in failure rate with time may be brought about by the morphologic alteration in collagen architecture and biochemical differences seen in biopsy specimens of failed allografts. This raises an interesting question concerning long-term viability and function. From these results it was concluded that meniscal allografts should be used only in select cases in symptomatic athletic young patients who do not have significant arthrosis or articular incongruity.

The Hospital for Special Surgery (New York, New York) recently reported early results of transplanted deep-frozen cryopreserved meniscal allograft in 14 patients (6). Only two of the 14 patients had isolated meniscal allograft reconstruction. Although all meniscal reconstructions were performed through arthrotomies, it is unclear how anchoring of the meniscal horns was performed (i.e., soft-tissue or bony technique). Seven of the 11 patients with more than 6 months' follow-up underwent second-look arthroscopy to evaluate the meniscal allograft. Five of the seven menisci showed complete healing to the periphery with no evidence of shrinkage. The authors note that this remains an ongoing prospective investigation. The ability of the meniscal allograft to slow the progression of osteoarthritis remains to be determined by long-term follow-up evaluation.

In the series of 47 cryopreserved meniscal allografts in 45 patients reported by Goble and Kane (16), 17 (94%) of 18 patients who reached 2 years' follow-up reported significant decrease in knee pain and improved function on a subjective evaluation. A second-look arthroscopy was performed on 13 patients, of which 10 (71%) had a well-healed and functional menisci. Four of the grafts demonstrated a noticable pattern of degenerative wear or peripheral detachment at the posterior horn. It was felt that the failure of healing at the posterior horn was secondary to inadequate surgical technique. Biopsy performed on 8 of 14 grafts reavealed a average of 80% viable meniscal tissue. Only one graft was judged to be a failure that required meniscal resection.

O'Hara and McNally (12) recently reported the results of a multicenter study looking at the 6-year trend in cryopreserved allograft meniscal transplantation. There have been 854 transplants in 831 patients with an average age of 35 years. The bone-fixation technique was utilized in 87% of the procedures performed. The data demonstrated a 90% graft-survival rate and a greater than 20% increase in graft survival if bone plugs and fixation were included in the meniscal implant procedure. There was no report of an adverse immunologic reaction in any of the patients. Inferior results were seen in those individuals with moderate to severe arthrosis and articular incongruity.

Attempting to draw conclusions by comparing the results of these preliminary studies is exceptionally difficult . Differences in patient selection, concomitant procedures, meniscal-substitute selection, surgical technique, graft fixation, rehabilitation, and length of follow-up make this nearly impossible. Although meniscal reconstruction remains an exciting, encouraging procedure, the operation should be limited to a select group of individuals who meet specific, well-documented inclusion criteria in prospective study groups and investigational protocols until long-term results are determined. Standardized methods for patient selection, operative technique, rehabilitation, and length of follow-up need to be determined to further define meniscal-replacement techniques. We remain cautiously optimistic that meniscal reconstruction remains a treatment for the future.

Meniscal reconstruction is in its infancy. Clinical reports have demonstrated that meniscal reconstruction is technically feasible and has a high rate of incorporation into the host; however, the long-term viability and function of the meniscal replacement substitute is unknown. Further research is required to determine if allograft tissue can survive for an extended period of time and provide meniscal function to enhance stability and retard or prevent further degeneration in the postmeniscectomy knee.

There are several questions that need to be answered for the future development of meniscal reconstruction techniques: 1) What are the specific indications for meniscal reconstruction? The answer to this question has yet be defined. It appears from reviewing the available literature that those patients who are ligamentously stable with only grade I or II articular disease are the best candidates for meniscal reconstruction. Those individuals with ligamentous insufficiency or advanced articular disease with articular incongruity have less predictable outcomes. 2) What material is best suited for meniscus replacement? Experimental work has verified that fresh, deep-frozen, lyophilized and gamma-sterilized, and cryopreserved menisci can be incorporated and function in animal models (17). Several studies of meniscal reconstruction in humans have been performed using fresh-frozen or cryopreserved allograft. The investigational use of a collagen meniscus template or scaffold is undergoing human trials after limited success in basic science laboratories. Stone et al. (22) recently reported their preliminary results in 10 patients who underwent implantation of the collagen scaffold for irreparable meniscal tears or significant segmental meniscal defects. Although this prospective study is ongoing, it appears that the collagen meniscus implant can support meniscal fibrocartilagenous regeneration. It is believed by the authors that further refinement in the implant to speed ingrowth and enhance durability will continue to improve the ability to induce regrowth of the human meniscus cartilage. This may include new methods of processing the graft or impregnating or coating it with cellular specific bioactive factors to promote a more robust biologic response. 3) What is the most optimal, cost-efficient method to preoperatively size a meniscus implant? At the present time most scientific investigators use either a plain radiographic technique or MR imaging. With further refinements in MR imaging software, this may become the method of choice of meniscal sizing. 4) Is anchoring of the meniscal horn using bone necessary? Early clinical experience seems to suggest that anchoring of the meniscal horn using a bone technique gives more predictable results than using soft-tissue techniques. It remains to be determined whether, in using composite bone–meniscus–bone grafts, a bone bridge as recommended by Garrett or bone plugs anchored in osseous tunnels give more predictable results. 5) How do concomitant orthopedic procedures affect the "isolated" outcome of the meniscal transplant. Most clinical series to date have involved complex knee surgery involving ligamentous, osteochondral, and meniscal replacement. It is unclear how these associated procedures affect the overall outcome of the meniscal allograft. Results may be significantly different in those individuals who undergo "isolated" meniscal reconstruction. 6) What is the inflammatory, immune, and wound healing response of the host to the reconstructed meniscus, and what is the possible interplay between the graft tissue and host response? At present there remains no report of an adverse immunologic response after implantation of a meniscal allograft. Recent studies seem to suggest that an immunologic reaction is present after performing ACL reconstruction using frozen nonirradiated allograft, but it is not known whether this mounted response is beneficial in terms of graft healing and incorporation or detrimental, with potential bony tunnel resorption and ligament failure. Until the existence and degree of the cellular and molecular mechanism of the immune response is better defined, the exact effect of an immunologic response in allograft meniscal surgery will remain undetermined.

References

1. Baratz ME, Fu FH, Mengato R. Meniscal tears: the effect of meniscectomy and repair on intra-articular contact areas and stress in the human knee: a preliminary report. *Am J Sports Med* 1986; 14:270–275.
2. Levy IM, Torzilli PA, Warren RF. The effect of medial meniscectomy on anterior-posterior motion of the knee. *J Bone Joint Surg Am* 1982; 64:883–888.
3. Fairbank TJ. Knee joint changes after meniscectomy. *J Bone Joint Surg Br* 1976; 30:664–670.
4. Milachowski KA, Weismeier K, Wirth CJ. Homologous meniscus transplantation. Experimental and clinical results. *Int Orthop* 1989; 13:1–11.
5. Garrett JC. Meniscal transplantation. In: Aichroth PC, Canon WD, Patel DV, eds. *Knee surgery: current practice.* New York: Raven Press, 1992:95–103.
6. Veltri DM, Warren RG, Wickiewicz TL, O'Brien SJ. Current status of allograft meniscal transplantation. *Clin Orthop* 1997; 303:44–45.
7. Garrett JC. Meniscal transplantation: A review of 43 cases with 2 to 7 year follow-up. *Sports Med Arthroscopy Rev* 1993; 1:164–167.
8. Noyes FR. Irradiated meniscus allografts in the human knee: a two to five year follow-up study. Presented at the Meniscal Transplant Study Group, AAOS Annual Meeting, Orlando, FL, February 1995.
9. Rosenberg TD, Paulos LE, Parker RD, et al. The forty-five degree posteroanterior flexion weight-bearing radiograph of the knee. *J Bone Joint Surg Am* 1988; 70:1479–1482.
10. Johnson DL, Swenson TM, Harner CD. Meniscal reconstruction using allograft tissue: an arthroscopic technique. *Operative Techniques in Sports Medicine* 1994; 2(3):223–231.
11. Bach BR, Jewell BF, Bush JC. Surgical Approaches for medial and lateral meniscal repair. *Tech in Orthop* 1993; 8(2):120–128.
12. O'Hara A, McNally RT. The five year trends in cryopreserved allograft meniscal transplantation. Presented at the Meniscal Transplant Study Group, AAOS Annual Meeting, Atlanta, GA, February 1996.
13. Jackson DW, Whelan J, Simon TM. Cell survival of cells after transplantation of fresh meniscal allografts: DNA probe analysis in a goat model. *Am J Sports Med* 1993; 21:540–550.
14. Johnson DL. Arthroscopy assisted technique for meniscal reconstruction using fresh frozen allograft. *Operative Techniques in Orthopaedics* 1995; 5(1):88–94.
15. Johnson DL, Swenson TM, Livesay GA, et al. Insertion-site anatomy of the human menisci: gross, arthroscopic, and topographical anatomy as a basis for meniscus transplantation. *Arthroscopy* 1995; 11:386–394.
16. Goble EM, Kane SM. Meniscal allografts. In: Czitrom AA, Winkler H, eds. *Orthopaedic allograft surgery.* New York: Springer-Verlag Wien, 1996:243–252.
17. Jackson DW, McDevitt CA, Simon TM, et al. Meniscal transplantation using fresh and cryopreserved allografts. An experimental study in goats. *Am J Sports Med* 1992; 20:644–656.
18. Rodeo SA, Wickiewicz TL, Potter HG, Warren RF. Magnetic resonance imaging of meniscal allografts: correlation with early outcome. Presented at the Meniscal Transplant Study Group, AAOS Annual Meeting, Orlando, FL, February 1995.
19. Dye SF, Chew MF. Restoration of osseous homeostasis after anterior cruciate ligament reconstruction. *Am J Sports Med* 1993; 21:748–750.
20. Zukor DJ, Cameron JC, Brooks PJ, et al. The fate of human meniscal allografts. In: Ewing JW, ed. *Articular cartilage and knee joint function: basic science and arthroscopy.* New York: Raven Press, 1990:147.
21. Kohn D, Wirth CJ. Meniscal allografts. In: Czitrom AA, Winkler H, eds. *Orthopaedic allograft surgery.* New York: Springer-Verlag Wien, 1996:243–252.
22. Stone KR, Steadman TR, Rodkey WG, et al. Regeneration of meniscal cartilage with use of a collagen scaffold. Analysis of preliminary data. *J Bone Joint Surg* 1997;79:1770–1777.

3

J. RICHARD STEADMAN
WILLIAM G. RODKEY
STEVEN B. SINGLETON
KAREN K. BRIGGS
JUAN J. RODRIGO
C. WAYNE McILWRAITH

Microfracture Procedure for Treatment of Full-thickness Chondral Defects: Technique, Clinical Results, and Current Basic Science Status

Articular cartilage defects rarely heal spontaneously (1–4). This observation is true whether the defects are acute, chronic, or degenerative in nature. Although some patients do not develop significant clinical problems as a result of an articular cartilage defect, most eventually develop degenerative changes associated with the cartilage damage. These degenerative changes are progressive, and they become irreversible if no intervention is applied. This problem is very significant, as evidenced by estimates that 32 to 37 million Americans of all ages have degenerative arthritis that has become progressive from either acute or chronic chondral injuries. Many of these patients become severely or completely disabled, and total joint arthroplasty becomes the only alternative.

In spite of the seemingly "sudden" interest in chondral defects, for over 250 years physicians have attempted to heal damaged or degenerative articular cartilage. Many techniques have been used in the past to include spongialization, abrasion, drilling, tissue autografts, allografts, and cell transplantation (1,2). Clinicians have taken a greater interest in treating chondral defects recently, in part because of a better understanding of cartilage biology and pathophysiology and because of advances in imaging techniques and arthroscopic surgery. Nonetheless, it seems that very recently attitudes have changed toward articular cartilage resurfacing, and greater emphasis now is placed upon it (1,2).

A procedure referred to as the *microfracture* technique has been developed by the senior author of this chapter to enhance chondral resurfacing by providing a suitable environment for tissue regeneration (1,2). This procedure was first used about 15 years ago, based on an intuition that it would provide certain advantages over other techniques, such as drilling smooth round holes. Specific advantages are described subsequently in this chapter. This technique has now been used in more than 1,200 patients, and it is described in detail here.

■ HISTORY OF THE TECHNIQUE

The general indication for microfracture is full-thickness loss of articular cartilage in either a weight-bearing area between the femur and tibia or an area of contact between the patella and trochlear groove. The presence of unstable cartilage overlying or down to the bone surface is also an indication for microfracture. Another indication is degenerative changes in a knee that has proper axial alignment. Although these changes may not be true osteochondral defects, they reflect loss of articular cartilage over the bone–chondral surface.

In these situations, consideration should be given to patient age, angulatory deformity, and activity level. If all of these criteria define someone who could benefit from chondral resurfacing, then the patient might be considered for microfracture.

■ INDICATIONS AND CONTRAINDICATIONS

Contraindications for microfracture include angulatory deformity, a patient unwilling to rehabilitate in the appropriate manner, partial-thickness defects, inability to use the opposite leg for weight bearing during the minimal weight-bearing time, and a relative contraindication for patients over 60 years old. The contraindication in patients older than 60 years of age is only relative: If the patient is able to meet all other criteria, then this procedure can be considered for those older patients.

With specific reference to angulatory deformity, the two radiographic measurements are the angle made between the femur and tibia on anteroposterior views, and the weight-bearing axis drawn from the central portion of the femoral head to the central distal tibia on longstanding radiographs. If the angle drawn between the tibia and femur is greater than 5 degrees different from the normal uninvolved side, this finding would be a relative contraindication for microfracture. If the weight-bearing axis is in the peripheral half of the plateaus, medial or lateral, this weight-bearing shift also would be a relative contraindication. Preferably the weight-bearing line should be in the central quarter of the tibial plateau of either the medial or lateral compartment.

One specific area in which further research is needed is the patient with the femoral condyle or tibial plateau that has developed sclerotic bone after loss of articular cartilage. The thickness of this sclerotic area may make the results of microfracture less successful, although this concern has not yet been addressed in our basic science or our clinical research.

■ SURGICAL
TECHNIQUES

Epidural anesthesia is the senior author's first preference. About 90 to 95% of patients select this form of anesthesia. The remainder undergo general or spinal anesthesia.

Three portals are made about the knee for use of the inflow cannula, the arthroscope, and the working instruments. No tourniquet is used routinely. A thorough diagnostic examination of the knee is performed. As a matter of routine, we carefully inspect the suprapatellar pouch, the medial and lateral gutters, the patellofemoral joint, the intercondylar notch and its contents, and the medial and lateral compartments, including the posterior horns of both menisci. In general, we perform other necessary intraarticular procedures prior to microfracture, with the exception of ligament reconstruction. This routine helps prevent loss of visualization from the fat droplets and blood that enter the knee from the small holes that form the "superclot." Additionally, particular attention is focused on soft tissues such as plicae and the lateral retinaculum, which could produce increased compression between cartilage surfaces.

Once the full-thickness articular cartilage lesion is identified (Fig. 3-1), the exposed bone is debrided of all remaining cartilage tags using a full-radius resector or Gator shaver (Linvatec, Largo, FL) or a curved curette. All loose or marginally attached cartilage from the surrounding rim of articular cartilage also is debrided to form a perpendicular edge of healthy, viable cartilage around the defect (Fig. 3-2). This prepared lesion provides a pool

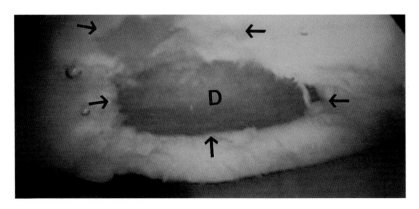

■ FIGURE 3-1

A full-thickness articular cartilage defect (*D*) on a femoral condyle. *Arrows* show the extent of the lesion.

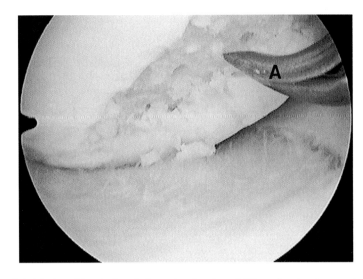

■ FIGURE 3-2

A chondral defect that has been debrided and is starting to be microfractured. The microfracture awl (*A*) can be seen penetrating the subchondral bone.

in which the superclot may form. The calcified cartilage layer that remains as a cap to many lesions is removed gently using a shaver or curette. We believe the removal of the calcified cartilage layer is extremely important, based upon our basic science research. In order to avoid excessive damage to the subchondral bone, care must be taken not to debride too deeply. An arthroscopic awl (Linvatec) then is used to make multiple holes, or microfractures, in the exposed subchondral bone plate. The holes are made as close together as necessary, but not so close that one breaks into another, thus damaging the subchondral plate between them (Fig. 3-3). This technique usually results in microfracture holes that are approximately 3 to 4 mm apart (or three to four holes per square centimeter). The appropriate depth has been reached if fat droplets are visualized emanating from the marrow; typically, this depth is about 4 mm. The arthroscopic awls produce essentially no thermal necrosis of the bone compared with hand-driven or motorized drills. We typically make microfracture holes around the periphery of the defect first, immediately adjacent to the healthy cartilage rim. We then work our way into the center of the defect. The arthroscopic irrigation fluid pump pressure then is reduced, and under direct visualization we observe

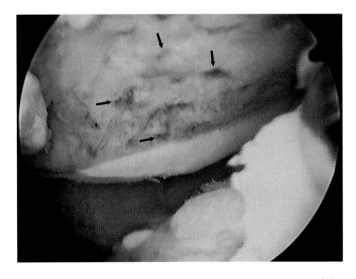

■ FIGURE 3-3

A chondral lesion after the microfracture procedure has been completed. *Arrows* point to some of the microfracture holes.

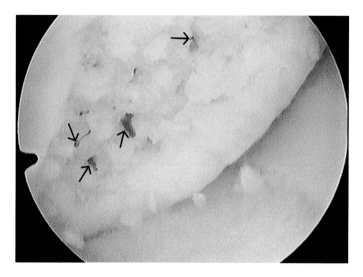

■ FIGURE 3-4

Blood and fat droplets (*arrows*) can be seen coming from the microfracture holes after the arthroscopic irrigation fluid pressure has been reduced.

the release of fat droplets and blood from the microfracture holes into the knee (Fig. 3-4). If the release of marrow contents is deemed adequate, all instruments are removed from the knee and the joint is evacuated of fluid. No drains are placed intraarticularly, because the goal is for a blood clot rich in marrow elements (a superclot) to form and stabilize, covering the lesion.

This technique of microfracture produces a rough surface in the lesion to which the superclot can adhere more easily, yet the integrity of the subchondral plate is maintained for joint-surface shape. In addition to eliminating thermal necrosis and providing a roughened surface for blood-clot adhesion, the different angles of arthroscopic awls available provide easier access to difficult areas of the knee. The awls also provide improved control of depth penetration. The key to the entire procedure is to establish the superclot to provide the optimal environment for a viable population of pluripotential marrow cells (mesenchymal stem cells) to differentiate into stable tissue within the lesion.

■ TECHNICAL ALTERNATIVES AND PITFALLS

Most patients progress through the postoperative period with little difficulty. Some, however, experience mild transient pain, most frequently following microfracture in the anterior portion of the knee. Small changes in the articular surface of the patellofemoral joint may be detected by a grating or "gritty" sensation of the joint, particularly if a patient initially is advanced out of the knee brace and begins normal weight bearing through a full range of motion. Patients rarely complain of pain at this time, and this grating sensation typically resolves in a few days or weeks.

Similarly, if a steep perpendicular rim has been made in the trochlear groove, patients may notice "catching" or "locking" as the apex of the patella rides over this lesion during joint motion. A few patients even perceive these symptoms in the continuous passive motion (CPM) unit. It has been our experience that these symptoms usually abate within 3 months. If this perceived "locking" is painful, then we treat the patient by limiting weight bearing and avoiding the symptomatic joint angle for an additional period of time.

On occasion, we have noted a recurrent effusion developing between 6 and 8 weeks postmicrofracture. Some of these patients present after beginning to bear weight on the injured leg following microfracture of a femoral condylar defect. This effusion often mimics the preoperative effusion, except that it usually is painless. We treat the painless effusion conservatively, and we have noted its resolution typically within several weeks after onset. Only on very rare occasions has a second arthroscopy been required for recurring effusions.

One alternative to microfracture is abrasion arthroplasty (5). This procedure involves arthroscopic use of a motorized burr or abrader to remove the sclerotic bone from the degenerative lesion. The burring goes deep enough to reach the blood vessels of the subchondral bone (5).

Another chondral-resurfacing technique that recently has attracted significant attention involves autologous cell transplantation (6). This technique involves two operative procedures. The first is performed arthroscopically, and normal articular cartilage is harvested for culture. After the chondrocytes have increased to a specific concentration in culture, the cells are implanted into the lesion and covered with a periosteal flap through open arthrotomy (6).

The rehabilitation program following microfracture for treatment of chondral defects in the knee is crucial to optimize the results of the surgery (7). The rehabilitation program should promote the ideal physical environment for the newly recruited pluripotential cells from the marrow to differentiate into the appropriate articular cartilage-like cell lines. We believe that the superclot provides the basis for the ideal chemical environment to compliment the physical environment. This cellular differentiation ultimately leads to the development and proliferation of a durable repair cartilage that fills the original defect (Fig. 3-5).

■ REHABILITATION

There are many important factors to consider in formulating the postoperative rehabilitation program following microfracture. The specific protocol that we recommend depends on two essential factors: that is, the anatomic location and the size of the defect. These factors are critical in determining the ideal postoperative plan (7).

For example, lesions on the weight-bearing surfaces of the femoral condyles are treated postoperatively with a CPM machine commencing immediately in the recovery room (2). The initial range of motion is 30 to 70 degrees; it is increased as tolerated by 10 to 20 degrees every 2 hours. The rate of the machine is usually one cycle per minute, but rate can be varied based upon patient preference. Many patients tolerate the use of the machine at night. For those who do not, however, our experience indicates that intermittent use during the day is equally beneficial. Regardless, the goal is to have the patient in the CPM machine for 6 to 8 hours every 24 hours. If the patient is unable to use the CPM machine, then instructions are given for passive flexion and extension of the knee, with 500 repetitions three times per day. Full passive range of motion of the injured knee is gained as soon as possible after surgery.

Crutch-assisted touchdown weight-bearing ambulation is prescribed for 6 to 8 weeks, depending on the size of the lesion. For most lesions, 6 to 8 weeks seems an adequate time to limit weightbearing. For lesions that are small (less than 1 cm in diameter), however, we

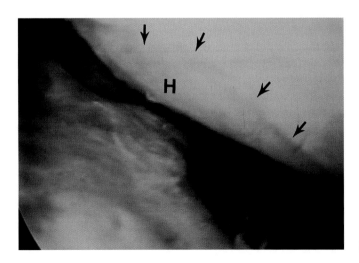

■ FIGURE 3-5

A treated lesion (*H*) that has filled in completely 7.5 months after microfracture. *Arrows* show the extent of the healed lesion.

may hasten weightbearing by a few weeks. Rarely do we use a brace for lesions on the femoral condyles or tibial plateaus. A brace is used for patellofemoral lesions. This brace is set at 0 to 20 degrees to limit compression of the regenerating surfaces. Passive motion is allowed with the brace removed.

Limited strength training also begins immediately. Patients perform double-leg one-third knee bends the day after surgery (7). Because they are touchdown weight-bearing, patients place most (75–80%) of their body weight on their uninjured legs to perform the exercise. Stationary biking and a deep-water exercise program are begun at 1 to 2 weeks postmicrofracture. The deep-water exercises include use of a kick board as well as a flotation vest for deep-water running. After 8 weeks, patients progress to full weight bearing and begin a more vigorous program of active motion of the knee. Elastic resistance cord exercises are begun at approximately 8 weeks after microfracture. A detailed description of use of the cord and the exercises has been published previously (7). The ability to achieve predetermined maximum levels for sets and repetitions of elastic resistance cord exercises is an excellent indicator for progressing to weight training. Exercises with free or machine weights are permitted if the patient has achieved the early goals of the rehabilitation program, but not before 16 weeks postmicrofracture. We strongly emphasize the importance of proper technique in beginning a weight program (7). Depending on the clinical examination, we may recommend a return to sports that involve pivoting, cutting, or jumping after 4 to 6 months.

For lesions of the patellofemoral joint, joint angles are noted at the time of arthroscopy to determine where the defect comes into contact with the patellar facet or the trochlear groove. These areas are avoided during strength training for approximately 4 months. This avoidance allows for training in the 0- to 20-degree range immediately postoperatively, because there is minimal compression of these chondral surfaces with this limited motion. Like those patients with lesions on the femoral condyles, patients with patellofemoral lesions are placed into CPM therapy immediately postoperatively. The regimen is similar to that described previously, with the same emphasis on obtaining pain-free full passive range of motion soon after surgery.

Weight bearing for microfractured lesions of the patellofemoral joint is as tolerated, but it should be limited to the angles of knee flexion at which the lesion is not compressed. Therefore, it is helpful to use a brace to prevent the patient from placing excessive shear force on the maturing superclot in the early postoperative period. Typically we lock the brace at between 0 and 20 degrees' range of motion to prevent flexion past the point at which the median ridge of the patella engages the trochlear groove.

If a knee brace is used, it is opened gradually or is discontinued between 4 and 8 weeks after surgery, depending on the clinical presentation and progress of the patient. At this point, strength training is advanced progressively.

We also prescribe cold therapy for all patients postoperatively. Our experience indicates that the cold helps control pain and inflammation, and most patients state that the cold provides overall postoperative relief. Cold therapy typically is used for 1 to 7 days postoperatively.

If other intraarticular procedures are performed concurrently with microfracture, such as anterior cruciate ligament reconstruction, we do not hesitate to alter the rehabilitation program as necessary. A full discussion of all of the possible variations of the rehabilitation program is beyond the scope of this chapter.

■ OUTCOMES AND FUTURE DIRECTIONS

Analysis of our long-term results in full-thickness articular cartilage defects of the knee treated with debridement and microfracture is ongoing, but 8-year follow-ups have been completed. We determined the functional results of arthroscopic debridement and microfracture, carried out long-term follow-up to document functional outcomes, and completed a year-to-year comparison for each patient versus that patient's preoperative status. All patients had a minimum of 2 years' follow-up, up to longer than 8 years. Our study protocol included a preoperative questionnaire completed by each patient. These patients then were provided annual questionnaires for subjective follow-up, in addition to routine clinical follow-up on as many patients as possible. Specific questionnaire parameters included pain, activities of daily living, sedentary work, strenuous work, and strenuous sports. Aggressive efforts were carried out to assure maximum patient follow-up. Our database entries also included information on demographics, primary and associated injuries, imaging and clinical examination findings, all surgical treatments performed, and any and all complications. The following results are from patients treated with microfracture between 1985 and 1992 for full-thickness chondral defects.

Patients followed for at least 7 years revealed that pain was the parameter with the greatest improvement. Similarly, at 3 and 5 years, 75% of patients were improved, 20% remained unchanged, and 5% were worse. Significant improvement also was noted for parameters of activities of daily living and strenuous work, with both showing 67% of patients improved, 20% unchanged, and 13% worse. Of patients involved with strenuous sports, 65% were improved. Finally, there was no change for the parameter of sedentary work, as might be expected.

We also determined whether there was a difference in results between those patients who had only isolated chondral defects versus associated injuries such as the anterior cruciate ligament or the meniscus. We observed a significant improvement for both groups through all years. The preoperative scores, however, were worse for isolated chondral defects. Interestingly, postoperative scores were consistently higher with combined injuries for the first 5 years, but the knee-function scores were similar from 6 years on.

We observed no complications directly related to the microfracture procedure. Overall in this study, it appears that the patients who did not improve had consistent finding of negative predictors that included chronic lesions, advancing age, preoperative joint-space narrowing, isolated chondral defects, and no CPM therapy following surgery. Many patients with one or two negative predictors, however, still showed improvement over their preoperative status.

Histologically, the microfracture-regenerated tissue appears to be a hybrid of articular cartilage and fibrocartilage. There are viable chondrocytes in lacunae with a uniform matrix (Fig. 3-6).

We believe that there are important future considerations for chondral resurfacing. It is important that we continue to gain a better understanding of the biology of articular cartilage. We must identify and understand endogenous biologic modulators of healing within the joint. Efforts should continue to examine the exogenous application of various factors to influence the cellular response and cartilage healing. The science of tissue engineering and the use of synthetic matrices are also likely to be critical to future success. Finally, we

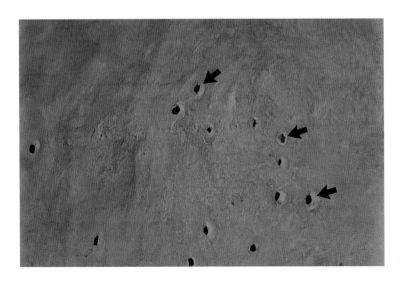

■ FIGURE 3-6

Histologic appearance of repair tissue approximately 8 years after microfracture. Note the chondrocytes within their lacunae (*arrows*).

must continue to attempt to gain a better understanding of the key role played by the calcified cartilage layer and the subchondral bone in both the formation of chondral defects as well as in cartilage healing.

We have made a concerted basic science effort to gain better understanding of the healing processes and how the microfracture technique may be beneficial. We have developed a large-animal model to study the repair of osteochondral defects using microfracture. We are doing this work in horses, examining the effect of microfracture through the subchondral bone plate on the long-term healing of full-thickness defects. In a recent study (8), 10 horses had full-thickness chondral defects made arthroscopically in both midcarpal and both femorotibial joints. Half of the lesions were treated by microfracture and the remaining half were left as untreated controls. Five of the horses were harvested at 4 months and the remainder at 12 months.

We found that the horse articular cartilage is quite similar to that of humans. We observed that the microfracture technique resulted in greater filling of defects both grossly and histomorphometrically. We also observed that the microfracture-regenerated tissue contained approximately 50% type II collagen, whereas the control tissue was only 30% type II collagen (8).

Grossly, the microfractured lesions healed with an average of 75% filling of the defects with regenerated tissue, compared with 45% filling in the control defects. This difference was statistically significant (8).

Histologically, the microfracture-regenerated tissue appeared to be attached better and more stably than the control tissue. This difference was most notable and consistent if all calcified cartilage was removed from the base of the lesion.

Twelve horses were operated on as part of a short-term study for which the objectives were to compare the healing of full-thickness articular cartilage defects (elimination of all calcified cartilage) with abrasion only compared to microfracture (C. W. McIlwraith, W. G. Rodkey, J. R. Steadman, et al., 1998, unpublished data). We evaluated the repair tissue qualitatively and quantitatively at 2, 4, 6, and 8 weeks postchondroplasty histologically, via molecular biology with polymerized chain reaction for gene expression, histomorphometrically, and by immunohistochemistry. At 2 and 4 weeks there was type I collagen in all defects, but no type II collagen. At 6 weeks we identified the mature form of type II collagen in the microfractured lesions, but there was none in the control lesions. Aggrecan expression also first was detected at 6 weeks. Aggrecan analysis at 8 weeks revealed a marked predominance of this marker for mature articular cartilage in microfracture versus control lesions. Likewise, there was a highly significant increase in type II collagen expression in microfracture compared with control lesions at 8 weeks. This finding confirms that the microfracture tissue is producing messenger RNA for the important components of mature articular cartilage as early as 6 weeks. Further analysis suggests that this tissue may be a cartilage "hybrid" that is a combination of hyaline cartilage and denser fibrocartilage. Based on our clinical observations as well as our 1-year horse data, we speculate that this hybrid cartilage may have durability comparable to normal articular cartilage but is smooth enough to function similarly to articular cartilage.

Other studies are ongoing using the equine model. We are assessing chronologic changes in cell population and cell activity in the superclot that forms following the microfracture procedure. We also are evaluating the presence and time of action of cytokine growth factors in the joint fluid. Another long-term study underway is designed to compare microfracture versus no microfracture if the other variable is the removal or the retention of the calcified cartilage layer. Overall, we believe this large-animal model will provide many clinically relevant answers to the biology of chondral resurfacing.

In summary, we believe that the advantages of the microfracture include that less heat, and therefore less necrosis, is produced than with drilling. The microfracture awls allow access to virtually the entire joint, whereas access is much more limited using a drill. The roughened surfaces produced by the microfracture provide surfaces to which blood clots can attach firmly. Although the subchondral bone plate is penetrated, its actual integrity as a structure (and therefore joint contour and shape) is maintained. Perhaps most important, this technique provides access to mesenchymal stem cells, not phenotypically mature chondrocytes that are used in cell transplants, and biologic modulators of healing.

References

1. Steadman JR, Rodrigo JJ, Briggs KK, et al. Long term results of full thickness articular cartilage defects of the knee treated with debridement and microfracture. *J Bone Joint Surg* (in review.)
2. Rodrigo JJ, Steadman JR, Silliman JF, et al. Improvement of full-thickness chondral defect healing in the human knee after debridement and microfracture using continuous passive motion. *Am J Knee Surg* 1994; 7:109–116.
3. Urrea LH, Silliman JF. Acute chondral injuries to the femoral condyles. *Operative Techniques in Sports Medicine* 1995; 3:104–111.
4. Singleton SB, Silliman JF. Acute chondral injuries of the patellofemoral joint. *Operative Techniques in Sports Medicine* 1995; 3:96–103.
5. Johnson LL. The sclerotic lesion: pathology and the clinical response to arthroscopic abrasion arthroplasty. In: Ewing JW, ed. *Articular cartilage and knee joint function: basic science and arthroscopy.* New York: Raven Press, 1990:319–333.
6. Brittberg M, Lindahl A, Nilsson A, et al. Treatment of deep cartilage defects in the knee with autologous chondrocyte transplantation. *N Engl J Med* 1994; 331:889–895.
7. Hagerman GR, Atkins JA, Dillman CJ: Rehabilitation of chondral injuries and chronic degenerative arthritis of the knee in the athlete. *Operative Techniques in Sports Medicine* 1995;3:127–135.
8. Frisbie DD, Trotter GW, Powers BE, et al. Arthroscopic subchondral bone plate microfracture technique augments healing of large osteochondral defects in the radial carpal bone and medial femoral condyle of horses. *Vet Surg* 1999; 28:242–255.

RONALD A.
NAVARRO
FREDDIE H. FU

4

Articular Autologous Chondrocyte Transplant

■ HISTORY OF THE
TECHNIQUE

The treatment of articular chondral defects, both acute and chronic in nature, long has been a daunting task for orthopaedic surgeons. Recently, new techniques have emerged that offer hope for patients with painful defects of the articular surface. At the Orthopaedic Research Society meeting in Atlanta, Georgia, in 1984, Peterson et al. (1) presented data that compared the effects of using periosteum alone with those of periosteum with autologous chondrocytes for the treatment of chondral defects. They showed that over a 1-year period, the periosteum alone produced a 30% fill rate of the defects; periosteum plus cells had a 90% defect fill rate. On histologic examination, the periosteum alone showed a very disorganized fibrocartilage. Periosteum plus cells produced a hyaline-like cartilage. Grande et al. (2) later published results of periosteal versus autogenous chondrocyte grafting in a rabbit model. Healing of the defect was seen in only 18% of subjects treated with periosteal grafting only, and in 82% treated with periosteum and autogenous chondrocyte grafting. Healing occurred in 16% treated with a sham operation.

Brittberg et al. (3) later reported on repairing deep cartilage defects in the knee in humans. Cultured autologous chondrocytes, isolated from the individual's own cartilage, were expanded *in vitro* and returned to the damaged site for repair of the articular defect. There were good to excellent results in 14 of 16 femoral condylar transplants and two of seven patellar transplants at 2 years' follow-up. Biopsies revealed hyaline cartilage in 11 of 15 femoral and one of seven patellar transplants. Because of this success, we have investigated this technique at our center and describe this technique as it has evolved for us.

■ INDICATIONS AND
CONTRAINDICATIONS

This technique is best suited for patients with isolated, well-localized defects of the articular surface of the knee. The cartilage defects may expose the subchondral bone, but lesions that include bony defects and bone loss usually are excluded from this procedure. In general, the upper limit of the size of each defect is 10 cm^2, and the age of inclusion ranges from the age at closure of physes to 55 years old. Other patients excluded from the procedure include those with gross malalignment of the femorotibial articulation, significant osteoarthritis, morbid obesity, and a history of anaphylaxis to penicillin, streptomycin, or bovine materials (materials used in fibrin sealant preparation). The procedure cannot be performed in the setting of infection or extreme malnourishment.

■ SURGICAL
TECHNIQUES (FIG. 4-1)

Arthroscopic Biopsy After general anesthesia, standard knee arthroscopy with typical portals is performed. Use of a tourniquet facilitates the procedure. The articular surfaces of the knee should be examined for any significant osteoarthritis that would make the transplantation contraindicated. The defect should be assessed with specific attention to the transition from injured to healthy tissue. The defect should be clinically significant and contained, preferably on the femoral condyle, with healthy surrounding tissue. If defects are located in the periphery of the condyle, one should be sure that a ridge of intact cartilage exists, so that eventually periosteal suturing can be performed.

The biopsy is taken from the non–load bearing area on the proximal medial femoral condyle during the staged arthroscopic procedure. Two or three long tubular ridges are

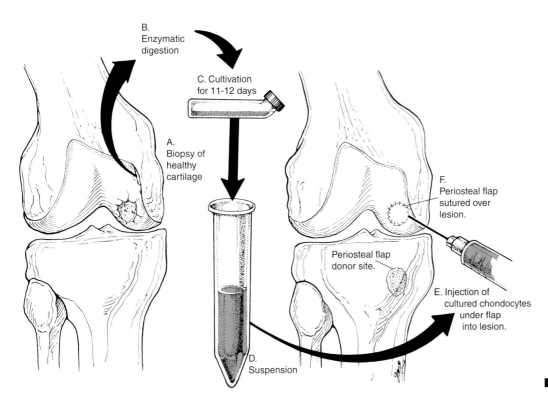

Diagram of chondrocyte transplantation in the medial femoral condyle. (Adapted from Brittberg M, Lindahl A, Nilsson A, et al. Treatment of deep cartilage defects in the knee with autologous chondrocyte transplantation. *N Engl J Med* 1994;33:889–895, with permission.)

taken using a ring curette, down to the subchondral bone, being careful not to puncture the subchondral bone plate. In a human, the normal articular cartilage is between 3 and 5 mm thick. Between 200 and 300 mg of healthy cartilage should be collected. The preferred technique is to create a "whittled dowel" with the curette. One should try not to detach the cartilage dowel when removing the curette. If a stump is left, it is easier to remove the cartilage biopsy with graspers. This saves time and the frustration of searching for it with the arthroscope. Alternatively, the biopsy can be obtained in the notch region, in which notchplasty is performed for anterior cruciate ligament reconstruction.

Cell Culture and Expansion   After the biopsy is removed, we place it in a specially designed transport container (Genzyme Tissue Repair, Boston, MA) in preservation media. It is sent for Carticel culturing and cellular expansion (Genzyme Tissue Repair). Carticel provides this service at a cost to the patient and holds the cultured cells until the patient's transplant date. Also, at this time the patient should give blood for procurement of cryoprecipitate to be used in the fibrin glue sealant.

Open Transplantation   After general anesthesia, a bump is placed under the hip on the side of the operation, and then a tourniquet high on the thigh. The entire lower extremity is draped and the limb exsanguinate in the usual sterile fashion. One should inflate the tourniquet and perform a parapatellar arthrotomy on the side of the lesion. Following arthrotomy, the lesion is debrided down to but not through the subchondral bone (Fig. 4-2); excessive subchondral debridement should be avoided. This is difficult in the setting of prior microfracture or abrasion treatment for the chondral defect. It is sometimes difficult to discern where reparative bone ends and true subchondral bone begins. Penetration of the subchondral surface must be avoided, and any subchondral bleeding treated immedi-

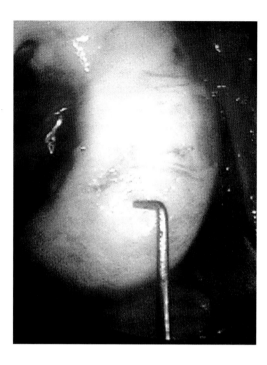

■   FIGURE 4-2

Probing a medial femoral condyle lesion that has undergone the microfracture technique previously.

ately with epinephrine and thrombin. The defect should have vertical walls, so that it can accept sutures and support the chondrocyte suspension (Fig. 4-3). An attempt should be made to create an oval shape for ease of suturing. Healthy cartilage should border the defect completely. No degenerative cartilage should surround the defect after the second debridement.

The defect is measured to create a suitably sized periosteal patch. In measuring the defect, one should oversize the dimensions by adding 2 mm to the height and width. Excess foil from the suture packages can be used to create a mold, which can be trimmed for placement on the donor periosteum.

To approach the donor periosteum, the incision can be enlarged distally to include the proximal tibia, or a separate incision can be made just below the pes anserinus on the an-

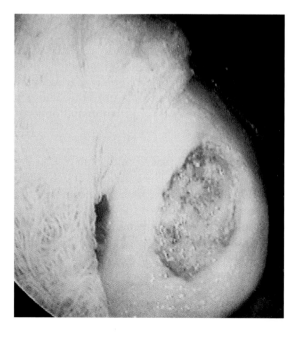

■   FIGURE 4-3

Medial femoral condyle lesion prepared and without bleeding.

terior medial tibia. The periosteal patch then is taken from the medial subcutaneous border of the proximal medial tibia. First the patch is measured. It is better to oversize the patch than to undersize it. The measurement outline can be marked with a marking ink pen. First, the incision is made sharply down to the bone with a no. 15 surgical blade, and then the superficial fat layer is removed. This can be done using the thumb to simply rub it off. Once incised, a wide wing-tip elevator can be used to lift it off gently (Fig. 4-4). The patch is kept moist with sterile saline while it is being removed and at all times, so that it does not become brittle and inelastic.

For suturing the periosteal patch over the defect, a 6.0 vicryl suture on a P1 cutting needle is used. The periosteal patch should have the cambium layer down toward the defect. The passage of the needle should be made through the periosteum and then into the cartilage. It is important that the cutting needle be pulled out in the line of its shape; otherwise, the needle may tear through the cartilage. This suture does not pass easily through the cartilage unless it is immersed in glycerin. The distance between the interrupted sutures should be approximately 5 to 6 mm, and the knots should be tied down firmly. The key to a good-fitting patch is to make sure that one goes to opposite sides in placing the sutures. A Z pattern is recommended (like tightening a drum, the graft is tightened evenly around the defect). In tying off the suture, the knots should be placed on the side of the periosteal patch and a small flap on the superior aspect of the defect left open to permit delivery of the chondrocyte cells. If no cartilage rim is available, one should stitch to the synovium, with the sutures approximately 3 to 4 mm apart to maximize the integrity of the seal.

A good way to make sure the closure is watertight prior to implantation of the cells is to inject 0.04 mL of either air or saline into the superior defect with a small (19-gauge) syringe. If leaks are visible, additional sutures should be added or fibrin glue applied to secure the edges. If the defect is adequately watertight, one can aspirate out all of the saline and prepare to inject the cells into the defect.

Use of fibrin glue in combination with the sutures is an optional technique to secure a water tight seal. The fibrin glue consists of two components: cryoprecipitate procured from the patient's own blood and bovine thrombin. Using a bifurcated syringe, the glue is applied around the edges of the patch. One should be sure that air has been injected under the patch before the sealant is administered, to ensure room for the cells. If the two components are mixed in open air they set in 10 to 15 seconds. The glue is applied in single

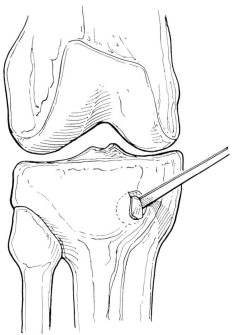

Elevator used to lift the measured periosteal patch.   ■ FIGURE 4-4

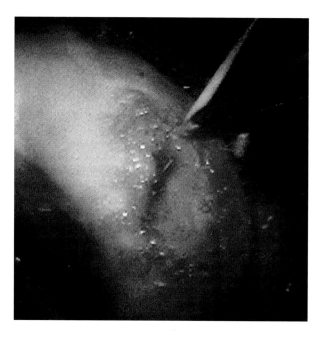

Cells injected into superior defect of sutured periosteal patch.

droplets in a 1:1 ratio between the two components only around the margins of the patch seal area. Too much glue on the patch affects its elasticity and permeability. One should have additional needles available in case the Y-needle gets clogged.

The chondrocytes are packaged in a small, nonsterile vial; (Only the inside of the vial is sterile.) Visual examination shows the chondrocytes as a yellowish pellet at the base of the vial. The cells can be resuspended in the media by agitating the vial. An 18- or 19-gauge needle is used to aspirate the cells from the vial; the cells and media contents are expelled gently and reaspirated several times until the cells are resuspended. The amount of cells provided per vial should be between 0.4 and 0.6 mL. Before injecting the cells, one also should aspirate air into the syringe and leave a column of air between the plunger and the cell media. This ensures that all of the cells are injected. The syringe cannot be inverted, or else it allows the air column to intermix with the cells. A blunt needle then is used to inject the cells into the defect. The catheter tip is advanced as far as possible to the distal border of the defect, and the cells are injected slowly and evenly over the defect (Fig. 4-5). Once an efflux is noted, the superior defect is sutured and the knee closed in the traditional layered fashion. The incisions are dressed under sterile conditions, and the patient is reversed from anesthesia. Routine parenteral and oral analgesics and cryotherapy are employed in the immediate postoperative period.

■ TECHNICAL ALTERNATIVES AND PITFALLS

Most of the published reports concerning chondral injuries and their treatment address the arthritic knee. This makes comparison of these reports with reports addressing results of treatment of acute chondral injuries difficult. Nonetheless, these reports can serve as a basis for understanding the difficulty of treating chondral injuries.

Nonoperative Treatment   Nonoperative treatment with regard to chondral injuries is variable but logically should include limited weight bearing and possibly controlled passive motion, although Salter's work (4) with partial-thickness chondral injuries showed no effect on the injury site. Treatment of chondral fractures is troublesome, because of the limited healing potential of the defects.

The avascularity of articular cartilage prevents a vascular response if there is cartilage injury alone. If the subchondral bone is injured, the inflammatory response produces mainly fibrocartilaginous tissue. This tissue is composed of mostly type I collagen rather than the type II seen in normal articular cartilage. The type I fibrocartilage is not durable and has been associated with eventual osteoarthritic degeneration. Articular cartilage is unique in that no vascular, neural, or lymphatic contribution is involved in its maintenance. Nourishment is dependent on the diffusion of nutrients. This creates difficulties if the reparative process is undertaken because of injuries. The chondrocytes do not migrate like other cells, and there is a slow regeneration rate of this cell type.

Debridement of the Joint In joint debridement, all loose bodies as well as meniscal fragments are debrided to a stable rim of hyaline cartilage. The side walls of a chondral lesion are fashioned to be perpendicular to the surface of the joint. Hubbard (5) found that 80% of patients treated with this technique had satisfactory results after 16 months.

The removal of cartilage and meniscal fragments can improve function and decrease severity of symptoms immediately. Magnuson (6) showed that 70% of patients can experience relief of symptoms. The efficacy of debridement for improving joint function, however, has not been established by prospective studies, nor do we know how long the benefits last. This procedure usually includes irrigation of the joint with a volume of fluid many times greater than the volume of the joint. This in itself could reduce the severity of the joint symptoms and pain. Jackson (7) compared his results with lavage alone to lavage and debridement and found little difference.

Both Kim et al. (8) and Mitchell and Shepard (9) have reported that debridement does not stimulate regeneration of an articular surface, nor does it halt the progression of the degenerative process. Removal of tissue debris and irrigation of the joint can decrease symptoms by decreasing the source of irritation to the synovial tissue. This procedure may be most helpful in young patients who have degenerative joint disease and no significant angular deformity or instability.

Abrasion Arthroplasty Abrasion arthroplasty is a technique in which a motorized burr removes sclerotic bone 1 to 2 mm in depth from the area in which a prior chondral injury has occurred. Blood vessel disruption and fibrin clot formation are the intended results. The joint must not bear weight for approximately 2 months because of the risk of fracture to the region that was burred. Johnson (10) recently described follow-up on 228 knees at 2 to 5 years. Although 75% had improved, 66% were still painful and 99% had restricted activity. No correlation existed between tissue regrowth at the injury site and eventual outcome.

The technique involves an intracortical abrasion (1–3 mm deep) into the subchondral bone. Cutting too deeply into the subchondral bone can result in worsening pain and a prolonged recovery period. The clinical outcomes from a number of different researchers have shown a variety of results. Ewing (11) reported that out of 223 patients, 163 had relief of pain and stiffness; Sprague (12) reported good pain relief in 51 of 69 patients. But Baumgaertner et al. (13) and Bert and Maschka (14) described less successful results. These variations in results could be attributed to a number of different factors: the severity of the degenerative tissue, the alignment of the joint, or perhaps the inability of the newly formed tissue to replicate the properties of hyaline cartilage. Friedman et al. (15) also noted that the age of the patient appears to influence the results of abrasion. Patients in their thirties had better results than older patients.

Subchondral Drilling or Microfracture Subchondral drilling or microfracture is used to stimulate bleeding similar to abrasion arthroplasty. The usual postoperative regimen allows for 8 weeks without weight bearing, with treatment with continuous passive motion (CPM). The microfracture technique has been suggested to be favorable because of its use of awls rather than drills to cause bleeding. Steadman (16) feels that the awls may cause less thermal injury to the bone immediately adjacent to the puncture site. Dzioba (17) found good results after 1 year in 69% of patients using this technique.

Drilling into the subchondral bone disrupts its blood vessels. This may lead to the formation of a fibrin clot. If the surface area is protected from excessive loading, a fibrocartilaginous repair tissue forms over the surface. The efficacy of this procedure in relieving pain and improving joint function is unpredictable. Some of the clinical reports show good symptomatic improvement after the procedure. (Childers and Ellood [18] reported 80% of their patients had excellent results.) In some reports it has been shown that the repair tissue functions relatively well as a load-bearing articular surface. Other reports, however, have shown little to no improvement from the procedure (19). One of the problems in trying to assess the efficacy of drilling into the subchondral bone is that none of the studies used outcome measures. The results were based primarily on subjective responses.

Perichondral Grafting   In perichondral grafting, autologous perichondrium is taken from the rib of the patient and grafted to the defect. Although this technique has been shown to yield hyaline-like cartilage, it is technically demanding and probably not reliably reproducible. Concerns about graft detachment, enchondral ossification of grafts, and durability have prevented widespread acceptance of this procedure.

Homminga et al. (20) have presented the only significant series of patients. A majority of the defects filled with hyaline-like cartilage, and 18 of 30 patients were pain free in followup. Although the Hospital for Special Surgery Knee score improved 17 points on average at 1 year of follow-up, 66% of the defects ossified with this technique.

Periosteal Grafting   Periosteal grafting is simply defect preparation and autogenous tibial periosteum sutured with the cambium layer oriented toward the joint. The objective is for the graft to stimulate chondrocyte growth from the bottom of the defect upward. Postoperatively, continuous passive motion is used, because it has improved results in a rabbit model.

O'Driscoll is the world's foremost expert with this technique and he and colleagues originally found improved results in immature rabbits with the use of continuous passive motion and the cambium layer oriented toward the joint (21). Type II collagen was seen in most of the specimens. In ongoing human trials at the Mayo Clinic and Foundation, others have not had the same success as O'Driscoll, implying a steep learning curve with this technique.

Osteochondral Autograft Transplantation and Mosaic Plasty   Three different groups recently have advocated this method as an alternative to other techniques. The basic technique involves taking donor osteochondral autograft cores from the notch or far lateral trochlea and placing them in the defect site, which has been prepared previously. Either motorized or manual cutting trephines perform the task of graft and donor site preparation. If more than one core is used, a mosaic pattern appears; hence the name *mosaic plasty*. This procedure can be performed completely arthroscopically and requires only one surgery. Of course, the specific cutting and insertion instruments must be available if the procedure is to be performed in the same sitting as the procedure that discovers the chondral injury. Magnetic resonance imaging will help in the future to define these injuries preoperatively with greater accuracy.

Bobi (22) described 12 patients in whom arthroscopic autograft transplantation was performed in conjunction with ACL reconstruction. The chondral lesions in this series measured from 10 to 22 mm in diameter. Three to five osteochondral cylinders were harvested from the notch region. At 2-year follow-up, 10 of the 12 patients had excellent response to the treatment. The first two continued to have pain, but the author attributed this to inferior instrumentation and inadequate surgical technique. Nine of the last ten cases had second-look arthroscopy at 1 year and had "normal shiny appearance and normal color of the grafted area" (22). Radiographs and magnetic resonance imaging confirmed graft integration in 10 of the 12 cases. Unfortunately, no patient-subjective follow-up data or biopsy data were presented.

As Bobi points out, with improvements in instrumentation this technique may find increased usage. In the setting of managed care, this operation has greater appeal.

The rehabilitation process is a critical component of the success of the procedure. Protocols must include early range of motion, flexibility exercises, strength training, and cross training. Weight bearing is introduced gradually over the first 6 weeks after surgery. Carefully guided rehabilitation affords patients the means necessary to regain functional use of the limb.

■ REHABILITATION

There are several important considerations in the proper design of an outcome assessment. Study design should aim to minimize potential bias. This is best accomplished using a randomized clinical trial with blinded assessment of results. Outcome assessment should follow a specific protocol, including standardized inclusion criteria, evaluation intervals, definitions of complications, and methods of assessment. An important proposed improvement of chondrocyte transplantation over other techniques of treatment of chondral defects is the ability to regenerate hyaline cartilage. Biopsy of treated lesions should be performed after healing to evaluate this issue. Peterson's (1) early results cannot be used as a definition of outcome, and only long-term studies can define the true efficacy of this procedure.

■ OUTCOMES AND FUTURE DIRECTIONS

Genzyme Tissue Repair is attempting to create a paste carrier for the cells and work out the details of an arthroscopic delivery system, which will make the procedure more attractive. The cost is still prohibitive, but our early results lend encouragement to our use of this technique in the setting of the problematic chondral injury.

The staff at Genzyme Tissue Repair in Boston, Massachusetts, graciously supplied material during our educational process that thoroughly details this procedure (23). Along with our own experience, that material was used to complete this chapter. Because this procedure is fairly detailed, a representative from Carticel will be available for technical support if the procedure is performed in any new setting. Neither author has received compensation for his efforts in preparing this manuscript.

■ ACKNOWLEDGMENTS

References

1. Peterson L, Menche D, Grande D, et al. Chondrocyte transplantation: an experimental model in the rabbit. In: *Transactions from the 30th Annual Orthopaedic Research Society, Atlanta, February 7–9, 1984*. Palatine, IL: Orthopaedic Research Society, 1984:218.
2. Grande DA, Pitman MI, Peterson L, et al. The repair of experimentally produced defects in rabbit articular cartilage by autologous chondrocyte transplantation. *J Orthop Res* 1989; 7:208–218.
3. Brittberg M, Lindahl A, Nilsson A, et al. Treatment of deep cartilage defects in the knee with autologous chondrocyte transplantation. *N Engl J Med* 1994; 33:889–895.
4. Salter RB. The biologic concept of continuous passive motion of synovial joints. *Clin Orthop* 1989; 242:12.
5. Hubbard MJS. Arthroscopic surgery for chondral flaps in the knee. *J Bone Joint Surg Br* 1987; 69:794–796.
6. Magnuson PB. Joint debridement: Surgical treatment of degenerative arthritis. *Surg Gynecol Obstet* 1941; 73:1–9.
7. Jackson RW. Arthroscopic treatment of degenerative arthritis. In: McGinty JB, ed. *Operative arthroscopy*. New York: Raven Press, 1991:319–323.
8. Kim HK, Moran ME, Salter RB. The potential for regeneration of articular cartilage in defects created by chondral shaving and subchondral abrasion: An experimental investigation in rabbits. *J Bone Joint Surg Am* 1991; 73:1301–1315.
9. Mitchell N, Shepard N. Effect of patellar shaving in the rabbit. *J Orthop Res* 1987; 5:388–392.
10. Johnson LL. Arthroscopic abrasion arthroplasty. In: McGinty JB, ed. *Operative arthroscopy*. New York: Raven Press, 1991:341–360.
11. Ewing JW. Arthroscopic treatment of degenerative meniscal lesions and early degenerative arthritis of the knee. In: Ewing JW, ed. *Articular cartilage and knee joint function: Basic science and arthroscopy*. New York, Raven Press, 1990:137–145.
12. Sprague NF. Arthroscopic debridement for degenerative knee joint disease. *Clin Orthop* 1981; 160:118–123.

13. Baumgaertner MR, Cannon WD, Vittori JM, et al. Arthroscopic debridement of the arthritic knee. *Clin Orthop* 1990; 253:197–202.

14. Bert JM, Maschka K. The arthroscopic treatment of unicompartmental gonarthrosis: A five-year follow-up study of abrasion arthroplasty plus arthroscopic debridement and arthroscopic debridement alone. *J Arthroscopy* 1989; 5:25–32.

15. Friedman JM, Berasi CC, Fox JM, et al. Preliminary results with abrasion arthroplasty in the osteoarthritic knee. *Clin Orthop* 1984; 182:200–205.

16. Steadman R. The 5th Annual Panther Sports Medicine Symposium, Pittsburgh, PA, 1992.

17. Dzioba RB. The classification and treatment of acute articular cartilage lesions. *J Arthroscopy* 1988; 4:72–80.

18. Childers JC, Ellwood SC. Partial chondrectomy and and subchondral bone drilling for chondromalacia. *Clin Orthop* 1979; 144:114–120.

19. Burks RT. Arthroscopy and degenerative arthritis of the knee: a review of the literature. *J Arthroscopy* 1990; 6:43–47.

20. Homminga GN, Bulstra SK, Bouwmeester PM, et al. Perichondral grafting for cartilage lesions of the knee. *J Bone Joint Surg Br* 1990; 72:1003–1007.

21. O'Driscoll SW, Keeley FW, Salter RB, et al. Durability of regenerated cartilage produced by free autogenous periosteal grafts in major full-thickness defects in joint surfaces under the influence of continuous passive motion. *J Bone Joint Surg Am* 1988; 70:595–606.

22. Bobi V. Arthroscopic osteochondral autograft transplantation in anterior cruciate ligament reconstruction: A preliminary clinical study. *Knee Surg Sports Traumatol Arthrosc* 1996; 3:262–264.

23. Bak P, George J, Chin I, et al. *Text for teaching slides for trained physicians.* Boston, Genzyme Tissue Repair, 1995.

5

Endoscopic Anterior Cruciate Ligament Reconstruction with Patellar Tendon Substitution

This chapter discusses the surgical technique for endoscopic or single-incision arthroscopy-assisted anterior cruciate ligament (ACL) reconstruction using patellar tendon substitution. The technique has been used by the author since October 1991 and evolved from a two-incision arthroscopy-assisted technique that had been used previously, beginning in 1986 (1–4). The technique discussed here was developed in anticipation of evolving to an outpatient ACL reconstruction technique, and to further reduce the incidence of early postoperative morbidity (5).

We recently had the opportunity to clinically review these two patient cohorts. Single- or double-incision arthroscopy-assisted ACL reconstruction with patellar tendon substitution is a predictable procedure for stabilizing the ACL-deficient knee. The clinical reviews comprised of 62, 105, and 109 patients, respectively. Modified Hospital for Special Surgery scores, Noyes knee rating scores, Tegner rating scores, and Lysholm scores have been comparable to previously reported series. The incidence of a negative pivot shift test for either technique at a 2- to 4-year interval has been between 90 and 92%, with patients generally demonstrating a grade 1 pivot shift phenomenon. We noted an 18% incidence of patellar pain in our initial 2- to 4-year follow-up of the two-incision technique (3). Patellar pain had a reduced incidence (12%) in our 5- to 9-year retrospective follow-up of the two-incision technique, and a 12% incidence in our prospective 2- to 4-year endoscopic follow-up. Arthrometry revealed a statistically significant ($P < 0.001$) reduction on maximum manual side-to-side testing for each group.

Our patients' subjective satisfaction has been extremely high in each of the three studies. Approximately 95% of the patients have been satisfied, as defined by being mostly or completely satisfied on subjective questioning and on visual analog scale analysis. Since May 1994 the author has performed the single-incision arthroscopy-assisted technique exclusively on an outpatient basis.

A decision to change to outpatient ACL reconstruction was based on our previous studies which evaluated hospitalization charges (5). Between 1989 and 1991, average hospitalization for patients undergoing the two-incision procedure was 2.9 days, with an average hospital charge of $15,500. Between 1991 and 1993, as our single-incision technique evolved, hospitalization was significantly reduced to an average of 1.6 days, with a reduction in cost to a mean of $13,500. In our main operating theater, the hospital charges are based on "*a la carte*" pricing rather than a fixed facility charge. As we evolved into outpatient ACL reconstructions, a transition was made to a hospital-owned surgicenter, which charges a fixed facility charge. In a previously published study, we demonstrated a significant reduction in hospital charges related to the outpatient ACL reconstruction technique. In that study, the fixed facility charge was $3,800, which represented a mean $5,000 charge difference if the outpatient ACL reconstruction was performed in our main operating room. Anesthetic advances including the use of propofol (Deprivan), ketoraloc tromethamine (Toradol), and periincisional and intraarticular bupirocaine hydrochloride (Marcaine) injection and im-

■ HISTORY OF THE TECHNIQUE

proved anesthetic techniques contribute to our ability to perform the procedure on an outpatient basis. Overall, the single- and two-incision techniques are functionally comparable.

■ INDICATIONS AND CONTRAINDICATIONS

Endoscopic single-incision ACL reconstruction using a patella tendon autograft is indicated for both primary and revision ACL surgery, providing the patella tendon has not been harvested previously. Patients who are candidates for acute reconstruction following ACL injury, and those with chronic ACL deficiency with functional instability should be considered for this technique. In patients undergoing revision surgery, graft availability may necessitate contralateral patella tendon harvest or the use of allograft patella tendon. Other graft sources, such as hamstrings or quadriceps tendons, require modification of fixation for the described technique.

■ SURGICAL TECHNIQUES

In contrast to the two-incision technique, in which we used a lateral thigh post with the leg held dependent off the side of the operating table, the single-incision technique is performed with an arthroscopic leg holder at the foot of the table drop. A well-padded thigh tourniquet is placed high on the proximal thigh. The waist of the table is flexed slightly to minimize lumbar spine extension, and the foot of the table is flexed enough to allow knee flexion to beyond 110 degrees. The contralateral leg is placed in a padded leg holder, which flexes the hip and knee, thereby protecting the common peroneal nerve. Duraprep is our standard antiseptic prep. As a prophylactic antibiotic, 1 g of cephalosporin (Ancef) is given preoperatively. Sixty milligrams of intramuscular ketoraloc tromethamine, 60 mg intramuscularly, is administered at the beginning of the procedure, and 30 mg is administered *en route* to the recovery room unless there are contraindications otherwise.

It is critical to examine the knee prior placing the extremity in the leg holder. The leg holder may negate or substantially reduce the pivot shift phenomenon. Both legs should be examined prior to positioning for comparison of the Lachman, anterior drawer, and pivot shift tests. Associated posterolateral laxity and assessment of collateral laxity should be assessed.

If the patient has demonstrable pivot shift with minimal degenerative joint disease, the patellar tendon graft is harvested prior to placement of the arthroscope. This is performed to expedite the procedure as well as for purposes of cosmesis.

Graft Harvest A 3- to 3.5-inch midline incision, approximately 3/8 inches from the midline is made. The skin is scored and infiltrated with 1 : 300,000 epinephrine, and the dissected section is carried down through the subcutaneous tissues to layer 1, which is incised and extended proximally and distally and retracted medially and laterally. Initially, Senn retractors followed by rake retractors are used to expose the patellar tendon, and Army–Navy retractors placed proximally in the wound for access to the distal patellar region. A single midline incision rather than miniincisions or two transverse incisions is preferred, to allow good visual exposure of the patellar tendon. The patellar tendon is measured distally, and its minimum width is documented in the operative report. A free central third graft is harvested after marking the distal pole and the tibial tubercle, and then we attempt to obtain 25-mm bone plugs on the tibia and the femur (Fig. 5-1). Bone plugs are outlined with a scalpel on the patella and distally extended into the patellar tendon and directed towards the tibial tubercle region. The author does not use double parallel blade graft-harvest knives, because the tendon has the tendency to taper towards the tibial tubercle. One also must be cognizant of different morphologies of the tibial tubercle. The very prominent tibial tubercle may result in less bone being harvested, rather than a more flattened tibial tubercle that allows a more ample harvesting of the tendon distally. Bone cuts are made in the patella and tibial tubercle with a no. 238 oscillating saw blade. The author prefers not to use an osteotome. The trapezoidal profile bone plug is harvested on the patella; a triangular bone plug is harvested on the tibial tubercle. The trapezoidal profile is selected on the patella to minimize the depth, thereby reducing the potential for stress fracture of the patella. In the tibial tubercle region, the rationale for obtaining a triangular bone profile is to maximize the amount of bone remaining for attachments of the medial and lateral thirds of the patellar tendon.

The middle third of the patellar tendon is harvested. A construct length of 90 to 100 mm usually is obtained. The patellar bone plug should be fashioned in a trapezoidal profile to minimize the depth of the cut on the patella. On the tibial tubercle site, the profile cut is triangular in shape. The patellar tendon may be harvested prior to arthroscopic placement if one has documented a pivot shift phenomenon and if one is convinced that there is not sufficient articular injury to preclude anterior cruciate ligament reconstruction. (From Bach BR. Endoscopic single incision ACL reconstruction. *Am J Knee Surg* 1992;5:146, with permission.)

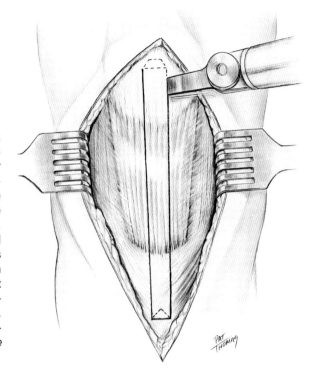

■ FIGURE 5-1

Graft Preparation   The graft is taken to a back table and prepared by an assistant. The total construct length is measured, including the lengths of the bone plugs and patellar tendon. The width is measured as well. The bone plugs are shaped and contoured and measured to slide through 10-mm sizing tubes, although we generally ream an 11-mm tibial tunnel (Fig. 5-2). The tendoosseous junction should be marked with sterile marking pen to

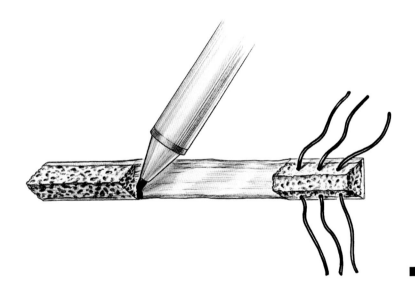

■ FIGURE 5-2

The tendoosseous junction is marked with a sterile marking pen to provide visual demarcation of this interval. This helps the surgeon judge the depth of graft placement on the femoral side. The shorter bone plug is prepared for placement on the tibial side to minimize the chance of construct tunnel mismatch. Three .062 K wire drill holes are placed parallel and immediately deep to the cortical surface of the graft. A suture passer will facilitate passage of no. 1 braided polyester sutures. (From Bach BR. Endoscopic single incision ACL reconstruction. *Am J Knee Surg* 1992;5:146, with permission.)

aid in visualization as the graft is passed, because generally we match the tendoosseous junction with the articular margin on the femoral side. In general, the longer bone plug is placed on the femoral side, and therefore two .062 mm K-wire drill holes are placed through the shorter bone plug for passage of either a number 5 Ticron suture or an 18-gauge wire passer. The advantage of the 18-gauge wire is that it will not be cut at the time of interference screw placement. The .062 K wire drill holes generally are placed parallel to the cortex, at the cortical cancellous interval of the graft, if number 5 Ticron sutures are used. If one prefers to drill perpendicular to the cortex, the author recommends use of an 18-gauge wire to preclude laceration of the suture. Following preparation, the graft is placed in a moist sponge and set aside. All personnel in the operating room should know where the graft has been placed, to preclude the inadvertent passage of the graft from the operating field.

The arthroscope is inserted via retracted skin edges through an inferolateral portal. The portal is made at the level of the distal pole of the patella with the knee flexed and adjacent to the lateral edge of the patellar tendon. The inferomedial portal is established similarly. The superomedial portal is established for the inflow pump, and intraarticular confirmation and intraarticular confirmation must be documented intraoperatively. If the fenestrations of the inflow cannula are not documented intraarticularly, marked extravasation of fluid can occur into the thigh or lower leg.

Diagnostic Arthroscopy   Diagnostic arthroscopy is performed in a systematic fashion. Clinical documentation of articular cartilage chondromalacia on the patellofemoral and the tibiofemoral joints is preferred. Assessment of partial-thickness meniscal tears, which commonly are noted in ACL deficiencies, should be made. Intercondylar notch osteophytes, the presence of a vertical strut (vertical scarring of the ACL to the posterior cruciate ligament [PCL]), or a lateral notch sign (chondral indentation of the lateral femoral condyle at the sulcus terminalis) should be documented. Finally, partial meniscectomy or repair should be performed prior to ACL stabilization.

Notch Preparation and Notchplasty   Notch preparation involves removal of residual ACL tissue. Frequently a vertical strut may be noted where the ACL has scarred to the adjacent PCL. The interval between the residual ACL tissue and the PCL should be defined, and to facilitate removal of the ACL tissue, tissue access channels can be created with arthroscopic scissors or an arthroscopic osteotome and then debrided with an arthroscopic shaver. The 30-degree arthroscope is placed in the inferolateral portal; the inferomedial portal is a working portal at this portion of the procedure. Residual tissue also is debrided from the lateral wall and also may be peeled from the wall with an arthroscopic osteotome (Fig. 5-3). Remnant ACL tissue on the tibial insertion site is smoothed until the bone can be assessed, which allows accurate placement of the tibial tunnel.

Notchplasty is performed with an arthroscopic shaver or burr. The author prefers a cylindrical 5.5-mm burr for ease of notchplasty (Fig. 5-4). In general, it is more difficulty to perform a left-knee notchplasty, because of the tendency of the torque of the burr towards the lateral wall. One should work from anterior to posterior and from top to bottom and be careful about proximal extension into the apex, because with hyperflexion the patella very closely approximates the intercondylar notch apex. There should be enough of a notchplasty performed to allow visualization for graft placement and to protect the graft from abrasion or impingement. There should be at least two burr widths between the lateral edge of the PCL and the lateral wall. Proper orientation of the arthroscopic camera is critical at this point, because rotation of the camera may result in misinterpretation of the notch configuration that is created with an arthroscopic notchplasty. Initially, one may use an arthroscopic osteotome to create the notchplasty, but the author prefers to do this under arthroscopic control with a burr, so that loose fragments do not require retrieval. The "over-the-top" top position must be confirmed arthroscopically, and one should be cognizant of a ridge that is in proximity to the PCL. In a fair number of failed ACL reconstructions referred to our center, anterior placement of the femoral tunnel is noted, and at subsequent revision surgery this ridge has been misinterpreted as the over-the-top orien-

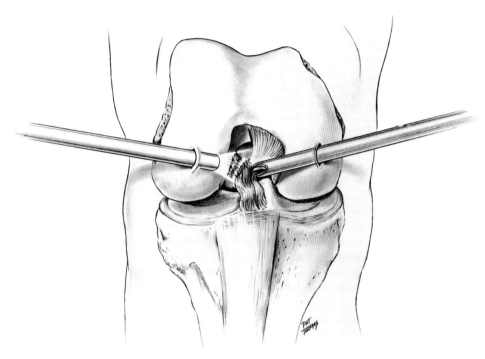

Intraarticular debridement of remnant anterior cruciate ligament tissue is performed with the arthroscope placed in the inferolateral portal. Attention is directed to debriding tissue on the insertion site as well as along the intercondylar wall. (From Bach BR Jr. Arthroscopy assisted patella tendon substitution for anterior cruciate ligament insufficiency: Surgical technique. *Am J Knee Surg* 1989;2 : 3–20, with permission.)

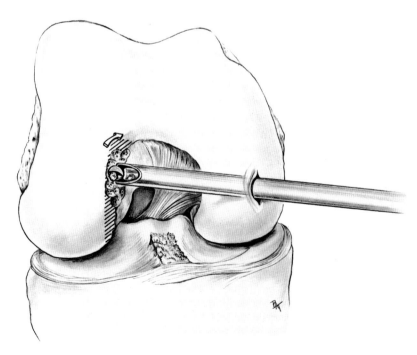

Notchplasty is performed with a 5- to 6-mm round motorized abrader to expand the wall to minimize graft abrasion postoperatively and to allow arthroscopic visualization of the "over-the-top" region. (From Bach BR Jr. Arthroscopy assisted patella tendon substitution for anterior cruciate ligament insufficiency: Surgical technique. *Am J Knee Surg* 1989;2 : 3–20, with permission.)

tation. To clearly define the over-the-top position, a curette or arthroscopic osteotome is used to clear the soft tissue so that the femoral guide may be slid over this position. The over-the-top position is clearly posterior to the PCL.

Tibial Tunnel Preparation   The first-generation tibial tunnel aimers selected a 40- to 45-degree angle from the horizontal plane for placement of the tibial tunnel (Fig. 5-5). This frequently resulted in graft construct mismatch with extrusion of the tibial bone plug. Subsequent aiming devices were developed to allow for variable angle determination for the tibial tunnel. In general, a 55-degree angle selected on a variable aimer allows for consistent ability to fixate the tibial bone plug with an interference screw. Several authors have recommended different formulas for determining the angle to be selected. For example, Miller (6) suggests that adding 7 mm to the soft-tissue length of the graft is a consistent method of determining the angle for tibial tunnel orientation. The entrance site on the tibial metaphysis is important. With the two-incision arthroscopy-assisted technique, this positioning is less important; however, the orientation on the femoral side is somewhat dependent upon the angle of the tibial tunnel with regard to the coronal and sagittal plane. One should select an entrance site that is midway from the posteromedial edge of the tibia and the tibial tubercle (i.e., midway within the tibia). This allows an 11 o'clock orientation on a right knee and a 1 o'clock orientation on a left knee if one flexes the knee and transposes a pin over the skin with the knee flexed in this orientation. An osteoperiosteal flap is created with electrocautery, with care taken to protect the remaining third medial patellar tendon, the pes anserine dis-

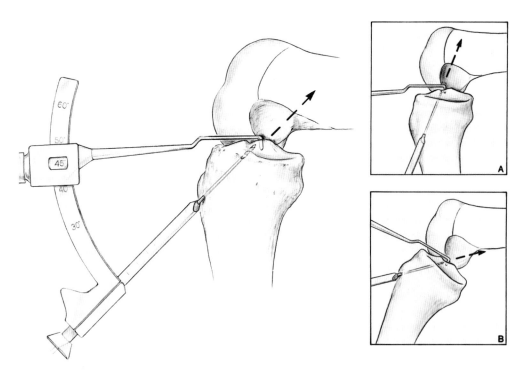

■ FIGURE 5-5

The tibial entrance site on the flare of the medial tibial metaphysis is slightly more proximal and horizontal than our previous technique description. The intraarticular entrance site for the tibial pin should be midway between the posterior edge of the anterior horn of the medial meniscus and the posterior cruciate ligament. In extension, this pin should be slightly posterior to the notch outlet. This schematic diagram demonstrates the importance of knee flexion position and orientation of the tibial pin. If the tibial tunnel is too steep, then the femoral tunnel placement may be made too anteriorly with the knee flexed at 90 degrees. A steep tibial tunnel may necessitate less knee flexion, at the risk of posterior cortex violation. Similarly, if an appropriate tibial tunnel angle is selected (50–55 degrees) but the knee is inadequately flexed, posterior cortical blowout may occur. (From Bach BR. Endoscopic single incision ACL reconstruction. *Am J Knee Surg* 1992;5:146, with permission.)

tally, and the superficial medial collateral ligament (MCL) medially. This medially based periosteal trap door is approximately 0.75 × 0.75 inches in size. The author uses the Acufex Protrak guide, which is placed through the inferomedial portal. In patients in whom patella alta is demonstrated radiographically, the soft-tissue bridge is lengthier, resulting in possible lifting of the arm of the guide from the horizontal plane. In these situations, one cannot easily place the stylet of the aiming device intraarticularly, in the appropriate position, while maintaining a steep tibial tunnel inclination. An accessory inferomedial portal is made immediately above the articular surface, and this can be dilated and the aiming device inserted.

In the mid- to late 1980s, the major focus of accurate tunnel placement was directed towards the femoral side; the tibial tunnel was thought to be less important. In fact, inaccurate tibial tunnel placement is equally as important, because anterior placement of the tibial tunnel may result in graft impingement on the anterior intercondylar notch region. An evolution has occurred to more posterior placement of the tibial tunnel. In the early years of arthroscopy-assisted techniques, many surgeons selected an anteromedial tibial tunnel placement. In the 1990s the transition has been towards a placement of the tibial tunnel in the middle third of the former ACL insertion site. General anatomic landmarks include the posterior edge of the anterior horn lateral meniscus, the posterior edge of the anterior horn medial meniscus, the intercondylar apex, the PCL, and the lateral intercondylar wall. The author selects a site that is in the coronal plane, in line with the posterior edge of the anterior horn lateral meniscus within the intercondylar eminence region. This also corresponds with the midpoint between the posterior edge of the anterior horn medial meniscus and the PCL. Other authors have developed a guide system that keys off the PCL and effectively brings the drill pin 7 mm from the it (7). Any of these methods allows accurate placement of the tibial tunnel within the middle third of the former ACL insertion site effectively placing the tunnel of the graft anatomically. The 3/32-inch pin is drilled under arthroscopic visualization and penetrates the articular margin by approximately 6 to 7 mm. The knee then is extended to assess the relationship of this pin to the intercondylar apex. Howell has demonstrated the importance of accurate tibial tunnel placement, and the pin should be 3 to 4 mm posterior to the intercondylar notch apex (8). This then is overreamed with an appropriately sized reamer. An 11-mm reamer is used for ease of passage of the graft. Prior to articular breakthrough, the arthroscopic inflow is turned off, which allows a more controlled collection of bone reamings for subsequent grafting of the distal patellar and tibial tubercle defects (9). One should drill directly through the articular margin, because the posterior edge often is irregular. A chamfer reamer and arthroscopic rasps are used to smooth the posterior and posterolateral aspect of the tibial tunnel (Fig. 5-6). An arthroscopic grabber and shaver may be placed through the inferomedial portal or through the tibial tunnel retrograde to clear the intraarticular eminence of residual debris.

Femoral Tunnel Preparation The trend has evolved away from of "isometric" to "anatomic" graft placement. The usage of an over-the-top off-set guide has allowed us to place the femoral tunnel consistently (Figs. 5-7 and 5-8). The guide is passed retrograde and positioned so that its "tongue" is engaged with the top position (Fig. 5-9). The drill pin is drilled 7 mm from the over-the-top position. Overreamed with a reamer 10 mm in diameter creates a 2-mm posterior cortical rim. The femoral offset guide is passed retrograde from the tibial tunnel with the knee flexed 80 ± 10 degrees. One should not drill this pin at less than 60 degrees of knee flexion. With the knee flexed in this position, subsequent drill pin placement and reaming preclude blowing out into the posterior compartment. Once the pin has been positioned preliminarily, it should be drilled approximately 1.5 inches into the femur. A 10-mm endoscopic reamer then is passed retrograde, and an initial footprint is created to a depth of approximately 8 to 10 mm (Fig. 5-10). This then is removed partially. The knee is irrigated, and the posterior cortex is assessed for correct placement relative to the over-the-top position. A thin 1- to 2-mm cortical bridge should remain (Fig. 5-11). Once the pin has been positioned on the femoral side, the knee should not be flexed, to avoid bending the pin. Reaming is completed approximately 5 to 10 mm longer than the length of the bone plug. The knee again is irrigated, and reamings are collected for subse-

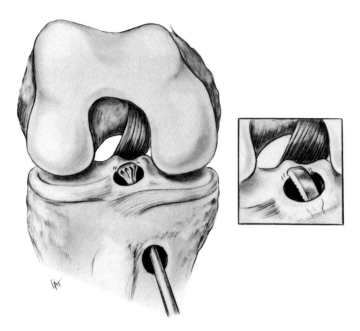

■ FIGURE 5-6

The motorized chamfer reamer is placed retrograde through the tibial tunnel to smooth posteriorly and posterolaterally. An arthroscopic rasp is used to smooth the posterior region of the tibial tunnel.

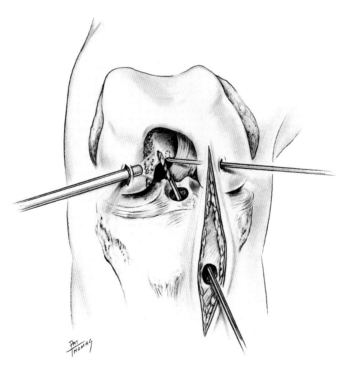

■ FIGURE 5-7

One may use a "freehand" technique to place the femoral pin, which is overreamed with a cannulated reamer. (From Bach BR. Endoscopic single incision ACL reconstruction. *Am J Knee Surg* 1992;5 : 146, with permission.)

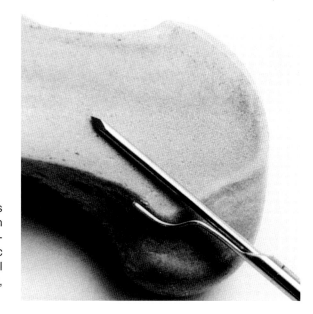

Femoral pin placement guide. This was developed to place the femoral pin 7 mm from the over-the-top location. Overreaming with a 10-mm diameter endoscopic reamer provides a 2-mm posterior cortical shell. (Courtesy of Arthrex, Portsmouth, New Hampshire.)

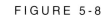 FIGURE 5-8

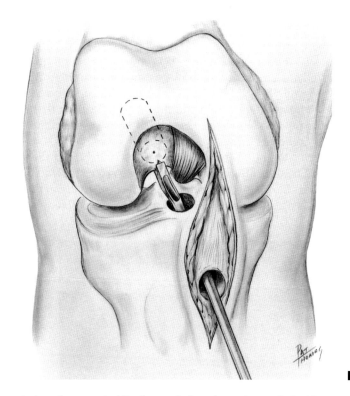

■ FIGURE 5-9

This anteroposterior schematic demonstrates placement of the femoral aimer in a retrograde fashion. The tongue of the aimer must slip over the posterior cortex. The knee is flexed usually between 75 and 90 degrees. (From Bach BR. Endoscopic single incision ACL reconstruction. *Am J Knee Surg* 1992;5:146, with permission.)

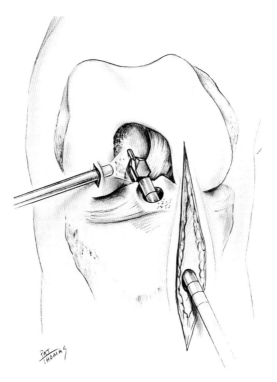

A 10-mm endoscopic reamer manually is inserted retrograde through the tibial tunnel up to the femoral region. This is reamed to a depth 5 to 10 mm deeper than the longest bone plug length on the patellar tendon construct. (From Bach BR. Endoscopic single incision ACL reconstruction. *Am J Knee Surg* 1992;5:146, with permission.)

quent grafting of the distal patellar and tibial tubercle defect. At this point, phase 2 notch-plasty is completed (Fig. 5-12). The anterolateral quadrant of the femoral tunnel is elipticized and smoothed to allow passage of the graft and femoral interference screw (Fig. 5-13). The wall, if needed, should be expanded laterally. In general, if the arc of the femoral tunnel violates the lateral wall, this is an indication that the lateral wall should be expanded. The roof also should be assessed, because roof height may vary from patient to patient and may require elevation.

Prior to graft passage, one should confirm that there is an intact femoral blind-end tunnel. Theoretically, one could create an accurate femoral tunnel, but if the angle at which the knee is flexed is inaccurate, one then could drill out through the posterior femur. Therefore, in all cases the entire femoral tunnel is visualized. This can be done easily by placing the

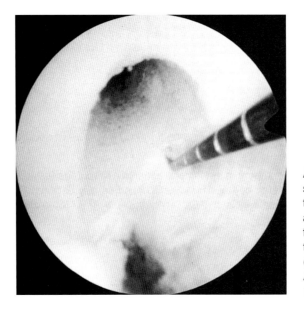

After femoral-tunnel reaming, the arthroscope probe is used to confirm that a posterior cortical has been maintained. The arthroscope can be placed either in the inferomedial portal or retrograde via the tibial tunnel to assist in visualization if needed. (From Bach BR. Endoscopic single incision ACL reconstruction. *Am J Knee Surg* 1992;5:146, with permission.)

■   FIGURE 5-11

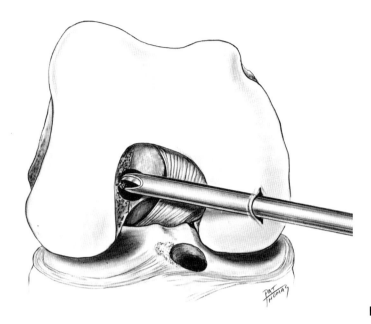

After reaming the femoral tunnel, phase 2 notchplasty is performed, and the inner edge of the femoral tunnel is smoothed. (From Bach BR Jr. Arthroscopy assisted patella tendon substitution for anterior cruciate ligament insufficiency: Surgical technique. *Am J Knee Surg* 1989;2:3–20, with permission.)

arthroscope retrograde from the tibial tunnel up into the femoral tunnel. This also allows for clearance of the femoral tunnel, which may become impacted with bone reamings.

Alternatively, O'Donnell and Scerpella (10) have placed the femoral aiming drill through an accessory portal rather than using retrograde tibial passage (Fig. 5-14). Using this modification requires hyperflexion of the knee prior to femoral pin placement. O'Donnell prefers this technique, which demonstrates improved parallel placement of femoral interference screws. I have used this modification selectively. It may be particularly useful in complex revision situations.

Graft Passage   The bone plug on the femoral side is oriented so that the cortex is directed posteriorly. This posteriorizes the soft-tissue component of the graft, thereby reducing the likelihood of soft-tissue graft injury with interference screw placement. Although there are methods using a Beath needle pull-through or a two-pin technique for graft passage, the au-

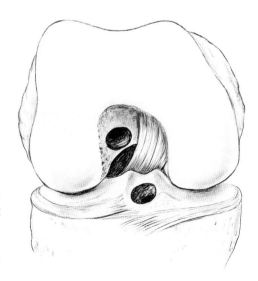

This schematic illustration depicts the femoral tunnel following reaming. The anterolateral quadrant may be ellipticized to facilitate graft and screw passage. (From Bach BR. Endoscopic single incision ACL reconstruction. *Am J Knee Surg* 1992;5:146, with permission.)

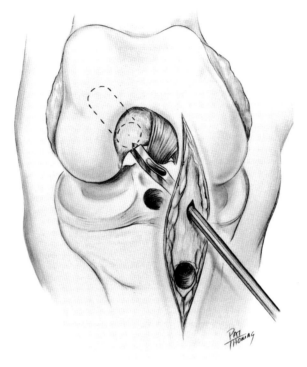

■   FIGURE 5-14

An alternative approach to femoral pin placement and reaming is through an accessory inferomedial portal rather than through a retrograde tibial tunnel.

thor has used a "push-in" technique, whereby an instrument is used to push the graft intraarticularly and a hemostat is used to grasp the graft and guide it into the femoral tunnel (Fig. 5-15). This can be facilitated by turning off the arthroscopic inflow. The tendoosseous junction is aligned flush with the articular margin, except in situations in which a graft is long and there may be a component of graft–construct mismatch. In these situations in which one anticipates a potential graft–tunnel mismatch, a portion of the bone plug is left initially prominent on the femoral side to act as a guide or skid for passage of the hyperflex Nitenol pin (Concept, Largo, FL) (Fig. 5-16). This pin is passed through the inferomedial portal and seated provisionally at a position between 11:30 and 12:30 on the clock, 3 to 5 mm deep, with the

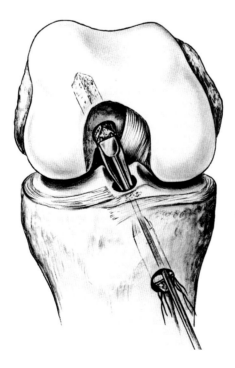

■   FIGURE 5-15

The graft is pushed retrograde with the assistance of a graft "pusher" through the tibial tunnel, intraarticularly, and in some situations directly into the femoral tunnel. An arthroscopic grasping instrument or hemostat is helpful in positioning the graft. If the cortical edge of the graft is placed posteriorly, graft injury is less likely during screw placement. (From Bach BR. Endoscopic single incision ACL reconstruction. *Am J Knee Surg* 1992;5:146, with permission.)

Endoscopic interference screw placement is facilitated with the placement
of a flexible 14-in Nitenol pin through
an accessory parapatellar tendon portal. The pin should be placed anterolaterally to the graft and initially seated,
the knee flexed further to 120 degrees,
and the pin further advanced. This
places the pin parallel to the graft. A
7 mm wide, 25 mm long cannulated
endoscopic screw is inserted via this
accessory portal. This lateral schematic demonstrates the relationship of
cannulated interference screw and
bone plug. Note that femoral bone plug
has been oriented with its cortex posterior to minimize soft-tissue injury. If
the bone plug is recessed, soft-tissue
injury is possible if the screw is not
placed in a parallel fashion.

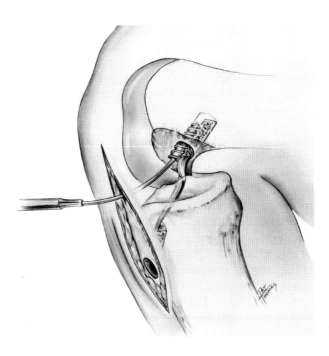

■ FIGURE 5-16

tunnel-plug interface. The knee then is flexed to approximately 100 to 110 degrees and the pin
further advanced. One should feel this pin bottom out in the depths of the femoral tunnel. The
author prefers to place the hyperflex Nitenol pin anterior to the bone plug rather than medial
or lateral to the graft. Once this has been seated, a cannulated interference screw is positioned.
A 7 × 25-mm cannulated screw almost always is selected for the femoral side. A soft-tissue
protector may be used to minimize injury to the graft when the screw is passed. After the
screw has been inserted half of its length, the hyperflex Nitenol pin is removed and the screw
then is completely seated (Fig. 5-17). At this point the sutures that have been placed on the tibial portion of the bone plug graft are grasped, tension is placed on the graft, and a "Rock" test
is performed to assess the graft screw tunnel fixation. Enough pressure is placed on these su-

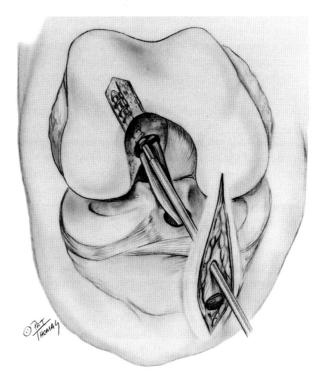

After the screw has been secured half
its length, the Nitenol pin is removed
and the screw advanced to the articular
margin or slightly recessed. (From
Bach BR. Endoscopic single incision
ACL reconstruction. *Am J Knee Surg*
1992;5:146, with permission.)

■ FIGURE 5-17

tures through the graft to oscillate the patient on the operating room table. Tension is placed on the sutures or the tibial plug, and the knee is flexed and extended to assess for any impingement and for "gross" isometry. One may place the thumb against the tibial tunnel and bring the knee into complete extension to assess for gross strain behavior of the graft.

The graft is secured on the tibial side with an interference screw in 95% of our procedures. In general, the screw is placed on the anterior aspect of the bone plug against the cortical surface. Mechanical testing has demonstrated that graft fixation is superior with cancellous-to-cancellous rather than cortical-to-cancellous apposition. Although some surgeons are concerned about possible soft-tissue injury resulting from placing the screw along the soft-tissue side of the graft, this problem has not been encountered in our experience. The graft is secured in complete extension, oriented anteriorly in the coronal plane. This effectively results in rotation of the graft fibers. If the bone plug extrudes by 5 to 6 mm, we still use an interference screw and burr down the extruded portion of the bone plug. If over 50% of the graft extrudes, we may consider creating a trough and securing this with two 3/8- or 1/2-in barbed staples. Fixation is performed with the knee in complete extension. A posterior Lachman force is not applied when the graft is secured. Once the graft has been secured, we assess for range of motion. The Lachman, anterior drawer, and pivot shift tests are performed and should be normal. To actually assess the pivot shift test, the strap on the leg holder must be released to allow freedom of the thigh; otherwise fixation of the leg within the arthroscopic leg holder dampens or eliminates even an abnormal pivot shift test.

At this point the knee is irrigated copiously, suctioned dry, and reevaluated arthroscopically. Graft tension is noted at varying degrees of knee flexion, and notch or lateral wall impingement is noted. Attention is directed towards closure.

With the knee flexed, the patellar tendon rent is closed with an absorbable suture. Bone reamings are packed into the distal patellar defect, and layer 1 is closed over the area with inverted absorbable sutures. If there is sufficient graft, the tibial tubercle also is grafted. The osteoperiosteal flap is closed. In the medial metaphyseal region of the tibial, one suture is cut longer to allow us to track into that region if we ever need to remove an interference screw, or for the remote possibility of having to perform a revision procedure subsequently. A drain generally is not utilized. Marcaine is injected copiously intraarticularly and into the surgical wound region. The subcutaneous tissue is closed with inverted absorbable sutures. The skin is closed with a running nylon subcuticular pull-out closure. Steristrips are applied loosely, with the knee flexed to minimize traction blisters; Owens gauze, dressings, an ice cryotherapy unit, an Ace bandage, and a drop-lock full range of motion brace are applied in the operating room. On the way to the recovery room, 30 mg ketoraloc tromethamine is administered.

■ TECHNICAL ALTERNATIVES AND PITFALLS

The endoscopic technique of ACL reconstruction differs in several ways from the two-incision technique. Because of this there are several pitfalls that can be encountered that require the surgeon to be able to make changes intraoperatively. As previously mentioned, the femoral socket needs to be positioned close to the lateral femoral cortex back wall. The lateral ridge on the lateral femoral cortex wall often is fairly prominent, and if not removed during the notchplasty it can give the surgeon an inaccurate landmark for femoral socket placement. It is therefore imperative in using the endoscopic technique that a complete notchplasty be performed and that the over-the-top position be clearly identified. Failure to do so results in anterior placement of the femoral socket and failure of the ACL reconstruction.

If the femoral socket is placed too posteriorly, however, one may perforate the back wall, resulting in femoral socket "blowout." If this happens, one must be prepared to obtain femoral fixation through other means. If the posterior cortex has been violated, fixation cannot be achieved with an interference fit screw. It is possible, however, to continue to drill the femoral socket and then with an additional lateral incision fix the graft to a post on the lateral femoral cortex or tie the sutures over a button laterally. One must recognize the fact that the posterior cortex has been violated and be willing to make these modifications so that adequate fixation on the femoral side is achieved at the time of surgery. In a similar vein, if one encounters significant osteoporosis or poor fixation with an interference fit screw, one should consider tying the no. 5 sutures from the femoral bone plug to a post that is placed in the lateral femoral cortex. Another option is to reinforce interference fixation that is felt to be inadequate by tying the sutures over a button over the lateral femoral cortex. One must not leave the operating room with inadequate femoral fixation.

Another pitfall that can be encountered is graft–tunnel mismatch. If the graft is too long and the tibial bone plug is outside of the tunnel, the options are several. As previously mentioned, a trough can be made on the anterior tibial cortex and the graft fixed with barbed staples. Alternative methods of dealing with this include deepening the femoral socket and then recessing the femoral plug, with fixation achieved by tying the sutures over a post on the lateral cortex or over a button on the lateral cortex of the femur. This allows for interference fixation on the tibial side. If the socket is deepened, interference fixation should be used only with caution, because of the danger of graft damage or cutting during placement the interference screw. Alternatively, the femoral socket can be left with an interference fixation, and the tibial sutures or wire can be tied over a post. In this situation a small trough in the tibial cortex should be made.

REHABILITATION

The patient is provided with a visual pain analog scale and a questionnaire to log all pain medications during the first 10 days postoperatively. The afternoon of surgery, the patient attends physical therapy and is taught removal and application of his or her brace and prone hanging, straight leg raising, and active range of motion exercises. With injection of Marcaine into the knee joint on the day of surgery, the patient generally is able to flex easily to 80 to 90 degrees; the patient should be informed that the following day he or she will have more discomfort. Patients are seen the day following surgery for a dressing change. The steristrips are removed and new strips applied to minimize the chance of skin traction blisters. Tincture of Benzoin is not advised. A formal supervised physical therapy program is recommended, and the author provides the patient with a protocol for rehabilitation that is similar to the accelerated rehabilitation program popularized by Shelbourne et al. (11) and modified at our institution (12). Sutures are removed 7 to 10 days postoperatively, and anteroposterior and lateral radiographs are taken at that time. Motion goals by 2 weeks after the operation are to have achieved complete extension and flexion to 90 degrees. Patients begin prone ankle hangs for extension immediately. The drop-lock brace is locked in extension for weight-bearing purposes. Patients are allowed to bear weight as tolerated and to discontinue crutches when comfortable. This generally is achieved by the end of the first week. The brace also is locked in extension for sleeping purposes, because most patients sleep with their knees flexed and this has been helpful in terms of maintaining extension during the first 6 weeks. A drop-lock extension brace is used to minimize the chance of traumatic injury to the donor site should the patient slip or fall during the first 6 weeks following surgery.

OUTCOMES AND FUTURE DIRECTIONS

Over the past decade, the author has evolved from an arthroscopy-assisted two-incision technique to a single-incision technique. The single-incision technique is fraught with a number of technical pitfalls unique to this procedure and should be performed, in my opinion, by experienced arthroscopic surgeons who understand the principles of knee-ligament surgery. In the majority of patients that I have seen for failed endoscopic techniques, there clearly has been a technical component contributing to the failure. In general, this is an anteriorization of the either femoral or tibial tunnel. Long-term results have not been reported for the endoscopic technique, but our early 2- to 4-year prospective study demonstrated results that were identical to those with the two-incision technique for stability assessed by physical examination and KT-1000 parameters, and slightly better for Lysholm, Hospital for Special Surgery, and Noyes ratings than two incision patients who were evaluated at a similar postoperative interval. Patients' subjective level of satisfaction for either technique was equally high, with 95% of patients indicating that they were "mostly" or "completely" satisfied.

References

1. Bach BR Jr. Arthroscopy assisted patella tendon substitution for anterior cruciate ligament insufficiency: Surgical technique. *Am J Knee Surg* 1989; 2:3–20.
2. Hardin GT, Bach BR Jr, Bush-Joseph J, et al. Endoscopic single incision ACL reconstruction using patellar tendon autograft-surgical technique. *Am J Knee Surg* 1992; 5:144–155.
3. Bach BR Jr, Jones GT, Sweet F, et al. Arthroscopic assisted ACL reconstruction using patellar tendon substitution: Two year follow-up study. *Am J Sports Med* 1994; 22:758–767.
4. Bach BR Jr, Jones GT, Hager CA, Sweet F. Arthrometric aspects of arthroscopic assisted ACL reconstruction using patellar tendon substitution. *Am J Sports Med* 1995; 23:179–185.
5. Novak PJ, Bach BR Jr, Bush-Joseph CA, et al. Cost-containment: A charge comparison of anterior cruciate ligament reconstruction. *Arthroscopy* 1996; 12:160–164.
6. Miller MD, Hinkin DT. The "N + 7 rule" for tibial tunnel placement in endoscopic anterior cruciate ligament reconstruction. *Arthroscopy* 1996; 12:124–126.
7. Morgan CD, Galinat BJ, Jones K. The tibial insertion of the ACL: Where is it? A rationale for reconstruction. Presented at the *58th Annual Meeting of the American Academy of Orthopaedic Surgeons*, San Francisco, CA, February 1993.
8. Howell SM, Taylor MA. Failure of reconstruction of the anterior cruciate ligament due to impingement by the intercondylar notch. *J Bone Joint Surg Am* 1993; 75:1044–1055.
9. Daluga D, Johnson JC, Bach BR Jr. Primary bone grafting following graft procurement for ACL insufficiency. *J Arthroscopy* 1990; 6:205–208.
10. O'Donnell JB, Scerpella TA. Endoscopic anterior cruciate ligament reconstruction: Modified technique and radiographic review. *Arthroscopy* 1995; 11:577–584.
11. Shelbourne KD, Nitz P. Accelerated rehabilitation after anterior cruciate ligament reconstruction. *Am J Sports Med* 1990; 18:292–299.
12. Williams JS Jr, Bach BR Jr. Operative and nonoperative rehabilitation of the ACL injured knee. *Sports medicine and arthroscopy review* 1996:4(1):69–82.

6

Endoscopic Anterior Cruciate Ligament Reconstruction using a Double Looped Hamstring Tendon Graft

The "ideal" anterior cruciate ligament (ACL) graft substitute should be free of any associated donor site injury, be readily available for use, and be capable of strong fixation with sufficient inherent strength to withstand an accelerated postoperative rehabilitation program. In addition, the long-term results of reconstructive procedures utilizing the ACL graft substitute should be favorable. Unfortunately, such an "ideal" graft material currently does not exist.

Use of the hamstring tendons for ACL graft material avoids disruption of the extensor mechanism and its associated problems, including potential fracture of the patella, patellar tendinitis, or development of anterior knee pain (1–4). Postoperative patellofemoral pain or crepitation is not limited to those reconstructions that utilize bone–patellar tendon–bone (BPTB) autografts but is found more commonly in such situations than after use of the hamstring tendons (4–7). Harvesting the hamstring tendons, however, is not without its own potential problems: Injury to either the saphenous vein or nerve may occur (8). Details of the pes anserine anatomy and its relation to the harvesting of these tendons have been described elsewhere (9,10).

Concerns regarding the use of the hamstring tendons as a graft material for ACL reconstruction include their strength, potential elongation of the graft during the postoperative period, less secure graft fixation, and a greater length of time necessary for incorporation into bone tunnels. Biomechanical data reported by Noyes et al. (11) demonstrated the relative strength of a 14-mm wide BPTB graft to be 168% of the reference ACL strength; the semitendinosus and gracilis tendons had relative strengths of 70 and 49% respectively. Two points should be made regarding this frequently cited study: First, most BPTB grafts used for ACL reconstruction are 10 or 11 mm in width rather than 14 mm; second, the semitendinosus and gracilis tendons that were tested were single-stranded.

More recently reported data (12), in addition to several as yet unpublished studies by Hecker et al. and Howell et al. (personal communications, 1997) have documented the increased strength obtained by utilizing either double- or quadruple-stranded hamstring tendon grafts. In addition, the stiffness of a hamstring tendon graft more closely approximates the normal ACL than does the significantly stiffer BPTB graft (11).

The healing process that occurs after placement of a soft-tissue graft within a bone tunnel has been detailed by several authors using animal models (13,14). In each of these studies, histologic examination demonstrated the formation and maturation of Sharpey-like fibers extending between the bone and soft tissue graft to occur between 4 and 12 weeks after graft placement. Biomechanical testing showed a progressive increase in the strength of the tendon–bone interface to occur over the first 12 weeks after the tendon transfer (13). The results demonstrated that as biologic incorporation of the graft took place between the bone tunnel and transplanted tendon on a histologic level, the structural weak point of the graft construct shifted from the fixation site to the inherent strength of the graft tissue it-self. These findings have important implications with regards to constructing specific components of a postoperative rehabilitation program following ACL reconstruction with a soft-tissue graft.

Macey (15) and Lipscomb (16) were some of the first surgeons to report on the use of a semitendinosus graft for an intraarticular ACL reconstruction. Mott (17) described a technique utilizing a graft composed of a double-looped semitendinosus tendon. Since that time, multiple reports have been published describing techniques in which the hamstring tendons serve as the ACL graft material during an intraarticular ACL reconstructive procedure (17–21).

In this chapter, an operative technique for ACL reconstruction is outlined that uses the semitendinosus tendon, with or without the gracilis, as the graft tissue. The reconstruction uses a quadruple-stranded hamstring tendon graft (two looped tendon strands) placed using an endoscopic technique. More traditional techniques using hamstring tendons have required the use of a second incision over the distal lateral femur. The technique presented here utilizes a commercially available device for femoral-sided fixation allowing for placement of ACL graft substitutes, including soft tissue grafts, in an endoscopic fashion (21). The EndoButton (Acufex Microsurgical, Mansfield, MA) is a 4 × 12-mm flat metallic anchor designed to be inserted endoscopically with simple instrumentation. The device is employed after graft insertion, anchoring onto the anterolateral femoral cortex. The author's experience with this technique has been very favorable, and it currently is the technique of choice for the majority of ACL reconstructions.

■ INDICATIONS AND CONTRAINDICATIONS

With an increasing number of individuals participating in both organized and recreational sporting activities, the incidence of major knee ligament injuries has grown. This is particularly true of the expanding number of female athletes who are involved in sports featuring high-risk cutting and pivoting. Because certain individuals with incompetent ACLs are able to remain involved in all of their desired activities, selection of operative candidates is a challenge in clinical judgement. The patient's preinjury type and level of activity are probably the most important factors in the decision concerning the appropriate treatment of a complete tear of the ACL (22).

Although no surgical indications are absolute, accepted indications for operative treatment of the ACL-deficient knee include symptomatic instability with activities of daily living or athletic participation, functional impairment in patients unwilling or incapable of altering their lifestyles, and failure of nonoperative management (23). In addition, the patient's willingness and ability to comply with a rigorous and time-consuming postoperative rehabilitation program are of critical importance. Without such a commitment, a less than satisfactory outcome surely will result despite even a technically superior surgical procedure.

■ SURGICAL TECHNIQUES

Patient Positioning and Preparation   The procedure is performed in an ambulatory setting. A general or regional anesthetic is provided, and the patient is positioned supine on the operative table. A systematic examination under anesthesia is performed, with comparison made between the injured and uninvolved lower extremities. Both the degree of translation and quality of the endpoint are noted for the Lachman and anterior drawer tests; in addition, the presence and magnitude of the pivot shift phenomenon should be assessed. Associated ligamentous laxity (e.g., collateral ligaments, posterolateral corner) also is assessed.

A well-padded pneumatic tourniquet is placed as proximally as possible on the thigh of the operative extremity. The nonoperative extremity is positioned in a well-padded leg holder with the hip and knee flexed and the hip both abducted and externally rotated. The foot of the operating table is dropped, and the operative extremity is placed in an arthroscopic leg holder at the level of the tourniquet. In this position, free unobstructed access to the entire operative extremity is possible, as is manipulation of the leg during the course of the procedure. The operative extremity is prepared and draped in a standard sterile fashion and exsanguinated and the pneumatic tourniquet elevated to an appropriate setting.

Diagnostic Arthroscopy   Anatomic landmarks are delineated on the skin with a marking pen and standard anteromedial and anterolateral portals are established on the joint line adjacent to the borders of the patellar tendon. An additional superolateral or superomedial portal also may be created for either inflow or outflow, depending on the surgeon's preference. A 30-degree arthroscope is inserted through the anterolateral portal and a thorough, systematic examination of the entire knee is performed. Evaluation includes assessment of the suprapatellar pouch, the patellofemoral joint (including patellar tracking and status of the articular cartilage), the medial and lateral gutters, and the medial and lateral compartments for any chondral or meniscal injury, as well as confirmation of the suspected ligamentous pathology. Instruments utilized during this diagnostic examination (i.e., arthroscopic probe, motorized shaver) are placed through the anteromedial portal. Occasionally, accessory portals (i.e., posteromedial, posterolateral) may be used for improved visualization or further inspection of a particular aspect of the knee; for example, a posteromedial portal may be used for the inspection and preparation of a peripheral tear of the posterior horn of the medial meniscus prior to repair. Passage of the arthroscope through the intercondylar notch as originally described by Gillquist et al. (24) also allows for better visualization of the posterior aspects of the knee joint. All pathology that is identified during the diagnostic evaluation of the knee is addressed as deemed appropriate by the operative surgeon. The specific sequence followed depends upon the particular combination of injuries that is present. For the purposes of this chapter, we assume that an isolated ACL reconstruction is to be performed.

Graft Harvest   The author prefers a vertical skin incision for harvesting the hamstring tendon or tendons. The incision is made in line with the anteromedial portal beginning just distal to the proximal margin of the tibial tubercle and extending 3 to 4 cm distally. Variation in the individual anatomy of the pes anserine insertion at times may necessitate slightly more distal extension of the incision. Alternatively, an oblique skin incision in line with the underlying gracilis and semitendinosus tendons can be made overlying the pes anserine inserion.

Dissection is carried down through the subcutaneous tissue until the sartorial fascia is encountered. Any infrapatellar branches of the saphenous nerve that are encountered are preserved if possible. Full-thickness subcutaneous flaps are raised in all directions, permitting retraction and improved visualization. Palpation of the sartorial fascia from proximal to distal permits the surgeon to identify the underlying semitendinosus and gracilis tendons. These tendons blend together as they approach their insertion onto the tibia, and the interval between them is more distinct proximal and posterior to their insertion. The sartorial fascia is incised over the interval between the semitendinosus and gracilis tendons and in line with the direction of the tendons themselves. This "window" in the sartorial fascia can be opened both proximally and distally as necessary, in order to isolate the underlying tendons (Fig. 6-1). Penrose drains are passed around both the semitendinosus and gracilis tendons. The semitendinosus is the more distal of the two tendons, so it may be captured by placing a right-angled clamp in the interval between it and the gracilis tendon and then passing it distally behind the semitendinosus tendon. A similiar maneuver is performed for the gracilis, except that the clamp is passed proximally from the interval. Again, the two tendons coalesce as they course to their insertion with the tibia, so it is much easier to isolate them from one another in a proximal location. By isolating both tendons, one can prevent injury to the gracilis as the semitendinosus tendon is being harvested.

Blunt and sharp dissection to free the semitendinosus tendon from all associated attachments is necessary for proper harvesting of the tendon. Great care is critical to ensure adequate release of all accessory fascial bands extending from the semitendinosus tendon to the fascia of the medial gastrocnemius (Fig. 6-2) prior to stripping the tendon, in order to avoid premature transection of the tendon (9,10). Prior to detaching the semitendinosus tendon from its distal insertion, a running whipstitch of no. 2 Ethibond suture is placed up one side of the tendon approximately 1.5 cm and then down the opposite side. The tendon

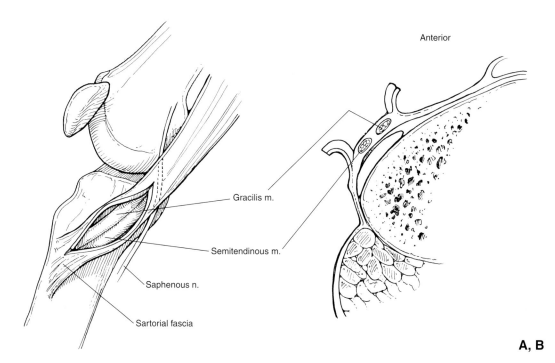

Anterior

Gracilis m.

Semitendinous m.

Saphenous n.

Sartorial fascia

■ FIGURE 6-1   **A, B**

A: Medial aspect of a right knee, depicting how opening of the sartorial fascia exposes the underlying gracilis and semitendinosus tendons. **B:** Axial cross-section of a right proximal tibia just above the level of the pes anserine insertion, demonstrating the same relationships of these structures. (Adapted from Pagnini MJ, Warner JJP, O'Brien SO, et al. Anatomic considerations in harvesting the semitendinosus and gracilis tendons and a technique of harvest. *Am J Sports Med* 1993;21:565–571, with permission.)

then is detached from its insertion with a portion of associated periosteum in order to maximize length. While tension is maintained on the sutures, blunt dissection about the tendon as it courses proximally into the posterior thigh is performed to ensure that no fascial connections remain. The sutures grasping the free end of the tendon then are threaded through a closed-ended tendon stripper. The tendon is harvested with the knee flexed and traction applied to the grasping suture. Great care is taken to run the instrument parallel to the tendon at all times; failure to do so may cause inadvertant premature tendon transection (Fig. 6-3). The tendon comes free from its myotendinous junction as the instrument is advanced proximally. Typically, a tendon measuring between 24 and 30 cm is obtained. If the free semitendinosus tendon is not of sufficient length to create a quadruple-stranded graft (see "Graft Preparation" below), the gracilis tendon is harvested in a similar fashion.

Graft Preparation   Muscle remnants at the musculotendinous junction are removed. The remaining thin tendinous tissue at the proximal portion of the graft is tubularized with an absorbable 2-0 Vicryl suture, and the length of the graft is measured. In the author's opinion, the minimum total tendon length necessary to allow for creation of an appropriate length quadruple-stranded graft is 26 cm. This measurement is based on the following calculations:

1. The average intraarticular graft distance is approximately 25 mm (intraarticular distance from opening of tibial tunnel to opening of femoral tunnel).
2. The minimum desired length of graft tissue to be contained within each bone tunnel (tibial and femoral) is 20 mm.

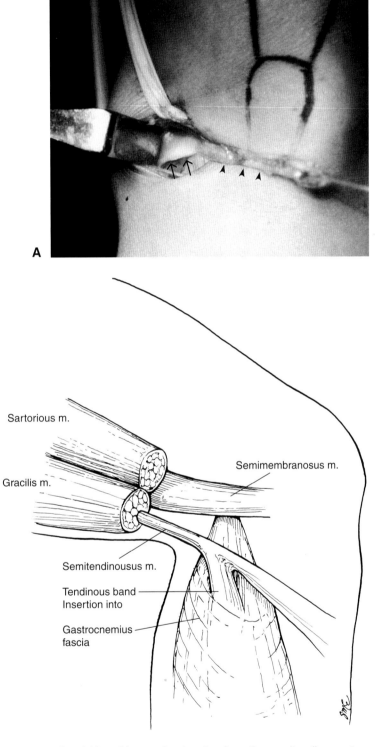

A: Clinical photograph of the accessory fascial band (*arrows*) extending from the semitendinosus tendon (*arrowheads*) to the fascia of the medial gastrocnemius. **B:** Line drawing demonstrating how the semitendinosus is tethered to the medial gastrocnemius fascia by this band. (Adapted from Ferrari JD, Ferrari DA. The semitendinosus: anatomic considerations in tendon harvesting. *Orthop Rev* 1991;20:1085–1088, with permission.)

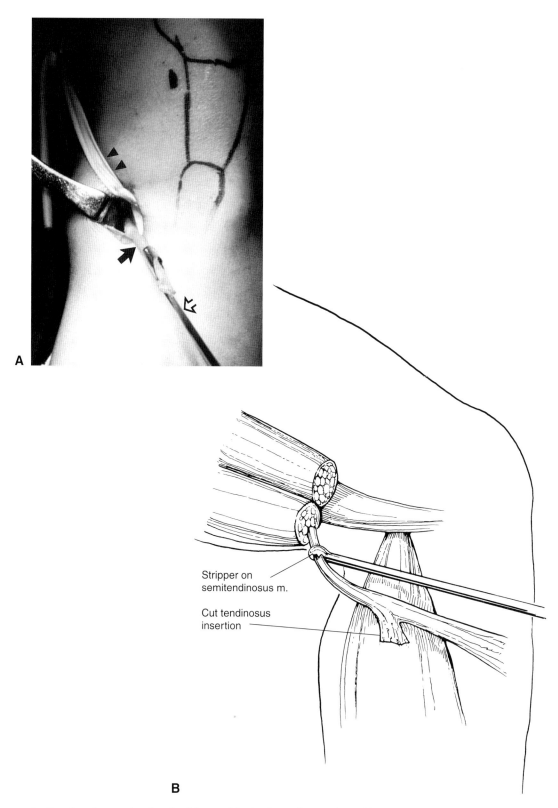

A: Semitendinosus tendon (*solid arrow*) just prior to harvesting with a closed-ended tendon stripper (*open arrow*). A Penrose drain is retracting the gracilis tendon (*arrowheads*). **B:** If the tendon stripper strays from the anatomic course of the tendon, premature transection may occur. (Adapted from Pagnini MJ, Warner JJP, O'Brien SO, et al. Anatomic considerations in harvesting the semitendinosus and gracilis tendons and a technique of harvest. *Am J Sports Med* 1993;21:565–571, with permission.)

3. The minimum total graft length equals 25 + (2 × 20) = 65 mm.
4. Four strands of 65 mm each equal 260 mm of total tendon length.

If the semitendinosus tendon is too short, then the gracilis tendon also is harvested, and the quadrupled graft is composed of a double strand of each tendon. The length of graft placed within the femoral tunnel is limited, by necessity, both by the size of the lateral femoral condyle and because this technique requires creation of a closed-ended tunnel. If both hamstring tendons are to be used, the total length of graft created and utilized depends on the surgeon's preference for tibial-sided fixation (i.e., suture around a post, or screw and spiked soft-tissue washer).

Utilizing the various clamps available with the GraftMaster preparation board (Acufex Microsurgical), running whip stitches extending up and down each of the remaining free ends of each tendon strand are placed using nonabsorbable no. 2 Ethibond suture. The length of tendon captured by the suture at each free end should be approximately 1.5 cm. A no. 5 Mersilene tape is passed around the looped portion of the graft, and the diameter of the graft is ascertained by passing the graft through commercially available cylindric sizers. Reamer size for creation of the tibial and femoral tunnels is selected based on the graft diameter. The smallest diameter that allows passage of the graft should be selected as the tunnel diameter. Because a quadrupled-stranded hamstring graft is cylindric in shape, the graft should fill the osseous tunnels and maximize soft tissue–bone contact, thereby providing an optimum environment for graft incorporation. Final graft preparation takes place after creation of the tibial and femoral tunnels.

Tunnel Placement and Creation   The ACL remnant is debrided using a combination of hand and mechanized instruments. On the tibial aspect of the knee joint, a "footprint" of the native ACL insertion may be left to assist with positioning of the tibial tunnel. Prior to creation of the tunnels, a notchplasty is performed to remove a sufficient amount of bone from the lateral and anterior aspects of the intercondylar notch to allow for placement of the ACL graft without subsequent lateral or anterior graft impingement. The amount of notchplasty or roofplasty that is necessary depends on the diameter of the ACL graft and the underlying anatomy of the notch.

The author prefers placement of the tibial tunnel in the posterior half and the medial lateral center of the native ACL tibial insertion. This position minimizes the risk of anterior graft impingement and allows for creation of the femoral tunnel in an endoscopic fashion. Landmarks that assist in proper positioning of the tibial tunnel include the anterior horn of the lateral meniscus (which inserts immediately adjacent to the anterior half of the ACL tibial insertion), the tibial spines, the anterior border of the posterior cruciate ligament, and the intercondylar roof. As mentioned, leaving several millimeters of intact native ACL fibers at the tibial insertion site during ACL remnant debridement also assists in proper placement of the tibial tunnel guide.

For creation of the femoral tunnel, it is critical to identify the posterior cortical margin of the lateral femoral condyle and to palpate the over-the-top position. Great care must be exercised to avoid the common error of mistaking "resident's ridge" for the posterior cortical margin. Failure to properly identify the over-the-top position may result in an excessively anterior placement of the femoral tunnel. It is important to place the femoral tunnel as posterior as possible at approximately the 10 o'clock position in a right knee (2 o'clock for a left knee); ideally, a 1- to 2-mm posterior cortical margin remains after creation of the femoral tunnel.

The tibial tunnel is created with a cannulated reamer of appropriate diameter, after placement of a guidewire using a commercially available guide system inserted through the anteromedial portal. The incision used for the harvest of the semitendinosus tendon is such that no additional incision is necessary for drilling of the osseous tunnels. The guidewire should enter the proximal medial tibia at approximately a 45-degree angle relative to the tibial shaft, at a point approximately halfway between the anterior tibial crest and the palpable posteromedial margin of the tibia. After creation of the tibial tunnel, the posterior margin of the tunnel entrance into the intraarticular aspect of the knee is debrided of overlying soft tissue and the cortical bone chamfered with a rasp to permit easy graft passage and to minimize abrasion at the graft–tunnel interface.

With the knee flexed to 90 degrees, the femoral tunnel is created in an endoscopic fashion after placement of a guidewire retrograde through the tibial tunnel into the center of the selected tunnel location; a handheld guide may be used for placement of the guidewire if desired. A cannulated, calibrated endoscopic reamer is used to produce a closed-ended femoral tunnel to a predetermined depth. The length of the femoral tunnel should equal the length of graft tissue that is to be placed within the tunnel plus an additional 6 mm to allow for turning or "setting" the EndoButton (see "Graft Insertion and Fixation" section). This additional depth provides the turning radius for the EndoButton, 6 mm being half the length of the device. The endoscopic reamer and guidewire are removed after creation of the tunnel, and bony debris is cleared using a mechanized shaver. The anterior cortical margin of the tunnel is chamfered again to minimize abrasion at the graft–tunnel interface.

The final step in preparation of the femoral tunnel is to penetrate the anterolateral femoral cortex. This is accomplished with the 4.5-mm calibrated channel drill from the EndoButton set placed retrograde through the tibial and femoral tunnels with the knee in a flexed position. Care is exercised to ensure that the direction in which the channel drill is aimed permits a beath pin used for graft insertion to exit out the distal lateral aspect of the thigh within the sterile field. A note should be made of the approximate measurement (in millimeters) on the channel drill at the point at which the anterolateral femoral cortex is broken through. A precise measurement of the entire channel length (distance from the opening of the femoral tunnel to the cortical breakthrough) is made with a depth gauge from the EndoButton system (Fig. 6-4). This measurement is used to determine the length of Mersilene tape needed to span the distance between the EndoButton and the looped portion of the semitendinosus graft; this length is the channel length minus the amount of graft to be contained within the femoral tunnel. For example, with a channel length of 60 mm with 25 mm of graft to be placed within the femoral tunnel, the length of the Mersilene tape should be 35 mm (Fig. 6-5). Tying a knot to leave the proper length of Mersilene tape can be done easily on the calibrated graft preparation board.

The EndoButton then is loaded onto the graft preparation board with a special clamp. The no. 5 Mersilene tape is looped through the central two holes of the EndoButton so that the two free ends are left in the interval between the looped portion of the ACL graft and the EndoButton itself. Two square knots (four throws only) are tied in the Mersilene tape; knots exceeding four throws may not pass through the 4.5-mm channel created in the distal femur. Through one of the two remaining peripheral holes a no. 2 Ethibond suture is passed, and through the other a no. 5 Ethibond suture (Fig. 6-6); these sutures are used to pass the graft into the knee and subsequently "set" the EndoButton on the anterolateral femoral cortex after graft insertion.

With the knee in a flexed position, a beath pin is passed retrograde through the tibial and femoral tunnels, through the channel in the distal femur, and out the skin of the distal lateral thigh in preparation for graft passage. If the tunnels have been created in appropriate positions, there should be no difficulty having the pin exit the distal thigh within the sterile field. The knee should not be flexed or extended further until the passing pin is removed.

Graft Insertion and Fixation   Prior to graft insertion, a circumferential reference mark is made on the ACL graft with a sterile marking pen. This mark is made at a distance from the proximal end of the graft equalling the length of the graft to be placed within the tunnel plus an additional 6 mm (the turning radius of the EndoButton). The graft is inserted into the knee in a retrograde fashion using the beath pin and the two Ethibond sutures that previously have been placed in the peripheral holes of the EndoButton. These sutures are looped through the beath pin, which then is withdrawn proximally, delivering the Ethibond sutures through both bone tunnels and out of the patient's distal lateral thigh. Tension then is applied to the no. 5 Ethibond suture in order to deliver the EndoButton lengthwise into the

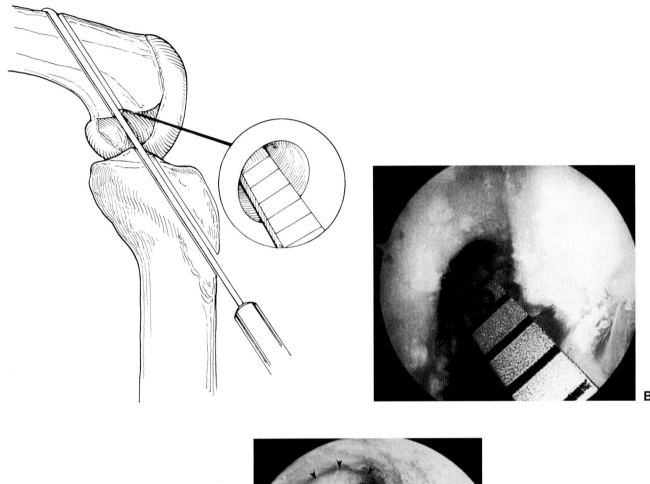

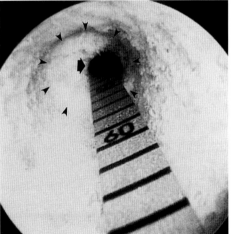

FIGURE 6-4

A: Calibrated depth gauge passed retrograde through the femoral tunnel and channel that has broken through the lateral femoral cortex to measure the total length of passing channel. (Adapted from Rosenberg TD, Graf B. *Endoscopic technique for ACL reconstruction with EndoButton® fixation.* Technical Manual. Mansfield, MA, Acufex Microsurgical, 1994, with permission.) **B:** Arthroscopic view of the calibrated depth gauge within the intercondylar notch, passing into the femoral tunnel. **C:** Arthroscopic view showing depth gauge within the femoral tunnel and entering into the channel (*arrow*) at the proximal portion of the closed-ended tunnel (*small arrowheads*).

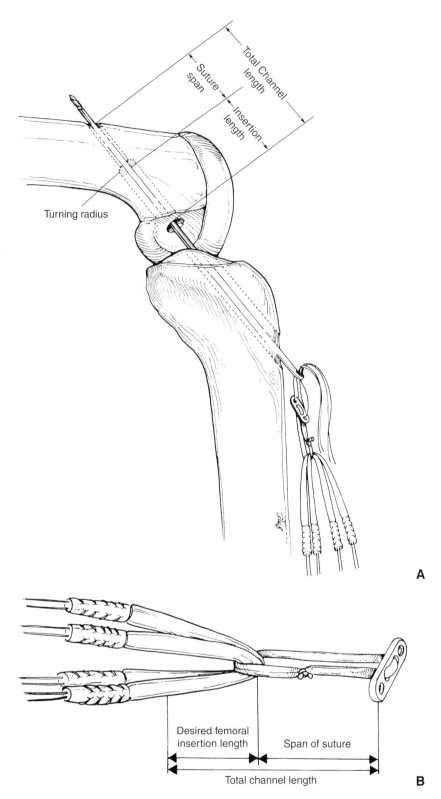

■   FIGURE 6-5

Line drawings depicting the various measurements that are made and used during femoral tunnel creation and graft preparation. **A:** Lateral view of a left knee. **B:** Completed double looped semi-tendinosus graft. (Adapted from Rosenberg TD, Graf B. *Endoscopic technique for ACL reconstruction with EndoButton*[R] *fixation.* Technical Manual. Mansfield, MA, Acufex Microsurgical, 1994, with permission.)

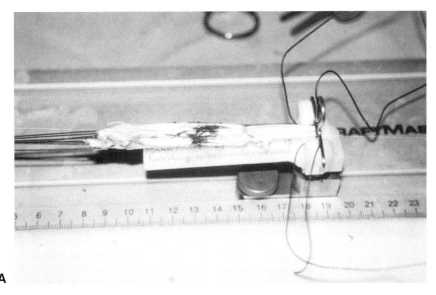

A

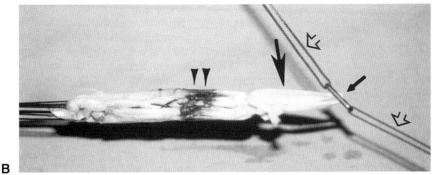

B

■ FIGURE 6-6

A: Calibrated graft preparation board with completed double looped semitendinosus graft. **B:** En-doButton (*small arrow*) with no. 2 and no. 5 Ethibond sutures peripherally (*open arrows*), no. 5 Mer-silene tape centrally (*large arrow*), and reference mark on graft (*double arrowheads*).

femoral tunnel and, subsequently, the channel. Slack in the no. 2 Ethibond suture is taken out gently during this process, but no significant tension is applied; this maneuver is criti-cal in order to maintain the EndoButton in a vertical orientation as it courses through the passing channel. Once the graft is delivered into the femoral tunnel to the level of the refer-ence mark, tension is released from the no. 5 Ethibond suture and maximal tension is ap-plied to the trailing no. 2 Ethibond suture. This maneuver rotates the EndoButton into a hor-izontal position and allows it to lie parallel to the shaft of the femur and bridge the 4.5 mm channel diameter, much as a toggle bolt is designed to function in a ceiling (Fig. 6-7). Max-imal tension then is applied to the sutures exiting the tibial tunnel, which sets the EndoBut-ton against the femoral shaft. If for some reason the EndoButton has not completely exited the femur and has lodged within the channel itself, it is pulled back into the knee at this point. If this were to occur, the above graft insertion process simply would be repeated so as to deploy the device properly. If any question exists as to whether or not the device is po-sitioned properly outside of the femur, an intraoperative radiograph may be obtained.

If the femoral tunnel has been created to a length greater than that necessary to equal the amount of graft to be left within the tunnel plus the additional 6 mm for turning the En-doButton, one should be cautious not to bring the graft into the femoral tunnel beyond the level of the reference mark. Pulling the graft too far within the femoral tunnel allows the EndoButton to pass out into the quadricep musculature, and when the EndoButton subse-quently is set, it may become entrapped within muscle tissue rather than resting on the

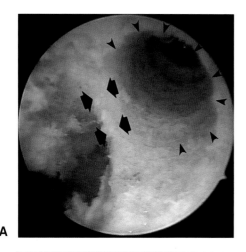

A

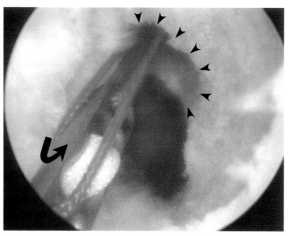

B

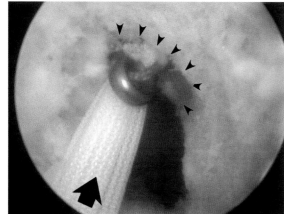

C

A: Arthroscopic view of a completed femoral tunnel (*small arrow-heads*) viewed from within the intercondylar notch. Note the very posterior portion of the tunnel, with only a 1-mm cortical bridge (*arrows*) between the posterior wall of the tunnel and the over-the-top position. **B:** Arthroscopic view of the EndoButton (*curved arrow*) being guided "head-first" into femoral tunnel (*small arrow-heads*) by Ethibond suture. **C:** Mersilene tape bridging between the EndoButton and the anterior cruciate ligament graft beginning to enter into the femoral tunnel. **D–F:** Line drawings depicting the EndoButton exiting from the femoral channel (**D**); being deployed into a horizontal position through use of the peripheral Ethibond sutures, thereby anchoring onto the anterolateral femoral cortex (**E**); and suspending the graft within the femoral tunnel (**F**). (Adapted from Rosenberg TD, Graf B. *Endoscopic technique for ACL reconstruction with EndoButton^R fixation.* Technical Manual. Mansfield, MA, Acufex Microsurgical, 1994, with permission.)

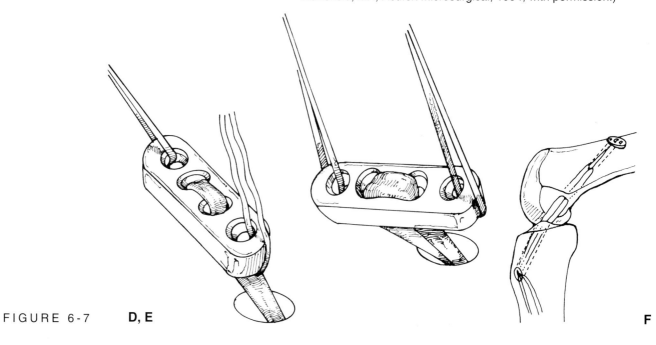

■ FIGURE 6-7   **D, E**

F

femoral cortex. This is not an ideal situation, because it may lead to loosening of the graft construct with time.

After the graft has been inserted and the EndoButton engaged, tension is placed on the sutures exiting the tibial tunnel, with the graft visualized arthroscopically. The knee is taken through a full range of motion to assess for any residual impingement present, particularly anteriorly. It is critical to restore full, symmetric knee extension without impingement of the graft (Fig. 6-8). If additional notchplasty is necessary, it should be done with caution to avoid damage to the graft.

Distal fixation is achieved by securing the sutures exiting the tibial tunnel around a post. The post should be a bicortical screw placed approximately 1 cm distal to the tibial tunnel and drilled in an anteromedial to posterolateral direction. The knee should be flexed to between 15 and 20 degrees while the graft is tensioned and secured. With a quadrupled-strand graft, two separate sets of sutures must be tied corresponding to the two loops of graft tissue. Sutures from the free ends of the same looped strand are to be tied to one another. While the first set of sutures is being tied, an assistant should be holding maximal tension on the opposite set of sutures. After both sets of sutures are tied, the post is seated fully into the tibia. The knee is taken through a full range of motion to ensure that inappropriate capturing of the knee has not occurred, and a Lachman test is performed to evaluate anterior tibial translation.

A layered closure is performed by reapproximating periosteum over the tibial tunnel and fixation post, followed by suturing of the subcutaneous tissues. The skin is reapproximated with a running subcuticular suture of 4-0 absorbable monofilament suture. Each of

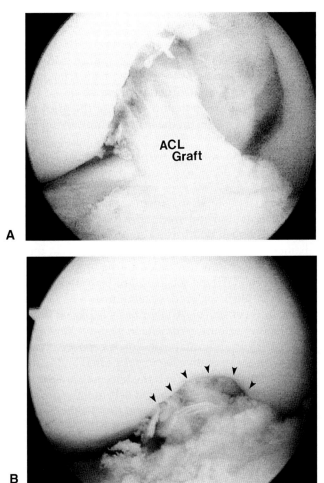

A

B   ■ FIGURE 6-8

With the anterior cruciate ligament graft in place, the knee is taken from flexion (**A**) to full extension (**B**) without impingement or restriction of motion noted.

the portals is closed with 4-0 nylon sutures. To assist with postoperative pain management, the portal sites and intraarticular space are infiltrated with 10 to 20 ml of 0.25% bupirocaine in addition to placement of 2 mg of morphine sulfate within the knee joint. A sterile dressing and cold compression device are applied to the knee, and the operative leg is secured in a long-leg hinged knee brace, which is locked in full extension; alternatively, a standard knee immobilizer may be utilized.

In the recovery room, the operative foot is elevated, leaving the knee and calf unsupported to allow for gravity-assisted full extension at the knee. The importance of maintaining full symmetric knee extension should be emphasized both pre- and postoperatively. The initial postoperative exercises are reviewed with the patient before discharge, and crutch-assisted ambulation is begun under the supervision of a therapist or nurse. The patient is seen in the office 48 hours after the procedure to change the dressings, inspect the knee, answer any questions or concerns, and again review the initial rehabilitation program expectations.

■ TECHNICAL ALTERNATIVES AND PITFALLS

Tibial-side fixation alternatives with a quadruple-stranded semitendinosus graft are quite limited because of the relatively invariable overall length of the graft. There are, however, several other commercially available devices for femoral fixation of a soft-tissue ACL graft. In addition, if both the semitendinosus and gracilis tendons are harvested and fashioned into a quadruple-stranded graft composed of a doubled loop of each tendon, the result is a much longer graft, allowing for further fixation options. With a graft of sufficient length to allow excess soft tissue to exit out of the tibial tunnel, fixation of the graft directly onto the proximal tibia can be accomplished with the use of soft-tissue staples, a fixation post and spiked soft tissue washer, or a combination of these methods. Interference fixation on both the tibial and femoral side with either bone plugs or specialized interference screws for use with soft-tissue grafts also have been advocated by some surgeons.

For those who prefer the use of a more traditional two-incision technique for ACL reconstruction, a quadruple-stranded hamstring tendon graft can be placed in the over-the-top position or within either an open- or closed-ended femoral tunnel. Femoral fixation is dictated by the position and length of the graft with alternatives including tying sutures over a post or button on the lateral femur, fixing the graft directly to the lateral femur with a post and spiked soft tissue washer, or interference fixation of the graft within the femoral tunnel itself. A familiarity with a number of surgical techniques and fixation options allows the surgeon to adapt to a variety of preoperative and intraoperative scenarios.

■ REHABILITATION

The initial postoperative management following ACL reconstruction is designed to control inflammation and swelling, rapidly restore full extension symmetric to the uninjured knee, reestablish quadriceps control and range of motion, and achieve normal gait mechanics (25). For the first postoperative week, the patient is allowed full weight bearing with the use of crutches and with the brace locked in full extension. Isometric quadriceps exercises (quadriceps sets, straight leg raises) are begun immediately. The patient is permitted to unlock the brace several times a day for self-administered active range of motion exercises (heel slides). An emphasis is placed on achieving early restoration of full extension. Loss of extension may have negative functional implications, leading to adverse outcomes such as abnormal gait, quadriceps weakness, andd patellofemoral pain (25). Prone lying with the operative leg unsupported and sitting upright with the heel of the operative leg supported on a chair and the knee free are encouraged, to assist with restoring full knee extension. The patient is taught self-mobilization of the patella and is encouraged to perform all of these exercises several times a day.

At 7 to 10 days postoperatively, the brace is unlocked if the patient demonstrates return of quadriceps control. Use of crutches is continued for a total of 4 weeks. The brace is discontinued after 6 weeks. Closed kinetic chain exercices are begun after the first postoperative visit. Hamstring-strengthening exercises are not begun until 8 to 10 weeks postoperatively, and hamstring stretching begins at 4 to 6 weeks. Further details of the postoperative protocol have been described elsewhere (25).

Anterior cruciate ligament reconstruction using autograft BPTB remains the "gold standard" to which other techniques typically are compared. If surgeons nationwide were to be polled as to their ACL graft of choice, those selecting BPTB would certainly outnumber those preferring hamstring tendons. Ever-improving methods for the use and fixation of the semitendinosus tendon, however, either alone or in conjunction with the gracilis tendon, are being developed. Because of concerns about increased incidence of operative and postoperative morbidity associated with the use of a BPTB graft, a growing interest in the hamstring tendon graft as an ACL substitute has mounted.

Several prospective studies comparing the outcome of ACL reconstructions performed using either BPTB or hamstring tendon autografts recently have been reported (5,6,26). Although minor differences in several postoperative parameters between groups were noted, overall results were comparable. Well-controlled, prospective studies reporting the long-term results (longer than 5 years) of ACL reconstructions using identical surgical techniques and postoperative protocols but different graft sources are necessary in order to make definite conclusions regarding the specific effect of the ACL graft material itself on surgical outcome.

The ability to achieve a successful outcome after ACL reconstruction goes far beyond simply choosing the "correct" graft tissue. A favorable outcome likely is more dependent on placement of a well-fixed biologic graft in an anatomic position in which graft impingement is prevented, followed by a well-conceived postoperative rehabilitation protocol, than on the specific graft material used for the ACL substitute. The technique presented here permits endoscopic placement of a strong autogenous graft with abundant collagen tissue for incorporation. It is a technique that is applicable for both primary and revision ACL surgery and is well suited for an ambulatory surgery setting.

■ OUTCOMES AND FUTURE DIRECTIONS

References

1. Christen B, Jakob RP. Fractures associated with patellar ligament grafts in cruciate ligament surgery. *J Bone Joint Surg Br* 1992; 74:617–619.
2. Graf B, Uhr F. Complications of intra-articular anterior cruciate ligament reconstruction. *Clin Sports Med* 1988; 7:835–848.
3. Hughston JC. Complications of anterior cruciate ligament surgery. *Orthop Clin North Am* 1985; 16:237–240.
4. Sachs RA, Daniel DM, Stone ML, et al. Patellofemoral problems after anterior cruciate ligament reconstruction. *Am J Sports Med* 1989; 17:760–765.
5. Aglietti P, Buzzi R, Zaccherotti G, et al. Patellar tendon versus doubled semitendinosus and gracilis tendons for anterior cruciate ligament reconstruction. *Am J Sports Med* 1994; 22:211–218.
6. Marder RA, Raskind JR, Carroll M. Prospective evaluation of arthroscopically assisted anterior cruciate ligament reconstruction: Patellar tendon versus semitendinosus and gracilis tendons. *Am J Sports Med* 1991; 19:478–484.
7. Warner JP, Warren RF, Cooper DE. Management of acute anterior cruciate ligament injury. In: Tullos HS, ed. *Instructional course lectures*, volume 40. Park Ridge, IL: American Academy of Orthopaedic Surgeons, 1991, pp. 219–232.
8. Sgaglione NA, Warren RF, Wickiewicz TL, et al. Primary repair with semitendinosus tendon augmentation of acute anterior cruciate ligament injuries. *Am J Sports Med* 1990; 18:64–73.
9. Ferrari JD, Ferrari DA. The semitendinosus: anatomic considerations in tendon harvesting. *Orthop Rev* 1991; 20:1085–1088.
10. Pagnini MJ, Warner JJP, O'Brien SO, et al. Anatomic considerations in harvesting the semitendinosus and gracilis tendons and a technique of harvest. *Am J Sports Med* 1993; 21:565–571.
11. Noyes FR, Butler DL, Grood ES, et al. Biomechanical analysis of human ligament grafts used in knee-ligament repairs and reconstructions. *J Bone Joint Surg Am* 1984; 66:344–352.
12. Steiner ME, Hecker AT, Brown CH, et al. Anterior cruciate ligament graft fixation: Comparison of hamstring and patellar tendon grafts. *Am J Sports Med* 1994; 22:240–247.
13. Rodeo SA, Arnoczky SP, Torzilli PA, et al. Tendon-healing in a bone tunnel. *J Bone Joint Surg Am* 1993; 75:1795–1803.
14. van Rens TJG, van den Berg AF, Huiskes R, et al. Substitution of the anterior cruciate ligament: A long-term histologic and biomechanical study with autogenous pedicled grafts of the iliotibial band in dogs. *Arthroscopy* 1986; 2:139–154.

15. Macey HB. A new operative procedure for repair of ruptured cruciate ligaments of the knee joint. *Surg Gynecol Obstet* 1939; 69:108–109.
16. Lipscomb AB, Johnston RK, Snyder RB. The technique of cruciate ligament reconstruction. *Am J Sports Med* 1981; 9:77–81.
17. Mott HW. Semitendinosus anatomic reconstruction for cruciate ligament insufficiency. *Clin Orthop* 1983; 172:90–92.
18. Gomes JL, Marczyk LS. Anterior cruciate ligament reconstruction with a loop or double thickness of semitendinosus tendon. *Am J Sports Med* 1984; 12:199–203.
19. Zaricznyi B. Reconstruction of the anterior cruciate ligament of the knee using a doubled tendon graft. *Clin Orthop* 1987; 220:162–175.
20. Larson RL, Burger RS. Acute ligamentous injury. In Larson RL, Grana WA, eds. *The knee: Form, function, pathology, and treatment*. Philadelphia, WB Saunders, 1993:554–565.
21. Rosenberg TD, Graf B. *Endoscopic technique for ACL reconstruction with EndoButton^R fixation*. Technical Manual. Mansfield, MA, Acufex Microsurgical, 1994.
22. Daniel DM, Stone ML, Dobson BE, et al. Fate of the ACL-injured patient: A prospective outcome study. *Am J Sports Med* 1994; 22:632–636.
23. Noyes FR, Matthews DS, Mooar PA, et al. The symptomatic anterior cruciate-deficient knee: Part II. The results of rehabilitation, activity modification, and counseling on functional disability. *J Bone Joint Surg Am* 1983; 65:163.
24. Gillquist J, Hagberg G, Oretorp N. Arthroscopic examination of the posteromedial compartment of the knee joint. *Int Orthop* 1979; 3:313.
25. Irrgang JJ. Modern trends in anterior cruciate ligament rehabilitation: Nonoperative and postoperative management. *Clin Sports Med* 1993; 12:797–813.
26. O'Neill DB. Arthroscopically assisted reconstruction of the anterior cruciate ligament: A prospective randomized analysis of three techniques. *J Bone Joint Surg Am* 1996; 78:803–813.

K. DONALD
SHELBOURNE
THOMAS E. KLOOTWYK

7

Two-incision Miniarthrotomy Technique for Anterior Cruciate Ligament Reconstruction with Autogenous Patellar Tendon Graft

A number of different surgical approaches are available for anterior cruciate ligament (ACL) reconstruction. These approaches include a miniarthrotomy through the patellar tendon defect, as well as arthroscopy-assisted and endoscopic techniques. Possible graft sources include autogenous tissue of the patellar tendon and semitendinosus and gracilis tendons and allograft tissue. Various fixation methods also exist, including metallic screws, metallic staples, screws and washers, bioabsorbable devices, and suture buttons. This report describes our approach to the reconstruction of the ACL with a miniarthrotomy technique with an autogenous patellar tendon graft and suture button fixation. Although this technique would be considered by many as the "old way" of performing an ACL reconstruction, we have found this technique to produce excellent results in over 3,500 reconstructions. The miniarthrotomy technique has remained our technique of choice because knee stability has been restored reproducibly, and patients have been able to participate in an accelerated rehabilitation program and return rapidly to activities of daily living and athletic activities after surgery.

■ HISTORY OF THE TECHNIQUE

The miniarthrotomy technique of ACL reconstruction with an autogenous patellar tendon graft is indicated for isolated and revision ACL reconstructions in addition to knees with multiple injured ligaments. If the patellar tendon has been harvested previously or injured significantly, we recommend using the opposite patellar tendon as a graft source. If neither patellar tendon is available for harvest, alternate graft sources such as the hamstring tendons must be considered. In nine cases we have reharvested the patellar tendon. The minimal length of time from the first harvest was 1.5 years. The quality of the reharvested tendon did not appear to be as good as the initial harvest, but all nine of these patients have done well to date.

■ INDICATIONS AND CONTRAINDICATIONS

We prefer the use of general anesthesia, but if circumstances dictate the procedure can be performed easily with the patient under a spinal or epidural block. Once the patient is under the effects of the chosen anesthetic, a careful examination of the knee is performed. A preoperative injection of 20 mL of 0.25% bupivacaine hydrochloride (Marcaine) with epinephrine is injected intraarticularly into the injured knee. The extremity then undergoes a standard alcohol and betadine preparation, followed by standard sterile draping.

An arthroscopy is performed immediately before the reconstructive procedure to evaluate for meniscal tears or chondral surfaces damage. We take an aggressive approach to meniscal preservation. Through tracking our 3,500 ACL reconstruction patients, we have been able to determine the types of meniscal tears most commonly associated with ACL

■ SURGICAL TECHNIQUES

tears. With this information we have been able to determine which meniscal tears are most likely to remain asymptomatic if left alone, which tears fare better if repaired, and which tears require partial meniscectomy. Once the necessary treatment of any meniscal lesions has been completed, the chondral surfaces are inspected and any large articular flaps are debrided. The joint surfaces and menisci are photographed for future reference.

Medial Miniarthrotomy   At the end of the arthroscopic procedure, a new extremity drape is placed on the knee, and a bump is placed under the involved thigh to bend the knee approximately 20 to 30 degrees. The tourniquet remains inflated from the beginning of the arthroscopic procedure. A 6-cm anteromedial skin incision is made proximally from the anteromedial arthroscopic portal site at level of the inferior pole of the patella to the level of the tibial tubercle. Sharp dissection is carried down to the level of the patellar tendon, and then sharp and blunt dissection is performed to develop the plane between the patellar tendon, anteromedial proximal tibia, and the subcutaneous tissue. This subcutaneous dissection allows for the miniarthrotomy and the eventual harvesting of the patellar tendon graft.

With electrocautery, a periosteal flap is created along the medial border of the patellar tendon extending approximately 4 cm below the joint line and then medially approximately 2 to 3 cm. The use of electrocautery helps control bleeding, because there is a large vein that lies along the medial border of the patellar tendon. A thick periosteal flap is preserved to provide a deep soft-tissue cover over the tibial button at the completion of the ACL reconstruction. The closure of this large flap has minimized the incidence of postoperative hardware removal in our patients to less than 1%.

Next, the medial miniarthrotomy is performed using the electrocautery. The capsular incision is started at the level of the tibia medial to the patellar tendon and carried proximally to the vastus medialis insertion into the patella. With the use of Slocum and Cushing retractors, the miniarthrotomy provides for unparalleled exposure of the tibial plateau and intercondylar notch. At no time during the reconstructive procedure is the patella dislocated from the trochlear groove.

Lateral Oblique Incision   The knee is placed into a 90-degree position by elevating the table height and dropping the foot of the table. An oblique lateral skin incision is performed approximately 2 inches above the superior pole of the patella. The skin incision is made oblique, in the plane of the skin lines of Langer. We have found that the oblique incision heals better, with fewer wound problems, than a traditional horizontal incision.

After the skin incision, dissection is carried down to the iliotibial band. The iliotibial band is split in line with its fibers. The soft-tissue plane underlying the vastus lateralis muscle is developed, and the muscle is lifted in mass. A Slocum retractor is placed under the vastus lateralis and over the anterior cortex of the femur, exposing the lateral femoral cortex. The periosteum is split with electrocautery and lifted with an elevator. This window of exposed cortex serves as the femoral tunnel exit site. The lateral wound is packed with a lap sponge, and attention is turned toward the anterior wound and the notchplasty.

Notchplasty   Exposure of the intercondylar notch is obtained by placing a Slocum retractor through the medial miniarthrotomy and around the lateral femoral condyle to retract the patellar tendon laterally. This provides excellent exposure of the intercondylar notch and tibial plateau for performing the notchplasty and drilling the bone tunnels.

The lateral aspect of the intercondylar notch is cleared of the ACL stump and remaining fibrofatty scar tissue. The lateral border of the posterior cruciate ligament (PCL) is used as a landmark, and all tissue lateral to this border from the intercondylar notch is removed. Initially the area is cleared, developing the plane along the lateral border of the PCL. A curette is used to aggressively clear all of the ACL scar tissue and stump. A gauze sponge is used to clean the lateral wall of the notch to aide in visualization of the posterior aspect

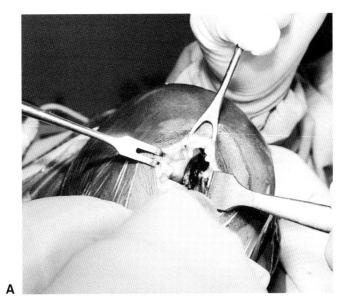

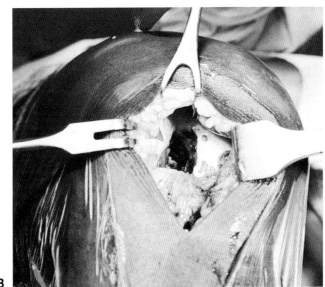

■ FIGURE 7-1

Adequate notch space is created lateral to the posterior cruciate ligament to ensure adequate space for the 10-mm anterior cruciate ligament graft. **A:** A lateral notchplasty is performed using a currette. **B:** A view after the notchplasty is performed.

of the notch for future drilling of the femoral tunnel. Often there are one or two bone bleeders from the area of the roof of the notch, which can be controlled easily with the use of suction and electrocautery. With the lateral aspect of the notch cleared, attention is turned to ensuring that the new ligament has adequate space within the notch.

The intercondylar notch measurements are done with calipers. Measurements are done to determine the space that was available for the native ACL (the space from the lateral femoral condyle to the medial border of the PCL) and the entire notch width. The notchplasty is performed with a curette, removing enough of the lateral wall of the notch to create at least a 10-mm space between the medial border of the PCL and the lateral femoral condyle border (Fig. 7-1). In addition, a portion of the notch roof is removed with a curette (roofplasty) to help prevent postoperative graft impingement. Postnotchplasty measurements are performed with the calipers. All measurements both before and after notchplasty are recorded.

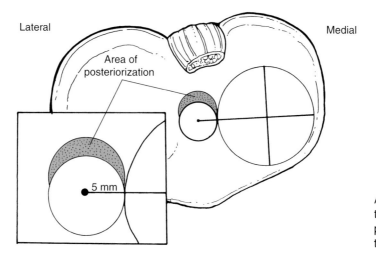

Lateral   Medial

Area of posteriorization

5 mm

A "clock face" is interposed on that portion of the medial tibial plateau that is visualized through the miniarthrotomy.

■   FIGURE 7-2

Bone Tunnels   The next step is the drilling of the bone tunnels. First, the tibial tunnel is created by drilling from an outside to inside utilizing a 3/32-inch guide pin and a 9-mm cannulated reamer. The guide pin is started on the anteromedial tibia in the area in which the periosteum previously was elevated. The guide pin positioning begins approximately 4 cm below the joint line and is directed to a predetermined target on the tibial plateau. It is now well accepted that the tibial tunnel needs to be placed more posterior than originally was recommended (1–3). A more anterior position of the tibial tunnel leads to an anterior graft, the need for a larger roofplasty, and possible graft impingement.

We recommend viewing the visible portion of the medial tibial plateau as a clock. In the clock model, the 9 o'clock position serves as the middle of the visible tibial plateau for a right knee, and the 3 o'clock position serves as the middle of the visible plateau for a left knee (Fig. 7-2). The center of the ideal tibial tunnel corresponds roughly to the a position just posterior to the 9 o'clock or 3 o'clock point, accordingly.

Using these guidelines, the point on the tibial plateau for the center of the tunnel is marked with a hemostat, and the guide pin is placed. A 3/32-inch Steinmann pin is started in the area of the anteromedial proximal tibia previously cleared of its periosteal lining. The tunnel is started 3 to 4 cm below the joint line to ensure adequate tibial bone tunnel length. Also, the guide pin is placed at least 10 mm medial to the medial border of the patellar tendon, to ensure adequate room for the 19-mm diameter fixation button utilized to secure the graft at the completion of graft passage. A guide pin is used to allow a change in placement of the pin position, if needed after first pass. After acceptable pin position is accomplished, a 9-mm end-cutting cannulated reamer is passed over the pin to create the tibial tunnel.

Bone reamings from the tunnel are saved for future grafting of the patellar and tibial bone plug areas. The tunnel exit site on the proximal tibia is cleared of any remaining soft tissue around the tunnel. The remaining stump of the ACL is cut sharply off the floor of the tibial plateau with a no. 15 scalpel on a long handle. At this time the final positioning of the tibial tunnel is performed. Curettes of sizes 4, 5, and 6 are used to place the tunnel in the final position. A size 4 curette corresponds to a 9-mm diameter. This curette is passed first, and the tunnel is placed more posterior by 1 to 2 mm (Fig. 7-3). The tunnel then is enlarged with curettes of sizes 5 and 6, which correspond to 10 and 11 mm. With the use of the curettes, the tibial tunnel is placed in a adequate posterior position as it enters the joint.

Next, the femoral tunnel is created. We believe that the femoral tunnel is the most difficult and most important part of the procedure. It is our opinion that a large percentage of ACL surgical failures result from improper femoral tunnel placement. The femoral tunnel that is placed "too shallow" in the notch can lead to two separate problems: capturing the joint, with resultant joint stiffness; or graft failure, if full range of motion is achieved.

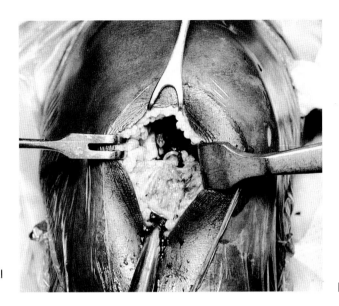

A curette is used to modify the tibial tunnel entrance into the joint.

■ FIGURE 7-3

With this technique of ACL surgery, the femoral tunnel is drilled completely independent of the tibial tunnel. That is, the femoral tunnel is drilled through the miniarthrotomy and not through the tibial tunnel, as is done with many other techniques. It is our opinion that the visualization of the important posterior aspect of the lateral wall of the notch is best if it is viewed through the miniarthrotomy. If the most posterior aspect of the notch can be visualized, the femoral tunnel can be placed in the appropriate posterior position, at the point at which the normal ACL attaches itself to the femur.

The knee is placed into a figure-four position to drill the femoral tunnel. The Slocum retractor is placed around the lateral femoral condyle to retract the patellar tendon, and a large two-prong rake is used to retract the medial aspect of the incision along with the fat pad. A 4 × 3 inch gauze sponge is used to dry and clear the posterolateral aspect of the notch again, and the position of the femoral tunnel is marked with a 3/32-inch guide pin. The blunt end of the guide pin is passed along the border of the PCL gently out the back of the notch, to identify the most posterior border of the notch. With the posterior wall referenced, the guide pin then is slid forward 6 to 7 mm and laterally 3 to 4 mm to the lateral border of the PCL. This position allows for a 1- to 2-mm posterior wall of the 10-mm femoral tunnel and placement of the ACL graft in appropriate position relative to the PCL. The guide pin then is drilled, aiming for the area of the previously cleared periosteum on the lateral cortex of the femur. Once the guide pin point has been determined inside the knee, it is helpful to take the free hand and place an index finger into the lateral wound and on the cleared area of the lateral cortex, and to aim the guide pin for that finger.

The guide pin is passed through the femur and out the lateral cortex. The position of the guide pin is accepted if the pin exits the femur in the area of the cleared cortex. If the position is not acceptable, the guide pin is redirected using the starting point in the notch previously determined. Once an acceptable position is accomplished, the guide pin is overdrilled with an Acufex 10-mm end-cutting cannulated reamer. The tunnel is drilled all the way through the lateral femoral cortex. The bone reamings from the tunnel are saved for future grafting of the patellar and tibial bone plug defects. The joint is irrigated with antibiotic solution, and the tibial and femoral tunnel positions are checked visually (Fig. 7-4).

As the last part of our reconstructive procedure, the patellar tendon is harvested. Although it has never been studied, it is our opinion that the less time the patellar tendon is away from its normal environment, the better. Our approach is to drill standard-sized tunnels and then harvest bone plugs to fit the tunnels.

The patellar tendon is harvested through the same anterior skin incision through which the miniarthrotomy is made. With the use of Cushing retractors, the skin is mobilized to

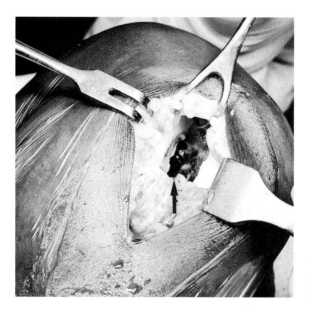

The femoral tunnel in the notch is shown in the appropriate posterior position and orientation.

■   FIGURE 7-4

expose the patellar tendon. The peritenon is split in the midline with metzenbaum scissors to fully expose the underlying patellar tendon. The width of the patellar tendon is measured and recorded. A 10-mm wide bone–patellar tendon bone graft is harvested. The initial incision in the tendon is referenced off the medial border, which is identified easily by the miniarthrotomy. A no. 10 scalpel blade is used to incise the tendon longitudinally. With the medial border of the tendon incised, the lateral portion of the graft is measured to ensure a 10-mm wide patellar tendon graft, and, with the scalpel blade, the tendon portion of the graft is completed. Also with the scalpel, the areas for bony block excision are scored. We prefer bone blocks that are 10-mm wide and approximately 25-mm long. Using a straight 1/4-inch osteotome and two or three strikes with a mallet, the ends of the bone blocks are marked. Next, the patellar and tibial bone blocks are harvested in a wedge-shaped fashion with an oscillating saw. With the bone plugs cut, they are removed from their bony beds with a curved 1/4-inch osteotome.

The bone plugs are contoured and measured so that they fit snugly through the bone tunnels. The tibial tunnel is usually 11 mm in diameter, and the femoral tunnel is always 10 mm in diameter. The bone plugs are shaped with a rongeur, and if needed an area of excessive soft tissue is removed with scissors. Three drill holes are placed in each bone plug, with a 1/16-inch drill bit. No. 2 Ethibond sutures are passed through the drill holes. The suture ends are evened and then cut, so that an equal portion of each suture strand is on either side of the bone plug. These sutures aide in graft passage and serve to secure the graft to the fixation buttons. Harvesting of the patellar tendon up to this point has been done with the patellar tendon still attached to the fat pad and its blood supply. At this time the tendon is removed from its final fat pad attachments. The graft is laid on the back table and measured in length and width. The excess fat pad is excised from the tendon with scissors, and the graft is passed into the knee.

The patellar bone plug with its slightly more curved shape is passed into the tibial tunnel with a suture passer placed from outside to inside and then brought out the front miniarthrotomy incision. The sutures passed through the patellar bone plug are passed through the loop of the passer and brought out the tibial tunnel. Using pickups, the patellar bone plug is guided into the tibial tunnel with the cancellous bone facing anteriorly. This anterior placement of the bone block puts the patellar tendon in a more posterior position, which further decreases the chance of notch impingement. Next, a ligament-fixation button is placed. Three suture ends each are passed through opposite holes of the ligament button and provisionally tied with two throws of the sutures. The button lies flat on the anteromedial tibial surface that was cleared previously. Next, the sutures of the tibial bone plug are placed through the loop of the suture passer for passage into the femoral tunnel. The suture passer is placed up the femoral tunnel and through the lateral cortex. Using the index finger passed under the vastus lateralis muscle and placed at the femoral tunnel exit hole at the lateral femoral cortex, the end of the suture passer is guided through the lateral skin incision. The sutures are removed from the suture passer loop, and the suture passer is withdrawn from the knee. The sutures are passed through the holes of the ligament-fixation button, and the button is tied down to the lateral femoral cortex. Two throws of the sutures are made, as well as a final check of the soft tissue around the button. Using a small elevator, the area for the button seating is cleared again, the previously two throws of sutures are retightened, and an additional three throws of sutures are made. In total, five knots are placed in the femoral fixation button sutures.

The advantage of ligament-fixation buttons is that they allow the surgeon to adjust graft tension without compromising the bone plug fixation. At this time the button tension is readjusted. A new impervious stockinette is placed, and a clean sheet is passed under the reconstructed extremity. The foot of the table is elevated so that the knee achieves a 30-degree flexion angle. The provisionally tied tibial sutures are adjusted. The tibial sutures are pulled so that the patellar bone plug is advanced in the tibial tunnel, which removes any slack in the femoral button fixation or graft. Next, the tibial button sutures are retied tightly with two throws of the sutures. The knee is moved through a full range of motion, including full hyperextension and full flexion. The tension of the tibial button sutures is checked. If the sutures have loosened they are retired, and the knee again is moved through a full range of motion. With the ability to adjust suture tension and check knee range of motion one is assured of not placing the ligament too tight and capturing the knee. Once the sutures are adjusted to the appropriate tension, the final three throws in the tibial sutures are placed, for a total of five knots (Fig. 7-5).

With the ligament fixation complete, attention is directed toward examination of the graft as the knee achieves full hyperextension. Through the miniarthrotomy the graft is well visualized in full extension. If any degree of roof impingement exists, additional roofplasty is performed with a curette. Next, a deep tissue injection of 0.25% bupivicaine with epinephrine is performed in both incisions, and both wounds are packed and the knee is wrapped with a 4-inch ace bandage. The tourniquet is deflated. With an uncomplicated arthroscopy at the start of the procedure, the tourniquet time for the arthroscopy and ACL reconstruction should be around 60 minutes.

The knee is allowed to stay wrapped for 3 minutes, and then the packing is removed. We have found that with this approach the need for electrocautery hemostasis is greatly di-

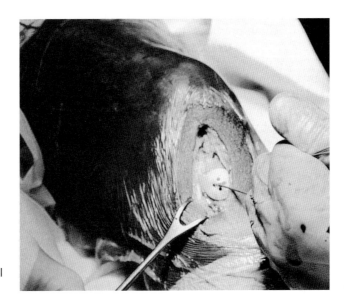

The sutures are tied over the tibial button.

■   FIGURE 7-5

minished. At this time any additional bleeding vessels are electrocauterized and both knee incisions are irrigated with a bacitracin antibiotic solution. Closure consists of no. 1 Vicryl to the patellar tendon defect in a running stitch. The bone reamings previously saved now are packed into the patellar and tibial bone plug areas, with closure over the bone reamings with soft tissue. The miniarthrotomy is closed with no. 1 Vicryl (Ethicon, Inc., Somerville, NJ) in interrupted fashion. Drains are placed in both wounds and brought out through separate stab wounds. The iliotibial band incision is closed with no. 1 Vicryl, and then both wounds are closed with 2-0 Vicryl subcutaneous stitch and a running 3-0 prolene subcuticular stitch. Steristrips, light bandages, and a compression stocking are placed, followed by a cold compression device (Cryo/Cuff; Aircast, Summit, NJ). The patient is transferred to the recovery room. We previously used a knee immobilizer for patient transport but have found that patients seldom wore it after the surgery. Therefore we no longer place patients in the immobilizer. After a short stay in the recovery room, patients are transferred to their hospital rooms to begin the postoperative rehabilitation program.

Postoperative pain management is an important part of the early rehabilitation of the reconstructed knee. We have utilized intravenous Toradol with excellent success. The patient receives an intravenous bolus of 30 mg in the operating room, followed by a continuous intravenous drip started in the operating room. This continuous administration is 90 mg of Keforalac tromethamine (Toradol) in 1,000 mL of fluid administered at 40 mL/h for 24 hours. This concentration and administration rate deliver 3.6 mg/h to the patient. With this protocol, our patients require administration of intravenous or intramuscular narcotics in less than 3% of cases, and the average number of oral narcotic doses administered in the first 24 hours postoperatively is two.

The postoperative ACL rehabilitation program starts once the patient arrives in his or her room after the reconstruction. He or she is placed into a continuous passive motion (CPM) machine that cycles from 0 to 30 degrees of flexion at a moderate rate. We have found that this provides a predictable means of knee elevation and also decreases the sensation of postoperative stiffness. Our postoperative surveys have found that patients consistently rate their CPM treatment as very important. The knee remains in the Cryo/Cuff during the cycling from 0 to 30 degrees in the CPM machine.

Extension work is started 1 to 2 hours after the patient arrives in the room. The Cryo/Cuff is removed, and the patient lifts his or her leg out of the CPM machine and props both feet on the end of the bed frame. It is important that the foot be elevated high enough so that the thigh also is elevated off the bed. This allows the knee to sag into full hyperextension. This hyperextension exercise is done for 10 minutes every hour from 8 AM until 10 PM. The Cryo/Cuff should be removed during this hyperextension exercise, because leaving the cuff in place prevents the knee from extending fully.

Flexion exercise also is started on the first postoperative day. We have found that the CPM machine provides an excellent means of comfortably achieving greater degrees of flexion. With the Cryo/Cuff off, the patient increases the flexion to 100 to 110 degrees. At this point the operation of the machine is paused, and the patient allows the knee to rest in this position for 10 minutes. The flexion exercise is done four or five times per day. Then the CPM machine is reset to 0 to 30 degrees and the Cryo/Cuff is placed back on the knee.

In addition to range of motion, our patients work on quadriceps-muscle leg control during the first week of rehabilitation. This is done by having the patient lift his or her own leg out of the CPM for the hourly extension work. In addition, in hyperextension the patient performs 10 isometric quadriceps-muscle contractions. Early leg control is important for a number of reasons, including mobilizing the patella, ensuring that the patellar tendon is brought to full length, and avoiding a possible patellar baja postoperatively. Also, the early return of quadriceps-muscle strength allows the patient to resume a normal gait pattern sooner.

With regard to gait, we allow our patients to engage in weight-bearing ambulation as tolerated, with the aide of crutches. They are instructed on heel-to-toe gait and are allowed off crutches as soon as they can resume normal gait patterns. Although we want our patients to bear full weight on the reconstructed leg after surgery, we also want to control swelling.

We have found that, in the first week after surgery, if patients are up for more than use of the bathroom or eating meals, the reconstructed knee has a tendency to become swollen. Swelling then limits the progress of range of motion and delays the overall rehabilitation process. Consequently, we instruct our patients to limit the amount of time that they are up out of bed for the first week after surgery.

We have not seen the need to pursue alternative techniques for ACL reconstruction. We acknowledge the injury caused by harvesting a graft from the central one-third of the patellar tendon, but it is our opinion that we can lessen the morbidity with an appropriate aggressive rehabilitation program with emphasis on full hyperextension and early return of quadriceps-muscle strength. We have not had experience with alternative graft sources. Because we use a two-incision technique, the length of our femoral tunnel is not an issue. We do not have a problem with graft–tunnel length mismatch. The lateral incision can have some problems with postoperative hematoma if care is not taken to ensure that all lateral vessels are coagulated at the time of tourniquet deflation before wound closure.

Although it is perceived as more invasive than an arthroscopy-assisted ACL reconstruction, we have not found the miniarthrotomy to be a limiting factor in the advancement of our accelerated rehabilitation program.

■ TECHNICAL ALTERNATIVES AND PITFALLS

Our patients return to the office 1 week after surgery. At this visit patients are monitored for full knee hyperextension, minimal knee swelling, good quadriceps-muscle leg control and flexion of 100 degrees. Most patients are still using crutches but are close to resuming normal gait patterns. Patients see the physical therapist at this time and are advanced in their rehabilitation programs. Prone hanging is added as an extension exercise. The CPM machine is returned at this visit, and thereafter flexion exercises are done with wall and heel slides. Patient activity is increased on a gradual basis, with the control of swelling being the guide for how much ambulation patients are allowed. A normal gait pattern is practiced, often in front of a mirror, because this gives the patient immediate visual clues as to how he or she is walking.

■ REHABILITATION

The patient again is seen at 2 weeks after the surgery. At this time the sutures are removed. Full hyperextension is confirmed, and we desire 110 and 120 degrees of flexion. The final degrees of flexion are achieved with heel slides. Quadriceps-muscle strengthening is advanced by adding quarter knee squats and stepups to the regimen. In addition, the exercise bicycle and stair-stepping machine are added to the rehabilitation activities. Activities of daily living return to normal after between 2 and 3 weeks.

At 4 weeks after reconstruction, the patient should have near full range of motion, and at this time we start some light agility and sport-specific activities. As long as the patient has good range of motion, additional weightroom exercises are added, including the hip sled and leg press. The agility drills are advanced as tolerated. The patient should be aware that it takes 2 to 3 months of sport-specific activities to become comfortable with the reconstructed knee. We often recommend that the initial postoperative testing at this time include KT-1000 and isokinetic strength testing.

The patient is advanced in activities as desired during these later stages of rehabilitation. Those patients who desire a rapid return to athletics are monitored closely and allowed to do so as long as they progress properly with their activities and continue with the final stages of rehabilitating their knees. We have never encouraged a player to return to sports at an early time after surgery. Likewise, if a player has full range of motion and good strength and has completed a functional progression program for their desired sport, we do not withhold them from participation based on a certain time schedule after reconstruction.

Our long-term results in 1,057 patients at an average of 4 years after surgery included a KT-1000 manual maximum side-to-side difference of 2.0 ± 1.5 mm. Isokinetic quadriceps-muscle strength testing showed that patients had an average of 93% strength compared with the opposite normal knee. The average modified Noyes score was 93 out of 100 points (4).

■ OUTCOMES AND FUTURE DIRECTIONS

We envision in the future a biologic ligament that will not require an autogenous harvest. The graft will need to allow an aggressive rehabilitation program and will be remodeled into a normal ligament by the body.

References

1. Arms SW, Pope MH, Johnson RJ, et al. The biomechanics of anterior cruciate ligament rehabilitation and reconstruction. *Am J Sports Med* 1984; 12:8–18.
2. Clancy WG, Nelson DA, Reider B, et al. Anterior cruciate ligament reconstruction using one-third of the patellar ligament, augmented by extra-articular tendon transfers. *J Bone Joint Surg* 1982; 64A:352–359.
3. Penner DA, Daniel DM, Wood P, et al. An in vitro study of anterior cruciate ligament graft placement isometry. *Am J Sports Med* 1988; 16:238–243.
4. Shelbourne KD, Gray T. Anterior cruciate ligament reconstruction with autogenous patellar tendon graft followed by accelerated rehabilitation: A two- to nine-year follow-up. *Am J Sports Med* 1997; 25:786–795.

JONATHAN B. TICKER
CHRISTOPHER D.
HARNER

8

Arthroscopy-assisted Posterior Cruciate Ligament Reconstruction

Surgical treatment of the posterior cruciate ligament (PCL)–deficient knee has progressed rapidly over the past 15 years, primarily as a result of innovations and application of arthroscopic techniques. More traditional approaches included a variety of open techniques, including primary repairs, nonanatomic reconstructions (i.e., with the medial head of the gastrocnemius or meniscus), and intraarticular reconstructions (i.e., with hamstring tendons) (1–3). In 1983, Clancy et al. (4) reported the use of a free graft to reconstruct the PCL, describing an open procedure using patellar tendon autograft. In 1985, Clancy and Pandya (5) reported that he began using an arthroscopy-assisted approach for these reconstructions, with the benefit of decrease morbidity and increased visualization. PCL reconstruction with a technique that is at least mostly arthroscopic is now well accepted; however, issues regarding timing of the reconstruction as well as treatment of associated instabilities are not well defined (6). Furthermore, the fate of the PCL-deficient knee that is not reconstructed is variable (7–11). This chapter details the current techniques for arthroscopic PCL reconstruction, highlighting the use of Achilles tendon allograft (12,13). To further their understanding of PCL injuries and treatment, in particular details on PCL anatomy and biomechanics, the clinical examination with static and dynamic tests, imaging, and treatment of avulsion fractures of the ligament insertion, readers are encouraged to review this material in the text *Knee Surgery* (14,15).

In the symptomatic PCL-deficient knee, the goal of surgery is to restore the principal function of the PCL as the primary static restraint against posterior translation of the tibia (16). On an individual basis, both subjective and objective factors, as well as the amount of time since the injury, need to be taken into account prior to indicating surgery. Subjective factors elicited from the history include complaints of instability or pain that have not been relieved with nonoperative measures.

Important clinical findings include an increased posterior drawer test (with the knee flexed to 90 and the hip flexed to 45 degrees), a decrease in the anteromedial tibial stepoff relative to the medial femoral condyle compared with the contralateral normal knee (with the knee at 90 degrees, usually about 1 cm), and a posterior sag of the tibia (with the knee and hip flexed to 90 degrees). The primary objective criterion from the clinical examination is the finding of the posterior drawer. The amount of posterior displacement is classifed as grade 1 (less than 5 mm), grade 2 (5–10 mm), or grade 3 (more than 10 mm). An essential function of the history and clinical examination is to distinguish an isolated PCL injury from a combined ligamentous injury, which usually has a posterior drawer of more than 12 to 15 mm. Instrumented laxity measurements play less of a role in diagnosis compared with their role in anterior cruciate ligament (ACL) deficiency, but they may be useful to study outcomes following PCL reconstruction.

With current techniques, in an isolated PCL-deficient knee, reconstruction should be considered for grade 3 instability, preferably in the acute setting. With a combined insta-

■ HISTORY OF THE TECHNIQUE

■ INDICATIONS AND CONTRAINDICATIONS

83

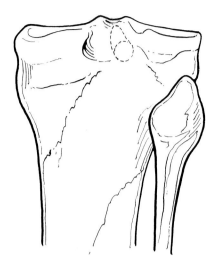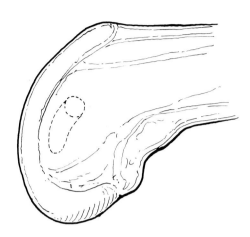

■ FIGURE 8-1

The posterior cruciate ligament tibial and femoral insertion sites and the preferred location for tunnel placement.

bility pattern (involving either the medial or lateral side) or knee dislocation, surgery preferably is performed in the acute setting to address all necessary ligament deficiencies. In the knee with combined ligamentous injuries with complete PCL rupture, posterior tibial sag (subluxation) is difficult to prevent and, as a result, surrounding torn capsular structures do not heal in the correct anatomic position, especially the posterolateral corner. Furthermore, these structures, which otherwise could be repaired primarily in the acute setting, may require a reconstruction if addressed in the setting of chronic instability. (These injury patterns are reviewed in more detail in the following chapters.) Although degenerative changes may develop in the PCL-deficient knee, the indications for surgical intervention to prevent this possibility are not well defined.

Contraindications to PCL reconstruction include neurovascular compromise that has yet to be addressed, an open wound, infection, and advanced degenerative arthritis.

In the chronic setting, significant motion limitations may be considered as a relative contraindication.

■ SURGICAL TECHNIQUES

Prior to undertaking any surgical reconstruction of the PCL, a few anatomic factors should be understood (17,18). These include a knowledge of the normal insertion sites, which are on the lateral aspect of the medial femoral condyle in an anterosuperior location in the intercondylar notch for the femoral insertion and in the sulcus of the posterior tibia between the condyles approximately 1 cm inferior to the level of the articular surface for the tibial insertion (Fig. 8-1). The normal PCL is wider and longer than the ACL, with a width averaging 13 mm and a length averaging 38 mm, and it is optimal for the graft to reflect this greater size. In addition, the PCL comprises different bundles, including the larger anterolateral and smaller posteromedial components, as well as the meniscofemoral components that are variable in size and not always present. The geometry and insertion-site anatomy of these bundles have been studied in detail (17). It is preferable to reconstruct the larger anterolateral component of the PCL with the current single-bundle reconstruction techniques. Because this component is tight in flexion, this should be the position of the knee during graft tensioning and fixation.

Arthroscopic instrumentation specifically designed for PCL reconstruction (Linvatec, Largo, FL) should be available (Fig. 8-2). Drill guide tips that aim the guide wire to the elbow of the drill guide, and not the very tip, provide a measure of safety in placing the guide wire for the tibial tunnel. A 70-degree arthroscope is quite helpful for visualization during preparation of the tibial insertion site and should be in the operative field. Tunnel dilators and sizers (Instrument Makar, Okemos, MI) are helpful in creating and preparing the tunnels.

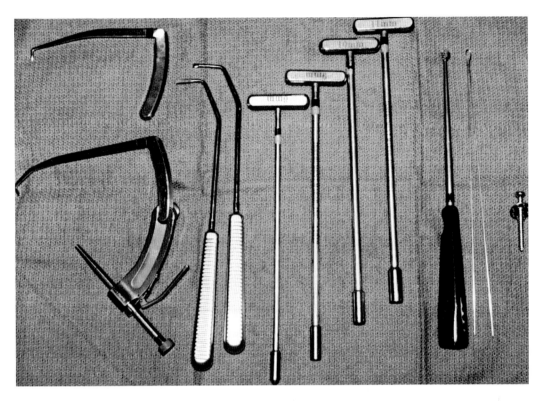

■ FIGURE 8-2

Instrumentation and devices used for arthroscopy-assisted posterior cruciate ligament reconstruction.

Although a number of grafts have been described for PCL reconstruction, an Achilles tendon allograft has a number of advantages. These include decreased tourniquet and surgical time, injury-free graft-site harvesting, easier passage because of a soft-tissue end, increased size of graft material, and ample graft length. Disadvantages include the potential for disease transmission and the requirement for soft tissue fixation at one end. With an Achilles tendon allograft, both interference screws and a screw with a spiked soft-tissue washer must be available for fixation. A staple may be used for supplemental fixation.

With the patient on the operating table in the supine position, general anesthesia is administered. A systematic examination under anesthesia is performed to confirm the pattern of instability. Both knees are examined to allow for side-by-side comparison. It is at this point that any additional instabilities must be recognized and planned for to achieve a successful outcome. A low-profile arthroscopic leg holder (Smith & Nephew Endoscopy, Mansfield, MA), a padded well-leg holder, and a tourniquet are used, and all down surfaces of the patient are padded. The foot of the operating table is brought down and out of the way. The operative extremity is prepared and draped in the usual sterile fashion, and a marker is used to outline planned portals and skin incisions. The leg is exsanguinated with an Esmark elastic wrap, and the tourniquet is inflated, usually to 350 mm Hg. Standard anterolateral and anteromedial portals are used for the initial diagnostic arthroscopy. The PCL disruption is confirmed, and meniscal or chondral pathology is addressed. While the ACL is being viewed, an anterior drawer is performed to reestablish the anteromedial tibial stepoff and restore the normal appearance of the intact ACL, which appears lax if the tibia is posteriorly subluxed.

Achilles tendon allograft preparation may begin on a side table (Fig. 8-3). The bone block is marked to obtain a final diameter of 11 or 12 mm and a length of 25 mm. An oscillating saw is used to make provisional cuts. The soft-tissue edges of the tendon are trimmed sharply. A ronguer and a bone biter are used to completely trim and shape the bone into a cylindric shape, without a curve in it. Compaction pliers (Instrument Makar) of the desired

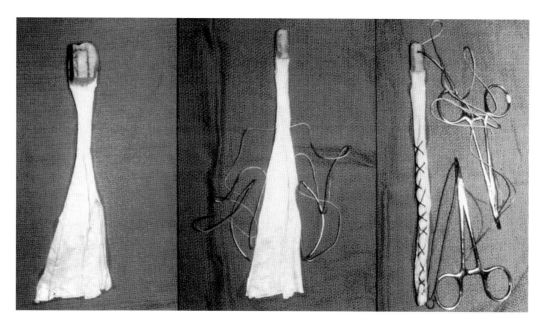

■ FIGURE 8-3

Achilles tendon allograft preparation.

diameter are useful in preparing the bone plug. A no. 5 nonabsorbable, braided suture, with needles on each end, is used to tubularize the tendinous portion of the graft. The suture ends are left long as they exit the end of the graft and are used during graft passage. The 11- or 12-mm sizing tube is used to assess ease of graft passage. Once this is completed, the graft is wrapped in gauze moistened with saline and safely placed on the table.

With the arthroscope in the anterolateral portal, a basket punch and mechanized shaver are introduced through the anteromedial portal, and the PCL midsubstance is debrided sufficiently to allow full appreciation of the femoral footprint and complete visualization through the notch. A 70-degree arthroscope then is used to visualize the PCL tibial insertion site and capsule in the posterior notch. A posteromedial portal is established under direct visualization and used as both a working and a viewing portal. An arthroscopic cannula may be used but is usually not necessary. A mechanized shaver is introduced through the posteromedial portal to debride the PCL at the tibial insertion. It is essential to visualize the tibial insertion and capsule fully during this phase of preparation. A 30-degree arthroscope now is placed in the posteromedial portal. An angled PCL rasp and curette are introduced alternately through the anteromedial portal to elevate the capsule and fully expose the distal and lateral aspect of the tibial footprint, which may be a few millimeters below the capsular attachment (Fig. 8-4). The tibial tunnel is centered in this portion of the tibial insertion site.

The arthroscopic PCL drill guide for the tibial insertion is set between 50 and 55 degrees and introduced through the anteromedial portal, with the tip seated in the distal and lateral aspect of the tibial footprint. The guide wire sleeve is advanced to leave a mark on the skin of the anteromedial proximal tibia at the midpoint between the anterior tibial crest and the posteromedial border of the tibia. The guide and sleeve are removed, and a 3-cm longitudinal skin incision is made. If ACL and PCL reconstructions are planned, the incision is extended 1 cm superiorly. The periosteum is exposed, incised, and elevated. The arthroscopic drill guide is replaced, with its position confirmed arthroscopically, and the guide wire sleeve is secured against the anteromedial tibia. Before drilling the guide wire into place, the angle of the proximal tibiofibular joint is marked. A well-placed tibial guide wire routinely follows the angle of the proximal tibiofibular joint and therefore is used to assist with guide wire placement. With this landmark noted, the guide wire is drilled into place under direct arthroscopic visualization. Care is taken to "feel" the second cortex, so that the

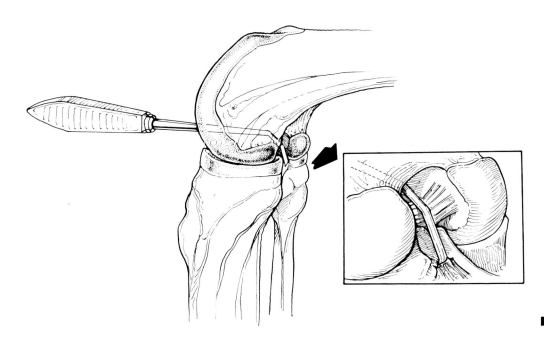

Angled instruments are used to clear the capsule to visualize the entire posterior cruciate ligament tibial insertion, in particular the distal and lateral aspect.

guide wire is not advanced inadvertently beyond the tip of the guide. The guide wire is advanced 5 to 7 mm with a mallet, and a lateral radiograph is obtained (Fig. 8-5). The error in guide wire placement usually is placing it too superiorly in the footprint. If ACL and PCL reconstructions are planned, the ACL guide wire is placed to ensure a 1-cm bone bridge on the anterior tibia between both tunnels, and the position of both guide wires can be assessed radiographically.

Once accurate guide wire placement is confirmed, the tibial tunnel is created with a cannulated reamer that measures the desired diameter to accommodate the graft. The PCL curette is placed over the tip of the guide wire, and the reamer is advanced under power. Perforation of the posterior cortex with the reamer is completed by hand for safety. Alternatively, the tunnel can be reamed to a smaller diameter and dilated up to the desired final diameter (Fig. 8-5). This serves to compress the cancellous bone in the tunnel to improve the bone stock. With the dilator perched at the intraarticular edge of the tunnel, soft tissue that would impede graft passage is debrided, with care taken not to remove capsular tissue. An aggressive round rasp is inserted up the tibial tunnel and used to chamfer the superior edge of the tunnel to create a smooth rounded surface to facilitate graft passage and limit graft abrasion. A plug then is placed in the entrance to the tibial tunnel on the anterior tibia to maintain fluid distention.

With the 30-degree arthroscope in the anterolateral portal, the PCL femoral insertion site is checked to ensure that its preparation is complete. With the arthroscopic instruments removed, a 2- to 3-cm modified medial parapatellar skin incision is made at the edge of the medial femoral condyle, approximately in the middle one third of the patella, with the knee flexed to 90 degrees. The vastus medialis is incised at the muscle–tendon junction to expose the articular edge of the condyle. The PCL femoral drill guide is set between 30 and 40 degrees and introduced through the anteromedial portal. The tip of the guide is placed 8 to 10 mm from the articular margin within the anterior portion of the PCL femoral footprint. With retractors utilized for exposure, the guide wire sleeve is secured against the medial aspect of the medial femoral condyle approximately 10 mm from the articular margin. The guide wire is drilled under arthroscopic visualization and tapped an additional 5 to 7 mm (Fig. 8-6). Once accurate guide wire placement is confirmed, the tunnel is reamed to the same diameter as the tibial tunnel. Care must be taken in perforating the second cortex in

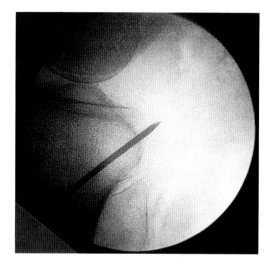

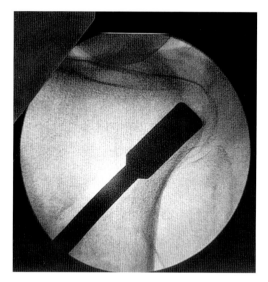

Placement of the tibial guide wire in the distal portion of the posterior cruciate ligament tibial footprint. The tunnel sizer clearly outlines the perimeter and location of the tibial tunnel.

■   FIGURE 8-5

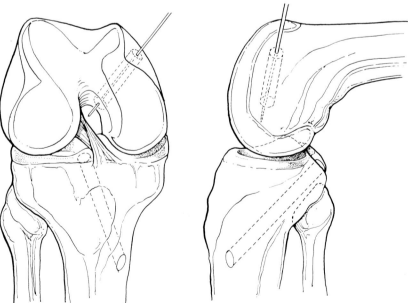

■   FIGURE 8-6

Femoral guide wire in the anterior portion of the posterior cruciate ligament femoral footprint at the desired angle.

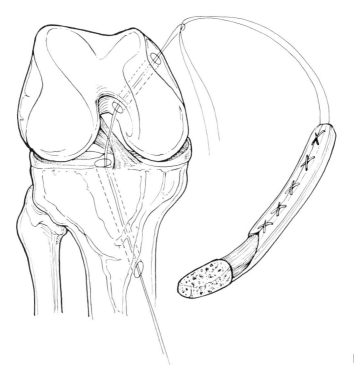

Femoral and tibial tunnels are demonstrated with the looped wire in place, in preparation for graft passage.

the intercondylar notch, because the intact ACL is at risk if the reamer "plunges" through this cortex. As with the tibial tunnel, the femoral tunnel alternatively can be reamed to a smaller diameter and dilated up to the desired final diameter, with the additional benefit of decreasing the risk for subchondral fracture. With the dilator perched at the edge of the tunnel, soft tissue that would impede graft passage or compromise the notch is debrided. An aggressive rasp then is inserted down the femoral tunnel and used to chamfer the posterior edge of the tunnel in the notch to create a smooth rounded surface to facilitate graft passage and limit graft abrasion.

   The Achilles tendon allograft must be passed from proximal to distal. In preparation for this step, a looped 18-gauge wire is advanced into the posterior joint in a distal-to-proximal direction, starting at the tibial tunnel. It is retrieved with a pituitary ronguer or similar device, and the loop is placed at the opening of the femoral tunnel. The pituitary ronguer then is placed down the femoral tunnel to grasp the loop of wire and bring it out through the femoral tunnel. The prepared Achilles tendon allograft is brought onto the field, and the suture ends are placed through the loop in the wire (Fig. 8-7). The end of the wire that remains out of the tibial tunnel is pulled, and the sutures are brought down the femoral tunnel, through the joint, and out the tibial tunnel. With traction on the suture ends, the tendinous portion of the graft is brought through the joint and out the tibial tunnel. The bone block is rotated with the cancellous side away from the articular margin and recessed in the femoral tunnel 1 to 2 mm below the medial cortex of the medial femoral condyle. A flexible guide wire for the cannulated interference screw is placed along the cancellous surface and the screw, 7 to 9 mm in diameter and 20 mm in length, is secured into place. With firm traction on the sutures and tendon coming out of the tibial tunnel, the knee is flexed repeatedly and extended to cycle the graft for pretensioning.

   At this point, preparation is made for distal fixation. This is accomplished by using a screw with a spiked soft-tissue washer (Linvatec, Largo, FL). After drilling, measuring, and tapping the hole in the tibia, a screw of the desired length with a washer is placed through a slit cut in the center of the graft and into the drill hole in the tibia. The knee is placed in

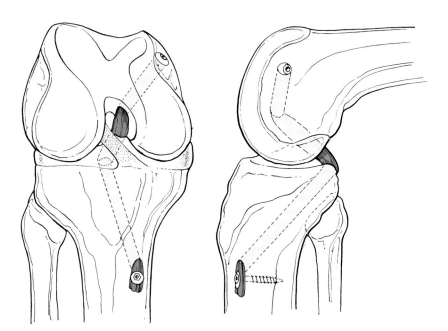

■   FIGURE 8-8

Achilles tendon allograft in place and secured with proximal and distal fixation.

70 to 90 degrees of flexion, and an anteriorly directed force is applied to recreate the normal anteromedial tibial stepoff of approximately 1 cm. With manual tension on the graft, the screw with spiked washer is secured firmly in place. Bicortical fixation with a 4.5-mm cortical screw is preferable to cancellous screw fixation in the proximal tibia. The completed reconstruction is checked by performing a posterior drawer, with the graft assessed arthroscopically (Fig. 8-8). Excess graft distal to the fixation on the tibia is excised sharply.

In the majority of cases, combined ligament reconstructions are performed in conjunction with PCL reconstruction. In these cases, fixation of the PCL on the tibial side is performed after the capsular and collateral repairs or reconstructions are completed. If a combined ACL and PCL reconstruction is planned, the PCL and the ACL tibial tunnels are drilled first, followed by the ACL and PCL femoral tunnels. The PCL graft then is passed and secured on the femoral side. The ACL graft, usually a patellar tendon allograft or occasionally an Achilles tendon allograft, is passed in an endoscopic fashion in most cases and secured on the femoral side. Capsular and collateral repairs or reconstructions then are performed as indicated. Final fixation for the PCL graft is completed on the tibial side with the knee in 70 to 90 degrees of flexion with an anterior drawer to recreate the normal anteromedial tibial stepoff of approximately 1 cm. The ACL then is fixed on the tibial side with an interference screw, with the knee in full extension. If the operating surgeon is uncomfortable with the tibial position after PCL fixation, an intraoperative lateral radiograph can be obtained prior to ACL fixation.

A meticulous layered closure is performed in the proximal and distal incisions, with no. 1 or 0 absorbable braided suture used for the deeper layer and no. 2-0 absorbable braided suture for the superficial layer. The skin and portals are closed with staples, or in a subcuticular fashion with a no. 3-0 absorbable monofilament suture as desired. A sterile dressing is placed, the tourniquet is deflated, and a cryocompression device (Aircast, Summit, NJ) is applied. The knee then is placed in a long-leg hinged brace locked in extension.

■ TECHNICAL
ALTERNATIVES AND
PITFALLS

Alternative positioning to perform arthroscopy-assisted PCL reconstruction is acceptable. This includes placing the patient in the supine position, with a lateral post and a sand bag to maintain the knee at 90 degrees of flexion. The arthroscope can be placed on a Mayo stand, which is positioned at the head of table. The procedure follows as described previously.

In addition to the Achilles tendon allograft, other grafts such as patellar tendon allografts, patellar tendon autografts, hamstring autografts, and quadriceps autografts have been used for PCL reconstruction (19). The patellar tendon grafts may be difficult to pass around the sharp angle at the intraarticular aspect of the tibial tunnel. This can be addressed by shortening the bone plug on the end of the graft that makes this acute turn as it is passed through the joint. Also, a straight instrument can be introduced through the posteromedial portal anterior to the passing sutures and used like a pulley to advance the entire bone plug out of the tibial tunnel before it turns toward the femoral tunnel. This problem also may be avoided by using a tibial inlay technique (20). The procedure is performed arthroscopically until final graft fixation on the tibial side, at which time the bone block is fixed to the PCL footprint through an open posterior approach. Finally, a hamstring autograft may be indicated for the smaller individual because of its smaller diameter (21). Certainly, there are advantages to being able to use more than one type of graft if the surgeon's preferred graft is not available. An Achilles tendon allograft alternatively can be passed from distal to proximal. In this setting, the tibial side is fixed first with an interference screw, with the proximal end of the bone plug advanced up the tunnel and flush with the edge of the posterior tibial cortex. The femoral side can be fixed with a screw and spiked soft-tissue washer or with a modified bone block technique, using a free bone plug wedged into the tunnel adjacent to the tendon with tension placed on the graft, and secured with an interference screw (13).

To summarize, the key steps to remember to avoid pitfalls are as follow:

1. Perform a thorough examination under anesthesia.
2. Preserve the footprint at both insertion sites.
3. Expose the distal and lateral aspects of the tibial insertion for tibial tunnel placement.
4. Use the posteromedial portal to facilitate preparation and tunnel placement of the tibial insertion.
5. Angle the tibial guide wire to approximate the angle of the proximal tibiofibular joint.
6. Confirm guide wire position with an intraoperative radiograph,
7. Create the femoral tunnel a sufficient distance from the articular margin.
8. Observe all guide wire placement arthroscopically.
9. Carefully prepare the tunnel edges to avoid graft abrasion.
10. Secure the graft in 70 to 90 degrees of knee flexion, with an anterior drawer performed to recreate the normal anteromedial tibial stepoff.

Some complications that could occur during or after PCL reconstruction are similar to those for other arthroscopic knee surgeries, such as infection, tourniquet-related problems, deep vein thrombosis, and pulmonary embolus (22). During any surgery such as this that requires a reconstruction with a graft, hardware failure and graft failure are potential complications. If an autograft is used, donor-site complications particular to that type of graft may be encountered. Technical errors may be associated with some of these problems, such as graft failure with poor tunnel placement or preparation of the tunnel edges. Stretching of the graft is prevented by avoiding posterior sagging of the tibia in the early postoperative period. For this reason, continuous passive motion devices are not used. Although stiffness can be found following other types of arthroscopic knee surgery, patients undergoing PCL reconstructions, particularly if performed with other ligament surgery, are at risk for motion loss, especially flexion. The location of incisions place the saphenous vein and nerve, as well as its infrapatellar branch, at risk. The popliteal nerve is at risk if a lateral repair or reconstruction is undertaken.

Other complications are inherent to arthroscopy-assisted PCL reconstruction (14,23). The neurovascular structures of the popliteal fossa, which are approximately 1 to 2 cm posterior to the capsule, are at risk during placement of the tibial guide wire and reaming the tibial tunnel. Therefore, during this portion of the procedure, instruments must be visualized continually as they are passed through the tibial tunnel. A posteromedial safety incision of 2 to 3 cm from the posteromedial portal extending inferiorly can be made to allow direct palpation of the tibial tunnel from an extracapsular approach, for further protection

(24). Maintaining the knee in a flexed position, using a drill guide that aims the guide wire to the elbow of the guide and not the tip, observing guide wire placement arthroscopically, covering the guide wire tip with a curette during reaming, and completing the reaming of the posterior cortex by hand to avoid "plunging" help to prevent injury to the neurovascular structures.

Avascular necrosis of the medial femoral condyle can present with femoral tunnel placement if the vascular supply is disrupted. In addition, if this tunnel is placed too close to the articular margin, the subchondral bone of the distal medial femoral condyle may fracture. Vascular complications following placement of the tibial fixation screw have been reported, and care must be taken to angle the initial drill hole away from neurovascular structures (22). In the acute reconstruction or if excessive capsular stripping is performed during preparation of the tibial insertion site and an arthroscopic pump is used, fluid extravasation may be increased and should not be overlooked. For this reason, gravity flow is used. At times, the knee is viewed with the arthroscope without fluid in the joint. Distal pulses should be checked at the completion of the procedure, and an arteriogram performed if pulses are diminished or not palpable.

■ REHABILITATION

The principles of rehabilitation following isolated PCL reconstruction to restore function begin with minimizing stress on the healing graft and avoiding posterior tibial translation, either by protecting against gravity or limiting hamstring activity. As this process progresses, restoration of motion, initially in a protected manner, and return of quadriceps function are essential. The patient must be counseled preoperatively regarding the expectations and limitations of the rehabilitation. The surgeon, patient, and physical therapist, as well as parents or an athletic trainer if involved, also should realize that full recovery following PCL reconstruction occurs more slowly than with ACL reconstruction, with a later return to sports. The following guidelines for rehabilitation are based on the protocol devised at the University of Pittsburgh.

Phase I is the first postoperative month and includes brace use in extension for the first week, with weight bearing as tolerated with crutches. At this point, assisted passive range of motion exercises begin, with caution taken to maintain an anteriorly directed force on the leg. Exercises that lead to posterior translation of the tibia are avoided. Quadriceps and hip exercises are instituted, along with calf exercises. Cryocompression is begun and continued throughout the rehabilitation. Phase II extends through the third postoperative month. The brace is unlocked for ambulation training and progressed for all activities, although its use continues until 8 weeks. Crutches are discontinued as quadriceps control and normal gait are demonstrated. Gains in range of motion to full extension and further flexion are pursued. Early strengthening exercises are begun, with efforts to minimize hamstring activity, and include the stationary bicycle and stairclimber. Hamstring flexibility, however, is added.

Phase III continues into the ninth postoperative month. Range of motion is restored, with recovery of full flexion occasionally as late as the fifth month. Therapeutic exercises and proprioception training are advanced, with progression to functional strengthening, with continued focus on the quadriceps. Phase IV extends until the patient has resumed desired activities. Sports-specific training is started toward the end of phase III and advanced in phase IV. Strength and endurance are maximized, and a maintenance program is reviewed with the patient.

■ OUTCOMES AND FUTURE DIRECTIONS

Nonoperative treatment of the isolated PCL-deficient knee can result in disabling pain, activity limitations including variable return to sports, and degenerative arthritis (7–11). As a result, PCL reconstruction is indicated in the symptomatically unstable PCL-deficient knee to limit the onset of these problems. Most series with allografts have reported a consistent decrease in the grade of instability, with good patient satisfaction and many patients returning to preinjury levels of activity (25–27). Furthermore, the results of acute reconstructions appear better than chronic reconstructions. It is clear, however, that more detailed studies are required to confirm the results of the limited number of studies in the literature.

Future directions for arthroscopic PCL reconstruction include further refinement of the arthroscopic technique. Two-bundle techniques are being developed, with separate femoral tunnels to recreate the anterolateral portion of the PCL, which is tight in flexion, and the posteromedial portion, which is tight in extension. In addition, direct fixation of the graft at the tibial insertion would avoid having the graft bend at the tibial tunnel. Although understanding of the structure and function of the PCL is progressing, the ideal graft material is not yet available. As the kinematics and proprioceptive role of the PCL-intact and -deficient knee are defined further, this procedure undoubtedly will evolve to a more anatomic reconstruction.

References

1. Hughston JC, Bowden JA, Andrews JR, et al. Acute tears of the posterior cruciate ligament: Results of operative treatment. *J Bone Joint Surg Am* 1980; 62:438–450.
2. Insall JN, Hood RW. Bone-block transfer of the medial head of the gastrocnemius for posterior cruciate insufficiency. *J Bone Joint Surg Am* 1982; 64:691–699.
3. Lipscomb BA, Anderson AF, Norwig ED, et al. Isolated posterior cruciate ligament reconstruction: Long-term results. *Am J Sports Med* 1993; 21:490–496.
4. Clancy WG, Shelbourne KD, Zoellner GB, et al. Treatment of knee joint instability secondary to rupture of the posterior cruciate ligament. Report of a new procedure. *J Bone Joint Surg Am* 1983; 65:310–322.
5. Clancy WG, Pandya RD. Posterior cruciate ligament reconstruction with patellar tendon autograft. *Clin Sports Med* 13; 1994; 561–570.
6. Covey DC, Sapega AA. Current concepts review: Injuries of the posterior cruciate ligament. *J Bone Joint Surg Am* 1993; 75:1376–1386.
7. Boynton MD, Tietjens BR. Long-term follow-up of the untreated posterior cruciate ligament-deficient knee. *Am J Sports Med* 1996; 24:306–310.
8. Cross MJ, Powell JF. Long-term follow-up of a posterior cruciate ligament rupture: A study of 116 cases. *Am J Sports Med* 1984; 12:292–297.
9. Fowler PJ, Messieh SS. Isolated posterior cruciate ligament injuries in the athlete. *Am J Sports Med* 1982; 10:553–557.
10. Keller PM, Shelbourne KD, McCarroll JR, et al. Nonoperatively treated isolated PCL injuries. *Am J Sports Med* 1993; 21:132–136.
11. Parolie JM, Bergfeld JA. Long-term results of nonoperative treatment of isolated posterior cruciate ligament injuries in the athlete. *Am J Sports Med* 1986; 14:35–38.
12. Schulte KR, Harner CD. Management of isolated posterior cruciate ligament injuries. *Oper Tech Orthop* 1995; 5:270–275.
13. Swenson TM, Harner CD, Fu FH. Arthroscopic posterior cruciate ligament reconstruction with allograft. *Sports Medicine and Arthroscopy Review* 1994; 2:120–128.
14. Miller MD, Harner CD, Koshiwaguchi S. Acute posterior cruciate ligament injuries. In: Fu FH, Harner CD, Vince KG, eds. *Knee surgery.* Baltimore: Williams & Wilkins, 1994:749–767.
15. Stuart MJ, Froese WG, Fowler PJ. Chronic posterior cruciate ligament injuries. In: Fu FH, Harner CD, Vince KG, eds. *Knee surgery.* Baltimore: Williams & Wilkins, 1994:769–785.
16. Butler DL, Noyes FR, Grood ES. Ligamentous restraints to anterior-posterior drawer in the human knee: A biomechanical study. *J Bone Joint Surg Am* 1980; 62:259–270.
17. Harner CD, Xerogeanes JW, Livesay GA, et al. The human posterior cruciate ligament complex: Ligament morphology and biomechanical evaluation. *Am J Sports Med* 1995; 23:736–745.
18. Miller MD, Harner CD. The anatomic and surgical considerations for posterior cruciate ligament reconstruction. *Instr Course Lect* 1995; 44:431–440.
19. Bach BR. Graft selection in posterior cruciate ligament surgery. *Operative Techniques in Sports Medicine* 1993; 1:104–109.
20. Berg EE. Posterior cruciate ligament tibial inlay reconstruction. *Arthroscopy* 1995; 11:69–76.
21. Shino K, Kakagawa S, Kakamura N, et al. Arthroscopic posterior cruciate ligament reconstruction using hamstring tendons: One-incision technique with Endobutton. *Arthroscopy* 1996; 12:638–642.
22. Marks PH, Harner CD, Fu FH. Complications of knee ligament surgery. In: Fu FH, Harner CD, Vince KG, eds. *Knee surgery.* Baltimore: Williams & Wilkins, 1994:897–910.
23. Veltri DM, Warren RF, Silver G. Complications in posterior cruciate ligament surgery. *Operative Techniques in Sports Medicine* 1993; 1:154–158.

24. Fanelli GC, Giannotti BF, Edson CJ. Arthroscopically assisted combined posterior cruciate ligament/posterior lateral complex reconstruction. *Arthroscopy* 1996; 12:521–530.
25. Bullis DW, Paulos LE. Reconstruction of the posterior cruciate ligament with allograft. *Clin Sports Med* 1994; 13:581–597.
26. Maday MG, Harner CD, Miller MD, et al. Posterior cruciate ligament reconstruction using fresh-frozen achilles tendon allograft: Indications techniques, results and controversies. Presented at the 60th Annual Meeting of the American Academy of Orthopaedic Surgeons, San Francisco, CA, 1993.
27. Noyes FR, Barber-Weston SD. Posterior cruciate ligament allograft reconstruction with and without a ligament augmentation device. *Arthroscopy* 1994; 10:371–382.

Additional Reading

Clancy WG, ed. The posterior cruciate ligament [Issue]. *Clin Sports Med* 1994; 13:509–682.
Cooper DE, ed. Posterior cruciate ligament injuries. *Operative Techniques in Sports Medicine* 1993; 1:86–158.
Fu FH, ed. Current management of PCL injury. *Sports Medicine and Arthroscopy Review* 1994; 2:73–175.

9

PETER T. SIMONIAN
ANSWORTH ALLEN

Acute and Chronic Injuries to the Lateral Corner: The Popliteus and the Lateral Collateral Ligament

Recognition of posterolateral rotatory instability (PLRI), identification of the anatomic structures of the posterolateral region of the knee, and understanding of their contribution to stability have been achieved relatively recently; therefore, surgical techniques to address these problems are evolving.

■ HISTORY OF THE TECHNIQUE

Several physical examination techniques have evolved to determine the presence of PLRI (1–4), as discussed in the "Indications and Contraindications" section. Seebacher et al. (3) in 1982 organized the structures of the posterolateral corner into three layers, which has helped standardize and clarify the regional anatomy. Several biomechanical studies have helped determine the contribution of each of the discrete anatomic structures to posterolateral stability (5–8). As discussed in the section on alternative techniques, surgical reconstructive sophistication has increased with improved clinical diagnostic ability as well as a better understanding of the anatomy and structural function of the region. This has culminated in the preferred technique of anatomic reconstruction of the posterolateral corner (9–11).

Surgical reconstruction of the lateral corner usually is necessitated by some form of PLRI. These injuries rarely are isolated to the posterolateral corner and most commonly result from significant trauma. They typically are part of multiligament injuries and almost always involve one or both cruciate ligaments. In rare circumstances PLRI can occur in patients with preexisting excessive external rotation who sustain relatively minor trauma.

■ INDICATIONS AND CONTRAINDICATIONS

Various physical tests have been described for assessing PLRI. The posterolateral drawer test demonstrates increased posterior translation of the tibia with drawer testing as the foot is rotated externally. Additionally, with the foot held in neutral, the lateral tibia moves posterior on the femur, but the medial side of the tibia does not change its position relative to the femur. If a posterior drawer is more marked at 30 degrees of flexion compared with 90 degrees, there probably is PLRI. The external rotation recurvatum test is performed by raising the feet and determining if the knee falls into varus and hyperextension. This test is more exaggerated if there is a combined cruciate ligament injury. The reversed pivot shift is done with the leg held in external rotation and the knee passively extended. The shift represents reduction of the posteriorly subluxated lateral side of the tibial plateau. Increased external rotation with the knee held in varying degrees of flexion also has been associated with PLRI. In the acutely injured knee, it can be difficult to determine which of these discrete structures are injured.

It is important to identify, as much as possible, the extent of the injured structures prior to surgery in order to plan the approach and sequence for reconstruction. This knowledge also helps determine the need for allograft tissue and possibly autograft tissue from the contralateral extremity. Magnetic resonance imaging can be a helpful adjunct to this determination; however, the posterolateral corner is the most difficult zone to assess by mag-

95

netic resonance imaging (12). Plain radiographs should be obtained with weight bearing, if possible.

If cruciate ligament injuries are identified in conjunction with posterolateral instability, they are reconstructed first using either an open or an arthroscopic technique. Arthroscopy also can be utilized to evaluate intraarticular and meniscal pathology, as well as injury to the popliteus tendon.

Assessment of the neurovascular structures needs to be pursued carefully in these patients prior to intervention and after surgery, especially if a knee dislocation is suspected to be the cause.

■ SURGICAL
TECHNIQUES

The following surgical techniques were developed at the Hospital for Special Surgery, and their description is adapted from Bowen et al. (11) and Veltri and Warren (9,10).

Anatomy   The anatomy of the posterolateral corner of the knee has not been well understood because of inconsistencies in terminology and variations in the anatomy. The principle structures of the posterolateral corner include the lateral collateral ligament (LCL), the arcuate ligament, the popliteus tendon, the popliteofibular ligament, the short lateral ligament, the fabellofibular ligament, and the posterolateral part of the capsule. Terminology describing these structures has been confusing: differentiation between the arcuate ligament and the arcuate ligament complex described by Baker et al. (13), which includes the arcuate ligament, LCL, popliteus, and lateral head of the gastrocnemius, must be recognized. Besides the variations in terminology, there are reported variations in the anatomy (3,14,15).

In an attempt to clarify and standardize the anatomy, Seebacher et al. (3) organized the structures of the posterolateral corner into three layers. Layer I includes the iliotibial tract with its expansion anteriorly and the superficial portion of the biceps with its expansion posteriorly. At the level of the distal femur, the peroneal nerve is deep to layer I and lies posterior to the biceps tendon (Figs. 9-1 and 9-2). It is often mandatory to identify the peroneal nerve in approaching structures in the posterolateral corner of the knee. In cases of acute injury, hematoma that is compressing the nerve should be relieved.

Layer II is formed anteriorly by the quadriceps retinaculum coursing anterolaterally adjacent to the patella. Posteriorly, layer II is incomplete and is represented by the two patellofemoral ligaments. The proximal patellofemoral ligament joins the terminal fibers of the lateral intermuscular septum. The distal patellofemoral ligament ends posteriorly at the fabella if the fabella is present, or at the femoral insertion of the posterolateral part of the capsule and the lateral head of the gastrocnemius (Figs. 9-1 and 9-2).

Layer III is the deepest layer of the posterolateral corner and forms the lateral part of the capsule. The capsular attachment to the periphery of the meniscus is called the *coronary ligament*. The popliteus tendon passes through a hiatus in the coronary ligament to attach to the femur anterior to the femoral attachment of the LCL. Posterior to the overlying iliotibial tract, the capsule divides into two laminae: superficial and deep. The superficial lamina encompasses the LCL. This superficial lamina ends posteriorly at the fabellofibular ligament or the short lateral ligament. If a fabella is present, the fabellofibular ligament is found coursing to the LCL from the fabella to the fibula, inserting posterior to the insertion of the biceps tendon. Kaplan (14) noted that if the fabella is absent the short lateral ligament may be absent or attenuated. If the short lateral ligament is present, it is found adjacent to the lateral limb of the arcuate ligament, running from the femoral condyle origin of the lateral head of the gastrocnemius to the fibula (Figs. 9-1 and 9-2).

The lateral inferior geniculate vessels lie between the superficial and the deep laminae of the posterolateral part of the capsule. The deep lamina of the posterolateral part of the capsule passes along the edge of the lateral meniscus to form both the coronary ligament and the hiatus for the popliteus tendon. This inner lamina terminates posteriorly at the Y-shaped arcuate ligament. If present, the arcuate ligament consists of a medial limb that arises from the posterior part of the capsule at the distal part of the femur and courses medially over the popliteus muscle to the oblique popliteal ligament. The lateral limb arises

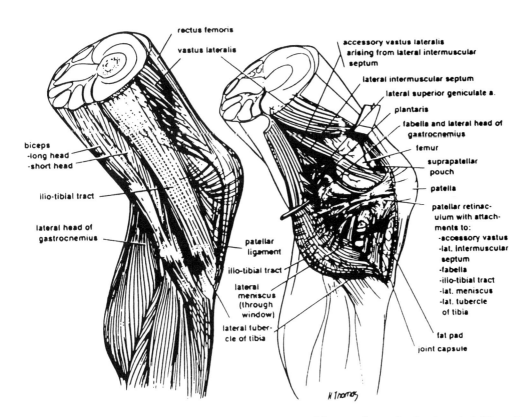

■ FIGURE 9-1

Posterolateral corner anatomy demonstrating layers I and II according to Seebacher et al. (From Seebacher JR, Inglis AE, Marshall JL, et al. The structure of the posterolateral aspect of the knee. *J Bone Joint Surg Am* 1982; 64:536–541, with permission.)

I - first layer
II - second layer
III - third layer

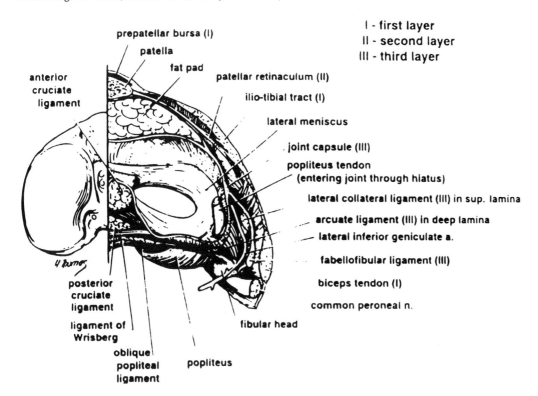

■ FIGURE 9-2

Posterolateral corner anatomy, coronal view, including layer III, according to Seebacher et al. (From Seebacher JR, Inglis AE, Marshall JL, et al. The structure of the posterolateral aspect of the knee. *J Bone Joint Surg Am* 1982; 64:536–541, with permission.)

from the posterior part of the capsule and courses laterally over the popliteus muscle and tendon, deep to the lateral inferior geniculate vessels, to insert on the posterior part of the fibula (Figs. 9-1 and 9-2).

The final component of layer III is the popliteofibular ligament. It also has been called the *popliteofibular fascicle* and the *fibular origin of the popliteus muscle* (15–17). This ligament is found deep to the lateral limb of the arcuate ligament. It arises from the posterior part of the fibula, posterior to the biceps insertion, and courses toward the junction of the popliteus muscle and its tendon. The popliteofibular ligament joins the popliteus tendon just proximal to its musculotendinous junction. The popliteofibular ligament was so named because it connects the fibula to the femur through the popliteus tendon. Therefore, the popliteus muscle–tendon unit is a Y-shaped structure, with a muscle origin from the posterior part of the tibia, a ligamentous origin from the fibula, and a united intersection to the femur (Fig. 9-3).

Acute Injuries

Popliteus   Surgical options for acute popliteus injuries include primary repair, advancement or recession, augmentation, and reconstruction. These injuries most often occur at the musculotendinous junction. A laterally based curvilinear incision can be utilized to expose the posterolateral corner. The iliotibial band is mobilized, and the posterior capsule is dissected posterior to the LCL and incised vertically posterior to the ligament. The posterior joint, popliteus muscle, and tendon are visualized. The tendon can be followed proximally to the point at which it travels beneath the LCL to its femoral attachment. Exposure of this femoral insertion is done by placing a clamp along the popliteus tendon beneath the LCL. An incision is made over the tip of the clamp, and the insertion site is visualized. It then is followed distally to its musculotendinous junction and the fibular and tibial insertions via the popliteofibular ligament. The musculotendinous unit then is examined to determine the extent of injury and the quality of the tissue for possible repair.

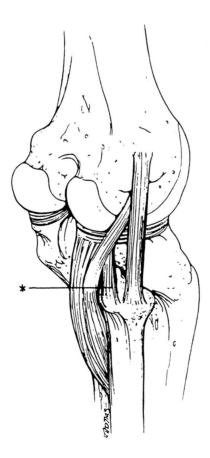

The popliteofibular ligament, arising from the posterior fibula, joins the popliteus tendon just above the musculotendinous junction. (From Veltri DM, Warren RF. Posterolateral instability of the knee. *Instr Course Lect* 1995; 44:441–453, with permission.)

■ FIGURE 9-3

In acute injuries in which the popliteus is intact but the tibial attachment is injured, an attempt can be made to restore tension by placing sutures in the tendon and pulling them distally through a drill hole from posterior to anterior. Alternatively, the tendon may be fixed to the tibia with a screw and washer. The bone bed must be prepared first and the foot rotated a few degrees internally prior to screw fixation. If the popliteus tendon is of insufficient quality, it can be augmented using a strip of the iliotibial band. Incorporating the incision made initially in the iliotibial band for exposure, a second longitudinal incision is made to create a 2-cm strip of iliotibial band. The strip is divided proximally and distally, leaving its insertion on Gerdy's tubercle intact. A drill hole sized to the fascia graft is made 1 to 2 cm below and parallel to the joint line from the anterolateral aspect of the knee. The exit site of the tibia should be in the area in which the popliteus crosses the proximal tibia. The iliotibial band graft then is passed through the drill hole and is secured to the remaining popliteus tendon with interrupted sutures (Fig. 9-4). Similarly, a strip of the biceps tendon can be used to augment the popliteofibular ligament. If the iliotibial band and the biceps are injured, one can reconstruct the tibial and fibular attachments of the popliteus with patellar ligament autogenous graft or allograft tissue.

Another approach to restore tension and dynamic function is to remove the popliteus insertion with a bone plug and advance and recess it into the femur. This is secured by passing sutures through the ligament and bone plug out through a drill hole to the medial side of the femur. The potential problem with this technique is that it relies on the competence of the popliteus muscle and tendon. If further failure and stretching occurs at the musculotendinous junction, the popliteus will not function properly. Conversely, the popliteus tendon may be fixed to the tibia using a screw and washer, thus converting the popliteus into a static stabilizer.

If there is inadequate tissue for repair, or the iliotibial band is damaged so that it is not available for augmentation, a bone–patella tendon–bone autograft or allograft or Achilles tendon allograft may be used as a substitute.

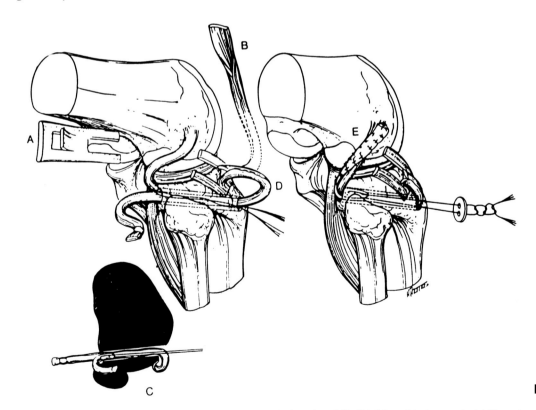

■ FIGURE 9-4

Popliteus augmentation with a strip of iliotibial band. A strip of iliotibial band is harvested (**A**) and rolled into a tube (**B**). It then is passed through the tibia from anterior to posterior (**C,D**), and is secured to the popliteus tendon with sutures (**E**). (From Bowen MK, Warren RF, Cooper DE. In: Insall J, ed. *Surgery of the knee.* New York: Churchill Livingston, 1993:505–554, with permission.)

Lateral Collateral Ligament   Similar to popliteal injuries, LCL injuries may occur as avulsions or interstitial injuries. Avulsions most frequently occur at the fibula attachment. Avulsions may be repaired with direct reattachment to the fibula. The peroneal nerve first must be identified and protected as it crosses the fibular neck. The ligament is prepared with Bunnel sutures, the tip of the fibula is prepared by making a trough, and drill holes are made anterolaterally about 1 to 2 cm down the fibular neck. The sutures from the ligament are passed through the drill holes into the bony trough and tied over the bone bridge. If there is a large enough bone fragment attached to the LCL, it can be fixed with an intramedullary screw and washer.

If the LCL does not reach the fibula or is ruptured interstitially, augmentation or reconstruction should be performed. The biceps tendon can be utilized to augment the LCL if it is not injured. A bone–tendon–bone autograft or allograft can be used if the biceps is injured at its attachment to the fibula.

To utilize the biceps tendon for augmentation, the central two thirds of the tendon is harvested by dissecting it from the muscle belly. The peroneal nerve is identified carefully and protected along the inferior aspect of the biceps tendon. The strip of tendon is extended proximally and incised at a length of about 12 cm. It is left attached to the fibula distally, and care is taken that pulling it into position does not put pressure on the peroneal nerve. The tendon is prepared with Bunnel sutures. The isometric point on the femur is then located. A K wire is drilled into the lateral femoral condyle near the attachment site of the LCL. A free suture is stretched from the LCL insertion site on the fibula up and over the K wire, and its position is marked on the suture. The knee then is brought from flexion to extension, and motion of the suture is observed. The femoral point is adjusted until there are no or minimal length changes in the suture through the knee range of motion. Once an isometric point is noted, the harvested biceps tendon is turned up and secured to the femur, using a ligament washer and screw. The knee then is brought through a range of motion and tested for varus stability (Fig. 9-5).

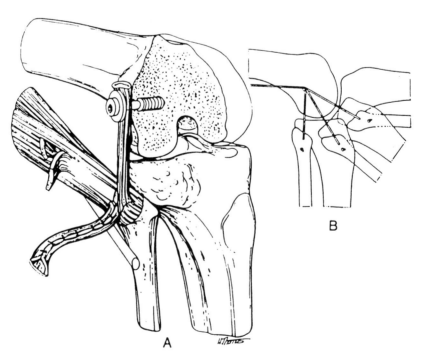

A   B

■ FIGURE 9-5

Lateral collateral ligament augmentation and repair using the biceps tendon. **A:** A strip of biceps tendon is dissected off muscle and used to create a new lateral collateral ligament. **B:** Drawing depicts assessment of isometry. (From Bowen MK, Warren RF, Cooper DE. In: Insall J, ed. *Surgery of the knee.* New York: Churchill Livingston, 1993:505–554, with permission.)

Combined Popliteus and LCL   A combination of the previous techniques of repair or augmentation is employed if possible. If the biceps and iliotibial band are not injured, they may be used to augment LCL and popliteus tears, respectively. If these structures are damaged, reconstructive techniques are utilized with autograft and allograft tissues. It may be possible to augment one of these; the other requires reconstruction.

Chronic Injuries

Popliteus   Evaluation begins with examination of the patient's static and dynamic lower-extremity alignment. If the patient has varus knee alignment and a lateral thrust in stance phase, a valgus proximal osteotomy is needed. If a reconstruction is done without addressing this type of alignment, the reconstruction will fail from the force of chronic repetitive stretching. The osteotomy may be performed as a staged or simultaneous procedure with the posterolateral reconstruction. The potential advantage of the staged approach is that sometimes the osteotomy alone resolves the symptoms of posterolateral instability.

For chronic popliteus insufficiency surgical options include advancement and recession of its bony insertion, distal advancement and tensioning of the tendon, reconstruction with a bone–tendon–bone patella tendon autograft or allograft, and reconstruction with an Achilles tendon allograft. Similar to the acute circumstance, chronic cruciate ligament injuries should be reconstructed first using an arthroscopic technique, followed by the same lateral curvilinear incision for reconstruction of the posterolateral corner. The procedure is performed by removing the popliteus insertion with a bone plug and advancing and recessing it into a tunnel created at the original insertion site. It is secured by passing sutures through the ligament and the bone plug and out through the drill holes to the medial side of the femur. The popliteus then is tensioned with the tibia in neutral rotation, and the sutures are tied over a button or bone bridge. The obvious advantage of advancement and recession of the popliteus is the use of native tissue and no graft requirement. The potential problem with this technique is the reliance on a competent popliteus muscle and tendon. If injury has occurred at the musculotendinous junction the popliteus cannot function properly. Therefore this is a viable alternative only if the popliteus tendon is robust and there is no evidence of injury at the musculotendinous junction. If it is not intact, there is a risk of failure because of stretching.

If injury at the musculotendinous junction is suspected but the popliteus tendon is robust, the preferred method is to tension the tendon by advancing it distally. This technique removes the dynamic restraint, because the tendon is fixed to the tibia. A screw and ligament are used to fix the tendon to a prepared site on the posterior tibia. The tibia is rotated internally at the time of fixation. Fixation may be accomplished by placing multiple sutures in the substance of the tendon as it passes from the tibia up toward its insertion on the femur. These sutures then are passed through a drill hole that is directed from the posterolateral corner of the tibia anterodistally. The sutures are tensioned over the anterior tibia with a button or a bone bridge if two drill holes are used. Again the tibia is internally rotated at the time of fixation.

Popliteus reconstruction is required if native tissues are insufficient or if the popliteus is attached to the tibia poorly. The graft choices include a bone–tendon–bone autograft from the ipsilateral or contralateral extremity or a bone–tendon–bone or Achilles allograft. The major factor that dictates the choice of graft material is the length that is required from the bone tunnel in the tibia to the tunnel in the femur. The distance is frequently longer than 5 cm, which is typically the greatest length that can be expected from the tendinous portion of the patella tendon graft. Therefore, Achilles tendon allografts are utilized more often for reconstruction of the popliteus tendon.

The tibial tunnel is prepared from anterior to posterolateral, similar to the preparation described for iliotibial band augmentation of an acute popliteus injury. Following exposure of the posterolateral corner of the tibia, a vector guide is used to place a guide pin and drill the tibial tunnel. The site on the lateral femoral condyle for the femoral tunnel is determined using an isometer suture and K wire as described previously. Once the isometric point is determined, the K wire is drilled across to the medial side of the femur, and an incision is made over it on the medial side. A cannulated reamer is passed over the guide wire from the lateral side to create a bone tunnel. Depending on the requirements of the graft, the tunnel is advanced either partially or completely through a femur. If the bone–tendon–bone graft is used, the tunnel is made just deep enough to recess the bone plug completely. Sutures through the bone plug are passed through the drill hole, allowing it to be advanced in the tunnel. The sutures then are tied over a bony bridge or button medially. An alternate fixation is an interference screw placed from the lateral side to secure the bone plug. If an Achilles tendon allograft is chosen, the bone plug is fit into the lateral femur and secured over a suture button or with an interference screw in the manner described previously. The tendon then is passed through the tibial tunnel and secured to the anterior tibia with a cancellous screw and washer (Fig. 9-6).

If there has been complete disruption of the tibial and fibular attachments, they should be reconstructed anatomically. A single split patellar ligament or Achilles allograft can be used to reconstruct both components of the popliteus. The popliteofibular ligament always should be reestablished, because it plays a critical role in the prevention of rotational instability (Fig. 9-7).

For either of the graft materials, the tension is set with the tibia placed in neutral rotation. Once the graft is fixed securely, the knee is put through a range of motion and is checked for external rotation at 30 and 90 degrees of flexion.

Lateral Collateral Ligament   For reconstruction of the LCL for chronic varus instability, surgical options include advancement and recession, biceps tendon augmentation or sub-

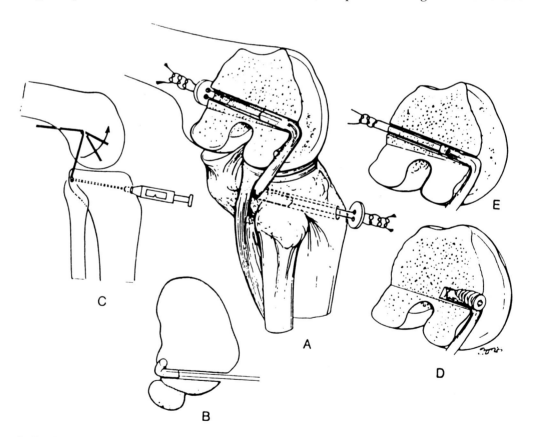

■ FIGURE 9-6

A: Popliteus reconstruction using a bone–tendon–bone graft. **B:** Tibial tunnel is placed from anterior to posterolateral. **C:** Isometric point on the femur is located using a K wire and suture. **D:** Interference screw fixation of bone plug in lateral femur. **E:** Fixation into femur by passing sutures to the medial side and securing them over a bony bridge. (From Bowen MK, Warren RF, Cooper DE. In: Insall J, ed. *Surgery of the knee.* New York: Churchill Livingston, 1993:505–554, with permission.)

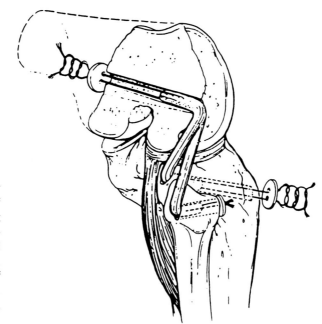

Reconstruction of the popliteofibular ligament and the tibial attachment of the popliteus with patellar ligament graft. The graft is placed into a common femoral tunnel and split into tibial and fibular tunnels. (From Veltri DM, Warren RF. Operative treatment of posterolateral instability of the knee. *Clin Sports Med* 1994; 13:615–627, with permission.)

■ FIGURE 9-7

stitution, or reconstruction using a bone–tendon–bone autograft or allograft. The native tissues first are assessed at the time of exploration. A recession may be performed by releasing the LCL from its femoral origin and advancing it into a bone tunnel with sutures placed through its substance or by securing it to its origin, using a ligament washer. If a bone tunnel is used to reconstruct the popliteus tendon, the LCL can be advanced into the posterior aspect of this same bone tunnel. This allows the ligament to remain close to its origin, as well as allowing the laxity to be removed. The free end of the LCL may be secured by passing the sutures in the ligament through drill holes either posteriorly in the lateral femoral condyle or across the femur to the medial side.

The biceps tendon can be used to augment or reconstruct the LCL in most patients. The details of the technique are described in the section on acute injuries to the LCL.

If the LCL is chronically deficient and the biceps tendon is not satisfactory, other tissue must be utilized. Autograft or allograft bone–tendon–bone preparations work well; however, other sources can be utilized. After carefully isolating the peroneal nerve from the the fibula, a slot to receive one bone plug is made in the top of the fibula, and two drill holes are placed distally. Sutures in the bone plug are passed through the holes in the fibula, and the graft is pulled distally into the tunnel in the fibula. Similar to the technique for chronic popliteus reconstruction, the isometric point on the femur is found with a suture and K wire as described previously. The bone plug or Achilles tendon is secured to the femur by drilling the isometrically placed K wire across from lateral to medial. An incision is made medially over the K wire, and the medial femur is exposed. An appropriately sized reamer then is used to create a tunnel sufficiently deep to recess the graft into the lateral femur; with the guide wire removed a looped wire is passed from medial to lateral, in order to bring graft sutures through the femur out the medial side. The graft first is secured to the fibula by tying the sutures distally. It then is placed under tension, and sutures coming out the medial femur are tied over a button; alternatively an interference screw may be used. The knee finally is checked for varus stability and range of motion (Fig. 9-8). Another option is to use an interference screw to secure the Achilles allograft bone plug to the fibula and isometrically secure the soft-tissue end of the graft to the femur with suture anchor devices.

Combined Popliteus and LCL Often both the popliteus and the LCL require stabilization. In reconstructing both the LCL and the popliteus, it is frequently difficult to fit and organize the grafts, particularly at their femoral attachments. Rather than drill two holes in the

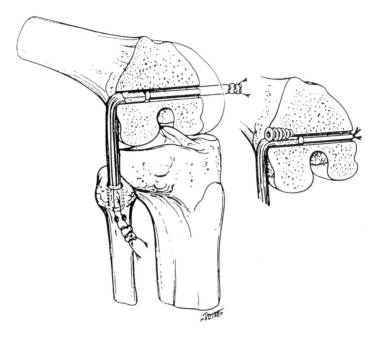

Reconstruction of the lateral collateral ligament using a bone–tendon–bone graft. (From Bowen MK, Warren RF, Cooper DE. In: Insall J, ed. *Surgery of the knee.* New York: Churchill Livingston, 1993:505–554, with permission.)

femur, one can use a split graft. By using one bone plug that is recessed into the femur at the site of the LCL and popliteus tendon, the reconstruction is simplified. This single bone plug is placed between the isometric points for the LCL and popliteus tendon and may be secured in the femur by drilling a hole partially or completely through to the medial side and tying sutures through the graft over a button, or an interference screw may be used. The graft then is split and passed through the respective tunnels. These are prepared in the same fashion as if the LCL and popliteus were being reconstructed alone. The distal arm of the split tendon should be used as the popliteus and passed under the proximal arm or the LCL. This approximates the anatomic orientation of the popliteus passing under the LCL (Fig. 9-9).

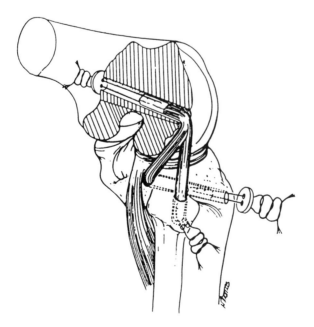

Reconstruction of the lateral collateral ligament and popliteus tendon using a split a bone–tendon–bone graft. (From Bowen MK, Warren RF, Cooper DE. In: Insall J, ed. *Surgery of the knee.* New York: Churchill Livingston, 1993:505–554, with permission.)

Several operations have been recommended to treat posterolateral instability. Reconstructive procedures typically involve either a tightening of lax lateral and posterolateral anatomic structures or the creation of a substitute restraint from the posterolateral corner of the knee to the anterior femoral epicondyle. These include popliteus tendon recession, arcuate advancement, biceps tenodesis, and popliteus tendon.

Recession of the popliteus tendon at its femoral insertion to restore posterolateral stability was recommended by Jakob et al. (18). This may suffice for mild instability but, as with advancement of the arcuate complex, proximal recession does not restore adequate tension to the popliteus if there is distal injury at the musculotendionous junction or injury of the popliteofibular ligament.

Some form of arcuate-complex advancement has been recommended in the following studies. Baker et al. (19) addressed acute posterolateral instability with repair of the injured structures. For acute injuries with insufficient tissue for primary repair and in chronic injuries, advancement of the arcuate complex was performed in the anterior and superior direction. If injury to the popliteus tendon and the posterolateral structures is distal to the joint, it was thought that femoral advancement alone would not restore adequate tension to the posterolateral corner. Hughston and Jacobson (20) also proposed distal primary repair and proximal advancement of the arcuate complex for chronic posterolateral instabilities. Depending on the technique, the advancement of the arcuate complex may shift the insertion sites of the popliteus and LCL anterior to the center of knee rotation. This may lead to stretching and failure of the reconstruction. Fleming et al. (21) reported 16 patients with chronic posterior and posterolateral treated again with an advancement of the arcuate complex. They also addressed the cruciate deficiencies and utilized a semitendinosus autograft reconstruction of the PCL and an Ellison iliotibial band extraarticular procedure for ACL deficiency.

Clancy (22) has advocated biceps tenodesis to reconstruct the posterolateral corner. The biceps tendon is transferred to the lateral femoral epicondyle; its distal attachment to the fibula is left intact. The biceps tendon is freed from the lateral head of the gastrocnemius and the peroneal nerve. It then is passed under the split of the iliotibial band and attached with a ligament screw and washer to the lateral femoral epicondyle. This transfer recreates an LCL and also may tighten the arcuate complex. Because this reconstruction does not recreate the popliteus tendon or the popliteofibular ligament, it only represents a partial reconstruction of the injured structures (23). Clancy reports (22) that this reconstruction is designed to contain only excessive external rotation and does not contain varus laxity. They perform a separate reconstruction of the LCL with autograft or allograft tissue if there is significant varus laxity (24). Wascher et al. (23) demonstrated in a cadaveric model that biceps tenodesis to a point 1 cm anterior to the insertion of the LCL on the femoral epicondyle can restore varus and external rotation stability to that of the intact knee.

Mueller (25) described the popliteus bypass procedure, which has not proven successful in the long term.

The optimal reconstruction would reestablish all the anatomy through repair of structures if possible and reconstruction of the remaining significant structures. Noyes and Barber-Westin (26) recently described the importance of anatomic reconstruction. They report utilization of allograft tissue in chronic injuries in which native autograft tissue is not available. They first reconstructed the LCL and performed either plication or advancement of the posterolateral structures, which also were sutured to the allograft LCL, producing a dense collagenous plate of tissues around the posterolateral corner of the knee. Biomechanical studies have demonstrated that the LCL and popliteus tendon are the major structures that prevent posterolateral instability (5,27). The popliteofibular ligament is an important component of the popliteal unit and its static stabilizing function to resist varus and external rotation. Therefore, in both acute and chronic posterolateral injuries, an attempt to repair or reconstruct the LCL, the popliteus tendon and its attachment to the tibia, and the popliteofibular ligament.

If posterolateral injuries are combined with cruciate ligament injuries, many recommend reconstruction of all injured ligaments. O'Brien et al. (28) documented that failures of ACL

■ TECHNICAL
ALTERNATIVES AND
PITFALLS

reconstruction can be caused by unrecognized and untreated posterolateral instability. Clinical series have reported that reconstruction of acute injuries is more successful than that of chronic posterolateral injuries. Acute reconstruction has been recommended for posterolateral instability both isolated and combined with a cruciate injury.

Complications from any of these procedures include recurrent instability, peroneal nerve palsy, stiffness, weakness, and hardware irritation (25).

■ REHABILITATION

Postoperative care for lateral knee augmentation or substitution is determined partly by whether or not a concomitant anterior or posterior cruciate ligament reconstruction has been performed. Patients are placed in a hinged postoperative brace and are begun on continuous passive motion therapy the first postoperative day. They are allowed to ambulate toe-touch weight bearing with the knee locked in extension. Assisted range-of-motion exercises are performed the second postoperative day. Weight bearing is restricted for 8 weeks. Bracing is continued for an additional 4 months.

■ OUTCOMES AND FUTURE DIRECTIONS

The trend for stabilization of the posterolateral corner has shifted towards more anatomic reconstructions, that is, attempts to recreate the known anatomic structures. This approach has evolved with a more thorough understanding of the anatomy and a better understanding of the biomechanical contribution of each of these discrete structures. Because these injuries are relatively uncommon, each creating unique damage to the other structures of the knee, evaluation of the different techniques is difficult. The need for randomized prospective protocols and standardized evaluation is clear.

References

1. Larson RL. Physical examination in the diagnosis of rotatory instability. *Clin Orthop* 1983:38–44.
2. Shelbourne KD, Benedict F, McCarroll JR, et al. Dynamic posterior shift test. An adjuvant in evaluation of posterior tibial subluxation. *Am J Sports Med* 1989; 17:275–277.
3. Seebacher JR, Inglis AE, Marshall JL, et al. The structure of the posterolateral aspect of the knee. *J Bone Joint Surg Am* 1982; 64:536–541.
4. Staubli HU, Jakob RP. Posterior instability of the knee near extension. A clinical and stress radiographic analysis of acute injuries of the posterior cruciate ligament. *J Bone Joint Surg Br* 1990; 72:225–230.
5. Gollehon DL, Torzilli PA, Warren RF. The role of the posterolateral and cruciate ligaments in the stability of the human knee. A biomechanical study. *J Bone Joint Surg Am* 1987; 69:233–242.
6. Meystre JL, Trouilloud P. [Postero-postero-external instabilities of the knee: experimental study of an extra-articular system to protect reconstructions]. *Rev Chir Orthop Reparatrice Appar Mot* 1994; 80:420–427.
7. Veltri DM, Warren RF. Anatomy, biomechanics, and physical findings in posterolateral knee instability. *Clin Sports Med* 1994; 13:599–614.
8. Skyhar MJ, Warren RF, Ortiz GJ, et al. The effects of sectioning of the posterior cruciate ligament and the posterolateral complex on the articular contact pressures within the knee. *J Bone Joint Surg Am* 1993; 75:694–699.
9. Veltri DM, Warren RF. Operative treatment of posterolateral instability of the knee. *Clin Sports Med* 1994; 13:615–627.
10. Veltri DM, Warren RF. Posterolateral instability of the knee. *Instr Course Lect* 1995; 44:441–453.
11. Bowen MK, Warren RF, Cooper DE. Posterior cruciate ligament and related injuries. In: Insall J, ed. *Surgery of the knee*. New York: Churchill Livingston, 1993:505–554.
12. Twaddle BC, Hunter JC, Chapman JR, Simonian PT, Escobedo EM. MRI in acute knee dislocation. *J Bone Joint Surg Br* 1996; 78:573–579.
13. Baker CL, Jr, Norwood LA, Hughston JC. Acute combined posterior cruciate and posterolateral instability of the knee. *Am J Sports Med* 1984; 12:204–208.
14. Kaplan EB. The fabellofibular and short lateral ligaments of the knee joint. *J Bone Joint Surg Am* 1961; 43:169–179.
15. Watanabe Y, Moriya H, Takahashi K, et al. Functional anatomy of the posterolateral structures of the knee. *Arthroscopy* 1993; 9:57–62.
16. Staubli HU, Birrer S. The popliteus tendon and its fascicles at the popliteal hiatus: Gross anatomy and functional arthroscopic evaluation with and without anterior cruciate ligament deficiency. *Arthroscopy* 1990; 6:209–220.

17. De Lee JC, Riley MB, Rockwood CA Jr. Acute posterolateral rotatory instability of the knee. *Am J Sports Med* 1983; 11:199–207.
18. Jakob RP, Hassler H, Staeubli HU. Observations on rotatory instability of the lateral compartment of the knee: Experimental studies on the functional anatomy and the pathomechanism of the true and the reversed pivot shift sign. *Acta Orthop Scand* 1981; 191(suppl):1–32.
19. Baker CL, Jr, Norwood LA, Hughston JC. Acute posterolateral rotatory instability of the knee. *J Bone Joint Surg Am* 1983; 65:614–618.
20. Hughston JC, Jacobson KE. Chronic posterolateral rotatory instability of the knee. *J Bone Joint Surg Am* 1985; 67:351–359.
21. Fleming RE Jr, Blatz DJ, McCarroll JR. Posterior problems in the knee: Posterior cruciate insufficiency and posterolateral rotatory insufficiency. *Am J Sports Med* 1981; 9:107–113.
22. Clancy WG Jr. Repair and reconstruction of the posterior cruciate ligament. In: Chapman MW, ed. *Operative orthopaedics*, volume 3. Philadelphia: JB Lippincott Co, 1993:2093–2108.
23. Wascher DC, Grauer JD, Markoff KL. Biceps tendon tenodesis for posterolateral instability of the knee: An in vitro study. *Am J Sports Med* 1993; 21:400–406.
24. Clancy WG, Meister K, Craythorne CB. Posterolateral corner collateral ligament reconstruction. In: Jackson DW, ed. *Reconstructive knee surgery*. New York: Raven Press, 1995.
25. Mueller W. *The knee form, function, and ligament reconstruction*. New York: Springer–Verlag, 1982.
26. Noyes FR, Barber-Westin SD. Surgical reconstruction of severe chronic posterolateral complex injuries of the knee using allograft tissues. *Am J Sports Med* 1995; 23:2–12.
27. Nielsen S, Helmig P. The static stabilizing function of the popliteal tendon in the knee. An experimental study. *Arch Orthop Trauma Surg* 1986; 104:357–62.
28. O'Brien SJ, Warren RF, Pavlov H, et al. Reconstruction of the chronically insufficient anterior cruciate ligament with the central third of the patellar ligament. *J Bone Joint Surg Am* 1991; 73:278–86.

JOHN C. L'INSALATA
PAUL A. DOWDY
CHRISTOPHER D.
HARNER

10

Multiple Ligament Reconstruction

■ HISTORY OF THE TECHNIQUE

Although generally considered an uncommon injury, the incidence of knee dislocation appears to be increasing. This is likely the result of a heightened awareness of "occult" dislocation with spontaneous reduction and of the limb-threatening potential of this injury. Although is agreed that prompt reduction of the dislocated knee and careful neurovascular evaluation is essential, the treatment of associated knee ligament injuries remains controversial (1–9).

Traditionally, treatment of knee dislocations consisted of closed reduction and cast immobilization. O'Donoghue (10) and Kennedy (11) reported the earliest series of surgical treatment of ligament injuries associated with knee dislocations. These and most subsequent reports on knee dislocations have reported the results for repairs of injured ligaments, with most authors recommending surgical treatment (1–4,7).

More recently, ligament reconstruction has become the standard treatment for cruciate ligament tears, particularly for those that occur within the midsubstance of the ligament. The current trend has been to apply this concept to the treatment of multiple ligament injuries. Most surgeons currently recommend cruciate ligament reconstruction as the cornerstone of treatment for multiple ligament injury following knee dislocations (5,6,8,12)

■ INDICATIONS AND CONTRAINDICATIONS

The diagnosis of a dislocated knee may not be obvious if the knee has reduced spontaneously. A high clinical index of suspicion should be present if examination reveals gross laxity in two or more directions. Initial evaluation includes a brief history, including mechanism of injury, followed by a thorough neurovascular examination. Special emphasis is placed on the assessment of peroneal nerve function and of pedal pulses, including comparison to the contralateral limb for symmetry. If the knee is dislocated, prompt reduction should be performed to reduce potential compression of the neurovascular structures, even prior to radiographic assessment. Following reduction, the neurovascular status should be reassessed and routine radiographs obtained to confirm reduction and to rule out associated fractures.

After reduction, if pedal pulses are absent or there is evidence of ischemia, a vascular consult is obtained and the patient is brought to the operating room, in which a one-shot arteriogram can be obtained and the injured vessels explored and repaired. If a vascular repair is performed, the stability of the knee is assessed in the operating room. If the knee is very unstable, an external fixator may be placed to maintain stability and protect the vascular repair. Postoperative management is dictated by the vascular repair and generally includes immobilization of the knee in extension. Ligament reconstruction usually is deferred for 10 days to 2 weeks following vascular repair (13).

If there is asymmetry of pedal pulses without discrete limb ischemia, a vascular consultation is made and an arteriogram performed to rule out intimal tears. If there is no evidence of ischemia and pedal pulses are normal, we generally obtain an arteriogram to rule out intimal tears; however, recent literature has suggested that serial examinations may be sufficient to detect arterial injuries requiring treatment (14).

Peroneal nerve injuries occur in approximately one quarter (range 9–49%) of knee dislocations and range from neuropraxia to neurotmesis (15). The risk of peroneal nerve injury is increased following posterolateral knee dislocation or with disruption of the lateral and posterolateral corner ligaments (15,16). Recovery of peroneal nerve function is unpredictable, with most series reporting no recovery in more than 50% of injuries (15). Early surgical intervention including exploration and neurolysis has not been shown to affect the outcome of peroneal nerve injury reliably. A recent report showed favorable outcome of operative decompression for peroneal nerve palsy, but none of the cases involved a knee dislocation (17). Thus, most authors currently recommend observation of nerve function for at least 3 months with bracing, and tendon transfers to restore function if recovery does not occur. The presence or absence of peroneal nerve injury does not affect the decision regarding treatment of associated knee ligament injuries.

Open knee dislocations occur in 20 to 30% of cases and require immediate surgical irrigation and debridement (8). Ligament reconstruction is usually delayed 1 to 3 weeks to allow control of the soft tissues and reduce the risk of infection. Associated fractures and extensor tendon ruptures are treated in standard fashion and should take precedence over ligament reconstruction.

Although ligament testing in the knee with multiple acute ligament injuries often is limited somewhat in the office setting, the presence of the normal medial tibial plateau stepoff in reference to the medial femoral condyle, Lachman examination, and collateral ligament stability usually can be assessed accurately. Magnetic resonance imaging has been very helpful in further evaluation of the knee, providing an accurate assessment of the status of the cruciate and collateral ligaments, menisci, and extensor mechanism and potentially identifying subtle fractures or bone bruises (18–20). This contributes to preoperative planning and allows improved discussion with the patient and family regarding the extent of injuries.

The goal of treatment of the knee with multiple acute ligament injuries is to restore stability and range of motion of the knee, allowing return to the preinjury level of function. Variables that may affect these goals and the overall treatment outcome include patient age and expectations, extent of the injuries, and the presence of associated injuries. Important surgical considerations include timing, approach, graft selection, and rehabilitation. With injuries of the collateral ligaments, surgery ideally is performed within 3 weeks to prevent excessive scarring, which may distort the normal anatomy, making ligament repair more difficult. We generally defer surgery for 1 to 2 weeks following injury to allow restoration of knee motion and capsular healing. Patients are placed in a long-leg hinged knee brace and begin preoperative rehabilitation emphasizing restoration of range of motion and quadriceps strengthening, possibly in the prone position to prevent posterior subluxation of the tibia.

Relative contraindications to acute surgical reconstruction include associated injuries that may preclude early ligament surgery. These include intraarticular or periarticular fractures, local issues such as the status of the overlying skin and soft tissues, and systemic or medical issues. Older physiologic age and the presence of knee osteoarthritis may favor a nonoperative approach initially, with subsequent knee arthroplasty if symptoms persist.

Anesthesia The selection of anesthesia type is made in conjunction with the anesthesiologist and patient. We generally recommend an epidural anesthetic, which provides both anesthesia and muscle paralysis and may reduce pain in the immediate postoperative period. Alternate anesthetic techniques include spinal and general anesthesia.

■ SURGICAL TECHNIQUES

Surgical Approach and Positioning Following anesthetic induction, the patient is placed supine on the operative table, and a thorough examination under anesthesia is performed to define the ligamentous injuries more completely. The contralateral knee always is examined for comparison. We have found that the most useful determinants of complete ligament tear and the need for surgical repair or reconstruction following knee dislocation are the following: in the posterior cruciate ligament (PCL), posterior sag and posterior drawer test results; in the anterior cruciate ligament (ACL), anterior drawer and Lachman test results; in the medial collateral ligament (MCL), valgus laxity test results in the extended knee; in the lateral collateral ligament (LCL), varus laxity test results in the extended knee; and in the posterolateral corner, posterolateral drawer test results.

The most common patterns of ligament injury following knee dislocation include combined injury of the ACL, PCL, and MCL and combined injury of the ACL, PCL, LCL, and posterolateral corner. Less commonly, the PCL remains intact or is torn only partially and does not require repair (4,21,22). Our approach is to repair or reconstruct all complete ligament tears; partial injuries generally do not require treatment. Avulsed ligaments and intrasubstance MCL tears may be repaired directly; intrasubstance tears of the cruciate and lateral ligaments generally are reconstructed. Peripheral meniscus tears and capsular avulsions are repaired directly.

With the patient supine on the operating room table, a well-padded tourniquet is applied to the upper thigh. We prefer not to inflate the tourniquet unless it is absolutely necessary, especially if a vascular repair has been performed or an intimal injury is present. We occasionally use the tourniquet to improve visualization during arthroscopic reconstruction of the ACL and PCL. The surgical approach is dictated by the involved ligaments, particularly the collateral ligaments.

Dislocation with Lateral Ligament Injury

Arthroscopy   If the cruciate and lateral structures are torn, attention is directed first to the arthroscopic cruciate reconstruction. An arthroscopic approach is advocated to avoid the need for both medial and lateral incisions, which may jeopardize wound healing. With the patient in the supine position, a lateral post is placed at the proximal thigh to allow a valgus stress to be applied to the knee as necessary. The operative leg is prepped and draped in the standard sterile fashion, and the skin incisions are planned and marked. These include a 2-cm incision at the anterior knee just medial to the articular edge of the trochlear groove and distal to the vastus medialis (for the PCL femoral tunnel); a 4-cm longitudinal incision beginning 1 cm medial to the proximal aspect of the tibial tubercle (for the ACL and PCL tibial tunnels); and a curvilinear incision beginning midway between the fibular head and Gerdy's tubercle and continued proximally to the lateral femoral epicondyle, paralleling the posterior edge of the iliotibial band for a total length of 12 to 15 cm (for the lateral reconstruction) (Fig. 10-1).

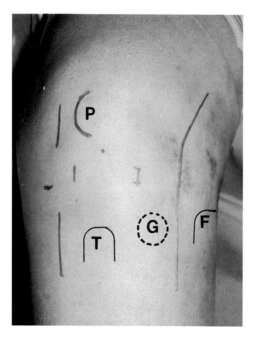

Skin incisions for combined arthroscopic anterior and posterior cruciate ligament reconstruction with open lateral or posterolateral reconstruction. *F*, fibular head; *G*, Gerdy's tubercle; *P*, patella; *T*, tibial tubercle.

■ FIGURE 10-1

Standard arthroscopic portals (anteromedial, anterolateral, and superolateral) are created, and the knee undergoes a systematic arthroscopic examination. In performing arthroscopy following a knee dislocation, it is important to avoid excessive fluid pressure within the knee to prevent extravasation of fluid. We use an arthroscopic pump setup with low or medium pressure and a continuous outflow cannula. The calf and thigh are observed throughout the procedure to ensure that excessive fluid extravasation has not occurred. If necessary for proper visualization, the tourniquet is inflated following exsanguination of the limb. After confirmation of intraarticular pathology, attention is directed to preparation for the ACL and PCL reconstruction. The ACL remnant is debrided, leaving a small stump of tissue at its tibial insertion, and a lateral notchplasty is performed for exposure using an arthroscopic burr and shaver.

Although most PCL injuries involve an interstitial tear of the ligament, occasionally there is a soft-tissue avulsion ("peel-off") of the PCL at its femoral insertion. If this is the case, a primary repair using a modified Marshall technique (23) is performed as described subsequently. For interstitial tears, the remnant of the PCL is preserved maximally to augment the reconstruction. Similarly, the meniscofemoral ligaments are preserved, if intact. To visualize the PCL insertion, a 70-degree arthroscope is placed through the anterolateral portal into the posterior aspect of the intercondylar notch adjacent to the medial femoral condyle. A posteromedial portal is created under direct visualization anterior to the saphenous vein and nerve. A small curette and a full-radius resector then are introduced alternately and used to separate the distal insertion of the PCL from the posterior capsule.

Cruciate Graft Preparation The ACL usually is reconstructed with a bone–patellar tendon–bone allograft, and the PCL with an Achilles tendon allograft. Allografts are used to reduce the surgical trauma associated with harvesting of autografts in the already traumatized knee. The fresh-frozen allografts are thawed at temperatures of less than 40°C in order to prevent denaturing of the collagen. The grafts usually are prepared by an assistant during the tunnel preparation. Otherwise they should be prepared by the surgeon at the beginning of the procedure, prior to inflation of the tourniquet.

For the patellar tendon allograft, the central portion of the tendon is marked carefully prior to cutting the bone plugs with an oscillating saw. An 11-mm graft with cylindric bone plugs generally is preferred. After the appropriate cuts have been made, the bone plugs are fashioned to fit through the desired graft sizer. The interface between the soft tissue and bone plug is tapered to allow smooth graft passage through the tunnels. Two no. 5 nonabsorbable braided sutures are placed through the patellar bone plug, and one suture is placed through the tibial bone plug that will be inserted into the femoral tunnel.

For the Achilles tendon allograft, the central portion of the tendon insertion into the os calcis is marked. The bone plug is cut with an oscillating saw and trimmed to a diameter of 11 mm and a length of 25 mm. Care should be taken to produce a tubular, bullet-shaped bone plug and avoid creation of a curved or banana-shaped plug. A single no. 5 nonabsorbable braided suture is placed through a drill hole in the bone plug. The tendon end of the graft is tubularized using a double-loaded no. 5 nonabsorbable braided suture. The final graft should pass easily through a graft sizer of appropriate diameter.

Cruciate Tibial Tunnel Placement An arthroscopic PCL tibial drill guide is inserted through the anteromedial portal, and its angle is adjusted to approximate the slope of the proximal tibia–fibula joint (40–60 degrees). Under direct visualization the guide is placed so that the guide wire will exit at the junction of the distal and lateral third of the tibial PCL insertion. The starting point of the guide wire at the anterior tibia should be approximately 2 cm distal and medial to the tibial tubercle to provide a minimum 1-cm bone bridge between the PCL and ACL tibial tunnels. A 4-cm longitudinal incision is created over the planned tunnel sites at the anteromedial tibia (Fig. 10-1). Dissection is carried down to the periosteum, which is incised and sharply elevated for later closure. The exit site of the guide wire posteriorly is visualized arthroscopically and protected during drilling to pre-

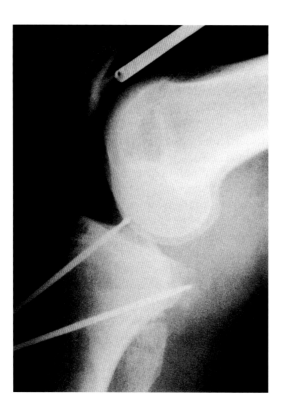

■ FIGURE 10-2

Intraoperative lateral radiograph confirming proper placement of anterior and posterior cruciate ligament tibial tunnels.

vent injury to the neurovascular structures. If the surgeon is uncomfortable with this technique, fluoroscopic imaging may be used to visualize the guide wire during insertion.

Next, the ACL tibial guide wire is inserted. The tibial guide is set at 55 degrees for a patellar tendon allograft (or 45 degrees for an Achilles tendon allograft) and positioned in the posteromedial aspect of the ACL footprint. The guide wire is drilled through the guide and checked for accurate placement. An intraoperative lateral x-ray routinely is obtained to confirm the proper location of the guide wires (Fig. 10-2).

The PCL guide wire then is overdrilled using a 10-mm cannulated drill. A curette is placed over the tip of the guide wire during drilling to prevent inadvertent advancement of the wire, which may injure the posterior neurovascular structures. As a further precaution, the posterior cortex usually is drilled by hand. The tunnel then is expanded to 11 mm using a bone tunnel expander (Instrument Makar, Kalamazoo, MI), for an 11-mm allograft. The superior edge of the tunnel is rasped to prevent graft abrasion, and any soft tissue at the entrance of the tunnel that may interfere with graft passage is debrided. The ACL tibial guide wire is overdrilled similarly with a 10-mm cannulated drill and expanded to 11 mm. The posterior edge of the tunnel is rasped to prevent graft abrasion and soft tissue at the tunnel entrance is debrided.

Cruciate Femoral Tunnel Placement   The ACL femoral tunnel is prepared using an endoscopic (single-incision) technique. Care must be taken to identify the posterior cortex of the intercondylar notch in order to prevent anterior placement of the tunnel, which may lead to graft impingement and failure. The guide wire is inserted through the tibial tunnel into the femur 5 to 6 mm anterior to the posterior cortex at the 10 o'clock position for a right knee and at the 2 o'clock position for a left knee. The knee is flexed to 100 degrees during placement of the guide wire, which then is overdrilled with a 10-mm cannulated intraarticular drill to a depth of 30 to 35 mm. The tunnel is expanded to 11 mm using a bone tunnel expander, the anterior edge is smoothed with a rasp, and debris is cleared from the tunnel entrance and notch. A 4.5-mm drill placed centrally within the tunnel is used to breach the lateral cortex of the femur.

Attention then is directed to creation of the PCL femoral tunnel, again approximating the anterolateral component of the PCL. A 2-cm skin incision is made over the anterior knee just medial to the articular edge of the trochlear groove and distal to the vastus medialus obliqus (VMO) (Fig. 10-1). The VMO is retracted superiorly, and the medial retinaculum and underlying synovium are incised, exposing the articular margin of the medial femoral condyle. The femoral drill guide is introduced via the anteromedial portal and positioned so that the guide wire will exit approximately 7 to 10 mm from the intraarticular cartilage of the medial femoral condyle distally, at the anterior half of the PCL footprint, corresponding to the anterolateral component of the PCL. On the extraarticular side of the medial femoral condyle, the guide wire should enter approximately 1 cm proximal to the articular cartilage margin and should be oriented so that the tunnel aims posteriorly toward the tibial insertion of the PCL. The guide wire is placed and overdrilled with a 10-mm diameter cannulated drill. The tunnel is expanded to 11 mm, and its posterior edge is rasped at the entrance into the joint to prevent graft abrasion.

For repair of avulsions of the PCL from the femur, several nonabsorbable sutures are placed within the avulsed ligament. Exposure of the medial femoral condyle and placement of a drill guide at the PCL femoral insertion site are performed as described previously. A 3/32-inch guide wire is used to drill two tunnels into the PCL insertion site. A suture passer is inserted, and the previously placed sutures are drawn out through the medial femoral condyle. The sutures are brought through a button but are not tied until just prior to final tensioning of the ACL graft and of the lateral reconstruction as described subsequently.

Cruciate Graft Passage   Both the PCL and ACL grafts are passed prior to fixation. The PCL graft is passed first. A looped 18-gauge wire is inserted from the PCL tibial tunnel and is grasped at its entrance into the joint posteriorly. It is delivered to the articular entrance of the PCL femoral tunnel, where it is grasped and brought out externally through the tunnel. The sutures at the tendinous portion of the graft are secured to the wire and advanced through the femoral tunnel into the tibial tunnel and exit anteriorly. The graft then is passed until the bone plug is flush with the femoral cortex.

A Beath pin is placed through the ACL tibial tunnel into the femoral tunnel and exits through the skin of the anterolateral thigh. Following the track of the Beath needle, the sutures from the tibial bone plug of the graft are pulled through the tunnels and out the skin of the anterolateral thigh. The graft then is pulled into the tibial and femoral tunnels, with care taken to orient the proximal bone plug anterior to the tendon prior to entering the femoral tunnel.

The femoral bone plugs of the ACL and PCL grafts are fixed while the tibial fixation is performed, after preparation of the lateral reconstruction. For the ACL, the guide wire for the interference screw is placed anteriorly, and a 7-mm screw is placed with the knee held in 100 degrees flexion. The PCL femoral bone plug is fixed with a 7-mm interference screw if a firm fit is present, or with a 9-mm interference screw if there is any gap between the bone plug and the tunnel edge. The knee is brought through a range of motion with the grafts visualized arthroscopically to ensure that there is no graft impingement. Prior to proceeding to the lateral reconstruction, the tourniquet is released if it was previously inflated, and hemostasis is obtained.

Lateral Reconstruction: Surgical Approach   The lateral structures then are approached using a curvilinear incision beginning midway between the fibular head and Gerdy's tubercle and continued proximally to the lateral femoral epicondyle, paralleling the posterior edge of the iliotibial band for a total length of 12 to 15 cm (Fig. 10-1). The peroneal nerve is identified proximally, posterior to the biceps tendon, and is dissected distally to the point at which it enters the anterior tibial muscular compartment. If there is a peroneal palsy and hematoma is present within the nerve, the epineurium is released. Dissection is continued between the posterior edge of the iliotibial band and the biceps tendon, and the iliotibial band is split longitudinally, allowing it to be retracted posteriorly and anteriorly for further exposure. A vertical capsular incision is made at the posterior border of the LCL, allowing visualization of the lateral meniscus and popliteus tendon.

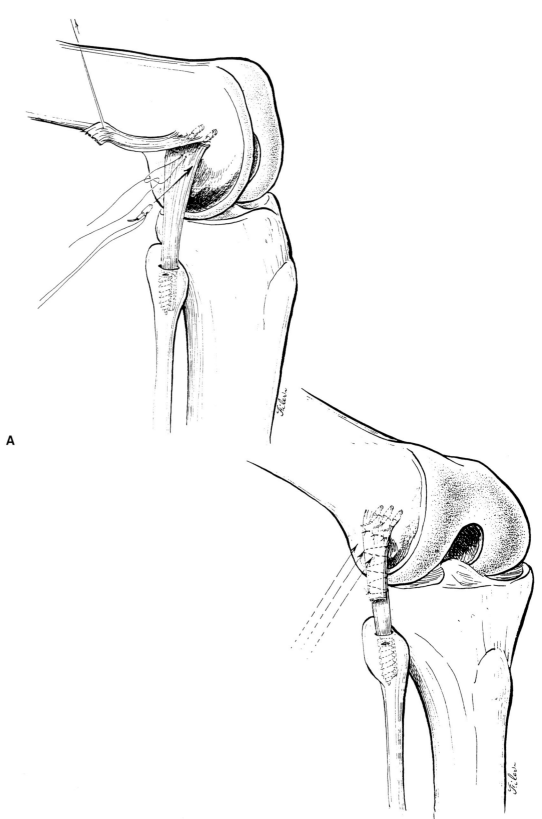

A

B

Illustration of lateral collateral ligament (LCL) reconstruction using Achilles tendon allograft. **A:** The torn or stretched LCL is detached and elevated from its fibular insertion, and the allograft bone block is fixed in a tunnel in the proximal fibula using an interference screw. The tensioned graft is fixed at the lateral femoral condyle using multiple suture anchors. **B:** The native LCL is tensioned and sutured to the allograft.

Each of the structures of the posterolateral corner then is evaluated systematically. Lateral meniscus peripheral tears are repaired using nonabsorbable sutures, and capsular avulsions are repaired using suture anchors. Avulsions of the LCL or popliteus are repaired directly. More commonly, interstitial injury occurs, requiring reconstruction.

Lateral Collateral Ligament Reconstruction   The LCL is reconstructed using an Achilles tendon allograft with a 7- to 8-mm bone block fixed at the fibula using an interference screw (Fig. 10-3). The allograft is prepared as described previously, except that no sutures are placed into the tendon or bone plug. The torn or stretched LCL is detached and elevated from its distal insertion. A 3/32-inch guide wire is inserted into the central portion of the proximal fibula and overdrilled with a cannulated drill of the appropriate diameter (7 or 8 mm). The bone plug is inserted into the proximal fibula tunnel so that it is flush with fibula cortex and fixed with a 7-mm interference screw. Fixation of the graft at the femur is performed following tensioning and fixation of the cruciate grafts as described subsequently.

Popliteus Reconstruction   If the popliteus is significantly injured, its static component via the popliteofibular ligament (24) is reconstructed using a double-looped semitendinosis autograft fixed anatomically on the femur using an EndoButton (Acufex, Boston, MA) (Fig. 10-4). Using the previously created anteromedial incision, the semitendinosis tendon is identified deep to the sartorius fascia. The fascia in incised parallel with the semitendi-

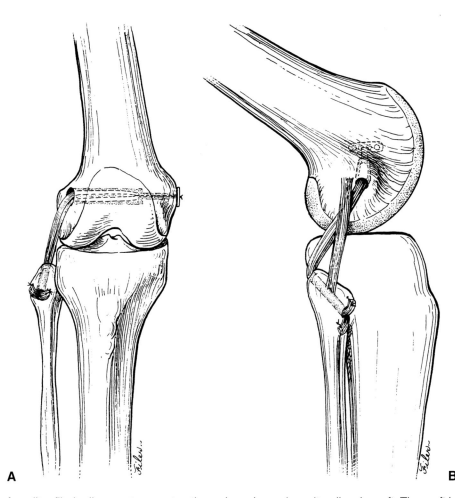

A   **B** ■ FIGURE 10-4

Illustration of popliteofibular ligament reconstruction using a looped semitendinosis graft. The graft is fixed into a tunnel in the lateral femoral condyle using an EndoButton set at the medial femoral condyle. It is passed deep to the lateral collateral ligament and through a tunnel in the fibula from posterior to anterior, where it is sutured to the soft tissues. **A:** Anterior view. **B:** Lateral view.

nosis, which is isolated and detached at its tibial insertion. A running whipstitch of no. 2 nonabsorbable braided suture is placed at the end of the tendon, and fascial attachments to the tendon are incised. A closed-end tendon stripper then is used to harvest the tendon, with the knee in the flexed position and tension applied to the tendon. The graft is prepared by an assistant. Any muscle remnants are debrided, and a whipstitch is placed into the proximal end of the tendon. The tendon is looped around a no. 5 Mersilene tape, which is threaded through the center two holes of an EndoButton (Acufex, Boston, MA).

With care to protect the peroneal nerve, the peroneus longus muscle is elevated subperiosteally at the proximal fibula. A tunnel of the appropriate diameter is created from posterior to anterior in the proximal fibula and at the femoral insertion of the popliteus tendon. The femoral tunnel is drilled to a depth of 26 mm in order to maintain 20 mm of graft within the tunnel. A 4.5-mm drill is used to drill from the base of the femoral tunnel out the medial femoral condyle, with care taken to avoid the intercondylar notch and trochlea. The femoral channel length (from the exit at the medial femoral condyle to the entrance at the lateral femoral condyle) is measured and used to determine the proper length to tie the Mersilene tape for the graft (channel length minus 20 mm). A Beath needle then is placed through the femoral tunnel out the medial femoral condyle and medial skin and is used to deliver the sutures for the EndoButton out medially. The EndoButton is delivered into the femoral tunnel and channel lengthwise and on exiting out the medial femoral condyle is "flipped" perpendicular to the channel. Tension is applied to the graft to "set" the EndoButton medially. The graft is then passed deep to the LCL graft and is brought through the fibular tunnel from posterior to anterior (Fig. 10-4). Tensioning of the graft and fixation at the fibula are performed after final tensioning and fixation of the cruciate grafts, as described subsequently.

Cruciate and Lateral Graft Tensioning and Fixation   After each of the ligament reconstruction grafts has been placed and fixed at one end, attention is directed toward final tensioning and fixation of each of the grafts. With tension applied to the tibial portion of the PCL and ACL grafts, the knee is brought through several cycles of motion. This provides a sense of the proper tension to maintain reduction of the joint and allows pretensioning of the grafts.

The PCL is fixed first. The knee is brought into 70 degrees of flexion, and the graft is tensioned to reproduce the normal anteromedial tibial "stepoff." A constant anterior drawer is applied. The graft is fixed at the anteromedial tibial using a bicortical screw and soft-tissue washer placed through a small longitudinal split made in the tendon. The graft is tensioned and fixed in flexion, because this is the position in which the anterolateral component of the PCL is under maximum tension (25), thus reducing the risk of overtensioning of the graft.

Next, the knee is brought into extension with tension applied to the ACL graft. The graft is fixed at the tibia using an interference screw. Attention then is directed laterally, where the LCL graft is tensioned and repaired at the lateral femoral epicondyle using suture anchors (Fig. 10-3**A**). The native LCL is tensioned and repaired to the graft (Fig. 10-3**B**). If the popliteofibular ligament has been reconstructed, the two limbs of the graft are tensioned at the fibula and sutured to the soft tissues (Fig. 10-4).

Closure   The knee is brought through a final range of motion to ensure full motion, and the knee stability is assessed. Any excess graft tissue is excised. Suction drainage is used for the lateral incision, and the wounds are closed in layers. Sterile dressings are applied, and the knee is placed into a long-leg hinged knee brace locked in full extension. A bolster is placed beneath the tibia to prevent posterior sagging of the tibia on the femur caused by gravity. Postoperative radiographs are obtained to confirm proper joint reduction and hardware placement (Fig. 10-5).

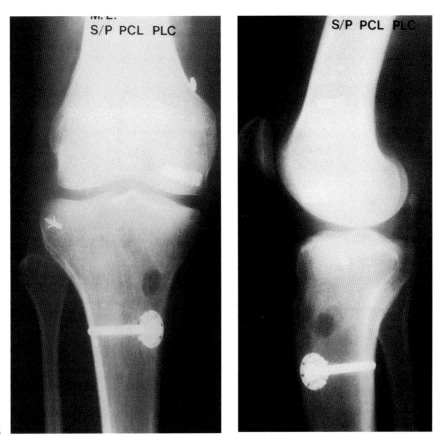

A   **B ■**   FIGURE 10-5

Postoperative radiographs following arthroscopic posterior reconstruction, with open reconstruction of the lateral collateral ligament and posterolateral corner. **A:** Anteroposterior view. **B:** Lateral view.

Dislocation with Medial Ligament Injury

Incision   If the cruciate ligaments and MCL are torn, a single medial incision is used to address each. We usually do not inflate the tourniquet. A medial "hockey stick" incision is made beginning at the level of the vastus medialis, continuing over the medial femoral epicondyle onto the anteromedial tibia 2 to 3 cm distal to the tibial tubercle (Fig. 10-6). This allows exposure of the MCL and medial joint line for capsular or meniscal repair (Fig. 10-7). Care should be taken to avoid injury of the saphenous nerve and its branches. Access to the knee joint is obtained via a short medial parapatellar arthrotomy through which the ACL and PCL are assessed and reconstructed.

Cruciate Reconstruction   The technique for cruciate ligament reconstruction is presented in detail in Dislocation with Lateral Ligament Injury. If performing the reconstruction via an arthrotomy, we find it useful to have the arthroscope available for illuminating and assisting visualization deep within the intercondylar notch. The locations of the PCL femoral and ACL tibial tunnels are identified easily via the arthrotomy. Proper location and drilling of the ACL femoral tunnel using the anteromedial incision are facilitated by hyperflexion of the knee. The location of the PCL tibial tunnel at the posterior tibial eminence is palpated through the intercondylar notch. This can be facilitated by anterior subluxation of the tibia on the femur. With injury of the posteromedial capsule, a finger can be inserted through the incision posteriorly to further confirm the proper location of the PCL tibial tunnel. Regardless of the technique used, it is essential that the tunnel site is selected and the neurovascular structures are protected during guide wire placement and tunnel drilling. Flu-

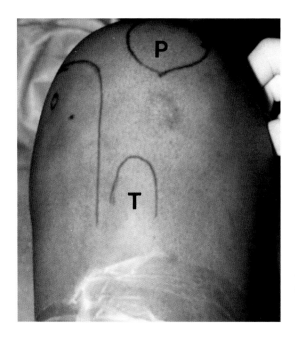

■ FIGURE 10-6

Skin incision for combined surgical exposure
of the medial collateral ligament, medial joint
line, and anterior and posterior cruciate ligaments. *P*, patella; *T*, tibial tubercle.

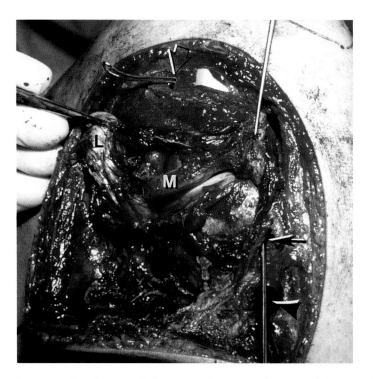

■ FIGURE 10-7

Intraoperative photograph demonstrating a complete tear of the superficial medial collateral ligament
(*L*; in forceps) with avulsion of the medial capsule and extrusion of the medial meniscus (*M*). The tibial and femoral tunnels for the anterior and posterior cruciate ligament reconstruction have been
drilled through a small parapatellar arthrotomy. In preparation for graft passage, a Beath needle has
been placed from the anterior cruciate ligament tibial tunnel (*solid arrow*) and exits the femoral tunnel (not seen), and a looped 18-gauge wire has been placed from the posterior cruciate ligament tibial tunnel (*solid arrowhead*) and exits the femoral tunnel at the medial femoral condyle (*open arrowhead*).

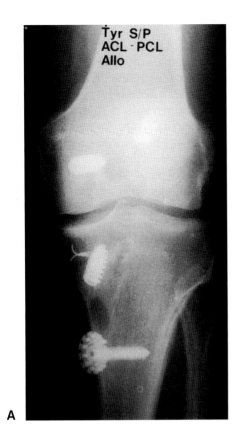
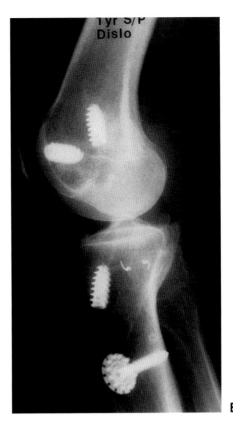

A   **B** ■ FIGURE 10-8

Postoperative radiographs following open reconstruction of the anterior and posterior cruciate ligaments and primary repair of the medial collateral ligament, medial meniscus, and medial capsule.
A: Anteroposterior view. **B:** Lateral view.

oroscopic imaging may be used if there is any uncertainty, and a lateral radiograph is obtained routinely to confirm the proper location of the tibial tunnels.

Medial Repair   If necessary, the meniscus is repaired with nonabsorbable sutures; capsular repair is performed with suture anchors. Avulsions of the MCL are reattached anatomically with suture anchors; intrasubstance tears are repaired primarily using nonabsorbable sutures. If the posteromedial capsule or posterior oblique ligament require repair,
this should be performed with the knee in extension to prevent overconstraining the knee
and potentially limiting full extension.

Closure   As is done laterally, the cruciate ligament grafts are tensioned and fixed prior
to final repair of the medial ligaments. The knee is brought through a complete range
of motion, and stability is assessed. Final hemostasis is obtained, a suction drain is placed,
and the wound is closed in layers. Sterile dressings are applied, and the knee is placed
into a long-leg hinged knee brace locked in full extension. A bolster is placed beneath the
tibia to prevent posterior sagging of the tibia on the femur caused by gravity. Postoperative radiographs are obtained to confirm proper joint reduction and hardware placement
(Fig. 10-8).

Prompt reduction of the dislocated knee, careful neurovascular evaluation, and emergent revascularization of the ischemic leg are accepted universally as the cornerstones of
acute treatment of the dislocated knee. Because knee dislocations are relatively uncommon
injuries, only a few published reports on the treatment of these injuries are available. Thus,
the most effective method of treatment has not been defined clearly.

■ TECHNICAL
ALTERNATIVES AND
PITFALLS

Several reports have presented results of nonoperative treatment of knee dislocations, with many reporting generally satisfactory results (8,9,26). As previously discussed, nonoperative treatment should be considered in physiologically older patients and those with preexisting osteoarthritis of the knee. Nonoperative treatment consists of initial immobilization of the knee in full extension for 2 to 4 weeks, followed by mobilization of the knee in a hinged knee brace. It is important to obtain radiographs regularly during this time to ensure that the knee has remained reduced. An external fixator should be used to maintain reduction of the knee if there is associated severe soft-tissue injury requiring muscle flaps or skin grafts for coverage, or if recurrent subluxation occurs.

Most published reports on the surgical treatment of ligament injuries following knee dislocation have reported the results of direct repair of injured ligaments (1–4,7,8,10,11,16,26). Although there are no definitive studies employing a prospective, randomized method, several authors have advocated surgical repair as superior to nonoperative treatment (1–4,7,16,26). We currently perform direct repairs of complete tears of the MCL and avulsions of the ACL, PCL, or LCL. For intrasubstance tears of the cruciate ligaments and LCL we perform ligament reconstruction using allograft, as described previously. This is based upon the current experience with isolated injuries of the ACL and PCL, in which ligament reconstruction has been demonstrated to provide superior results to ligament repair.

Another treatment alternative is to perform a limited ligament reconstruction or repair. Shelbourne et al. (6) currently recommend autograft reconstruction of the PCL and repair of the MCL and lateral structures; they do not treat tears of the ACL. They have reported satisfactory results with this approach and believe that potential stiffness associated with concurrent ACL reconstruction may be avoided; reconstruction of the ACL may be performed later if ACL instability develops (6). Isolated reconstruction of the ACL (without PCL reconstruction) generally is not advocated, because it may contribute to posterior subluxation of the tibia (6).

Several potential pitfalls are present in the treatment of ligament injuries following knee dislocations. In planning the surgical approach in the acutely injured knee, we attempt to avoid combined medial and lateral incisions, which may interfere with wound closure or healing. Thus, if a lateral approach is necessary to repair the lateral or posterolateral structures, we perform the cruciate reconstruction arthroscopically in order to avoid a medial incision and arthrotomy. In performing the arthroscopy it is important to maintain a low intraarticular fluid pressure in order to prevent extravasation of fluid, which could compromise the vascularity of the leg. The calf and thigh should be palpated intermittently so that fluid extravasation may be detected if present and the arthroscopic portion of the procedure aborted immediately.

A thorough understanding of the anatomy of the ACL and PCL insertions is necessary for proper tunnel placement. We routinely obtain an intraoperative lateral knee radiograph to confirm proper placement of the PCL tibial guide wire, often in conjunction with the ACL tibial guide wire (Fig. 10-2). A radiograph may be obtained to confirm proper placement of the ACL femoral guide wire, particularly if it is inserted via an anteromedial arthrotomy. In placing the ACL and PCL tibial guide wires, it is essential that they be started in the tibia at least 2 cm apart from one another, so that a minimum 1-cm bone bridge is present following drilling of the tunnels. In placing the PCL tibial guide wire and drilling the tunnel, it is important to protect the neurovascular structures and to visualize or palpate the posterior cortex during the arthroscopic or open procedure, respectively. If the surgeon is uncomfortable with this technique, fluoroscopy may be used during placement of the guide wire and drilling of the tunnel.

During the lateral procedure, it is important to visualize and protect the peroneal nerve, particularly when drilling the fibula. If the anatomic femoral insertion of the LCL is unclear, a K wire may be placed at the estimated location to test isometry after placement of the fibular portion of the graft. The femoral end of the graft is looped around the K wire, and the knee is brought through a range of motion while inspecting for graft isometry. The K wire can be adjusted to obtain the most isometric femoral insertion site.

During the medial approach, the saphenous nerve should be identified and protected. Because arthroscopy is not performed, it is important to examine and if necessary repair the peripheral aspect of the medial meniscus, which frequently is avulsed from its insertion via the deep MCL and capsule. In repairing the MCL and posterior oblique ligament, the tissues should be repaired anatomically without imbrication, and subsequent range of motion of the knee tested to prevent overconstraint and limitation of motion.

In securing the ligament grafts, it is important to tension and secure the PCL graft first, in order to restore the normal medial stepoff of the tibial plateau. The medial or lateral ligament repair or reconstruction is tensioned and secured after final tensioning and fixation of the ACL graft, in order to ensure proper reduction of the tibiofemoral joint.

■ REHABILITATION

The knee is maintained in full extension for 2 to 4 weeks and patients using ambulate feather-touch weight bearing of the limb with crutches to protect the collateral repair. Passive range of motion then is begun under supervised physical therapy to prevent posterior subluxation of the tibia; the brace may be unlocked for ambulation and sleeping. Ambulation is progressed to weight bearing as tolerated unless a posterolateral repair or reconstruction was performed, in which case ambulation remains feather-touch weightbearing for a total of 3 months. Quadriceps isometrics are begun immediately postoperatively, but active hamstring exercises are avoided for 4 months to avoid posterior translation stresses. If at least 90 degrees of flexion is not obtained by approximately 2 months following surgery, a manipulation under anesthesia is performed.

■ OUTCOMES AND FUTURE DIRECTIONS

There are very few published reports available on multiple ligament reconstruction following knee dislocations. Shapiro and Freedman (5) reported satisfactory functional results in six of seven patients who had allograft reconstruction of the ACL and PCL following knee dislocation. Three patients had rare or occasional giving way of the knee (5). Shelbourne and colleagues (6) reported satisfactory results in three patients who had isolated reconstruction of the PCL following knee dislocation.

We recently evaluated 18 patients at an average of 3 years following a knee dislocation treated with multiple ligament reconstruction using the techniques described herein. No patient lost more than 3 degrees of extension; four patients lost more than 15 degrees of flexion (minimum flexion 110 degrees). Five patients had a Lachman test result more that 2 mm different, and four had a posterior drawer test result of more than 5 mm different, compared with their opposite knees. Using the International Knee Documentation Center (IKDC) Rating Form, the patients' subjective assessment of their knee was normal for six, nearly normal for nine, and abnormal for three patients. Using IKDC guidelines, the overall knee ratings in seven were nearly normal, in six abnormal, and in five severely abnormal. We found that multiple ligament reconstruction following knee dislocation provided satisfactory subjective functional assessment, range of motion, and stability; the ability of patients to return to high-demand sports and manual labor was less predictable.

References

1. Frassica FJ, Sim FH, Staeheli JW, et al. Dislocation of the knee. *Clin Orthop Relat Res* 1991; 263:200–205.
2. Jones RE, Smith EC, Bone GE. Vascular and orthopedic complications of knee dislocation. *Surg Gynecol Obstet* 1979; 149:554–558.
3. Meyers MH, Harvey JPJ. Traumatic dislocation of the knee joint: A study of eighteen cases. *J Bone Joint Surg Am* 1971; 53:16–29.
4. Meyers MH, Moore HM, Harvey PJ. Follow-up notes on articles previously published in the journal: Traumatic dislocation of the knee joint. *J Bone Joint Surg Am* 1975; 57:430–433.
5. Shapiro MS, Freedman EL. Allograft reconstruction of the anterior and posterior cruciate ligaments after traumatic knee dislocation. *Am J Sports Med* 1995; 23:580–587.
6. Shelbourne KD, Porter DA, Clingman JA, McCarrol JR, Rettig AC. Low-velocity knee dislocation. *Orthop Rev* 1991; 20:995–1004.
7. Sisto DJ, Warren RF. Complete knee dislocation: A follow-up study of operative treatment. *Clin Orthop Relat Res* 1985; 198:94–101.

8. Taft TN, Almekinders LC. The dislocated knee. In: Fu FH, Harner CD, Vince KG, eds. *Knee surgery*, volume 1. Baltimore: Williams & Wilkins, 1994:837–857.
9. Taylor AR, Arden GP, Rainey HA. Traumatic dislocation of the knee: A report of forty-three cases with special reference to conservative treatment. *J Bone Joint Surg Br* 1972; 54:96–102.
10. O'Donoghue DH. An analysis of end results of surgical treatment of major injuries to the ligaments of the knee. *J Bone Joint Surg Am* 1955; 37:1–13.
11. Kennedy JC. Complete dislocation of the knee joint. *J Bone Joint Surg Am* 1963; 45:889–904.
12. L'Insalata JC, Harner CD. The dislocated knee: Approach to treatment. *Pittsburgh Orthopaedic Journal* 1996; 7:32–36.
13. Montgomery JB. Dislocation of the knee. *Orthop Clin North Am* 1987; 18:149–156.
14. Treiman GS, Yellin AE, Weaver FA, et al. Examination of the patient with a knee dislocation: The case for selective arteriography. *Arch Surg* 1992; 127:1056–1063.
15. Good L, Johnson RJ. The dislocated knee. *Journal of the American Academy of Orthopaedic Surgeons* 1995; 3:284–292.
16. Shields L, Mohinder M, Cave EF. Complete dislocations of the knee: Experience at the Massachusetts General Hospital. *J Trauma* 1969; 9:192–212.
17. Mont MA, Dellon AL, Chen F, et al. The operative treatment of peroneal nerve palsy. *J Bone Joint Surg Am* 1996; 78:863.
18. Dowdy PA, Vellet AD, Fowler PJ, et al. MRI of the partially torn ACL: An in-vitro animal model with correlative histopathology. *Clin J Sports Med* 1994; 4:187–191.
19. Speer KP, Spritzer CE, Bassett FH, et al. Osseous injury associated with acute tears of the anterior cruciate ligament. *Am J Sports Med* 1992; 20:382–389.
20. Vellet AD, Marks PH, Fowler PJ, et al. Occult post-traumatic osteochondral lesions of the knee: Prevalence, classification, and short-term sequelae evaluated with MR imaging. *Radiology* 1991; 178:271–276.
21. Cooper DE, Speer KP, Wickiewicz TL, et al. Complete knee dislocation without posterior cruciate ligament disruption: A report of four cases and review of the literature. *Clin Orthop Relat Res* 1992; 284:228–233.
22. Shelbourne KD, Pritchard J, Rettig AC, et al. Knee dislocations with intact PCL. *Orthop Rev* 1992; 21:607–611.
23. Marshall JL, Warren RF, Wickiewicz TL. Primary surgical treatment of anterior cruciate ligament lesions. *Am J Sports Med* 1982; 10:103–107.
24. Veltri DM, Deng X-H, Torzilli PA, et al. The role of the popliteofibular ligament in stability of the human knee: A biomechanical study. *Am J Sports Med* 1996; 24:19–27.
25. Stone JD, Carlin GJ, Ishibashi Y, et al. Assessment of posterior cruciate ligament graft performance using robotic technology. *Am J Sports Med* 1996; 24:824–828.
26. Almekinders LC, Logan TC. Results following treatment of traumatic dislocations of the knee joint. *Clin Orthop Relat Res* 1992; 284:203–207.

11

Technique of Lateral Retinacular Release and Anteromedial Tibial Tubercle Transfer

In the past, lateral release was used as a routine operative procedure in the hope of relieving anterior knee pain in patients with evidence of lateral tightness of subluxation. In the 1980s, this procedure was performed commonly and often without much hesitation. It became evident then that the procedure does not always work and can cause increased complications in some patients. Currently, therefore, there is an appropriate reluctance to perform a lateral release without specific indications (1).

If nonoperative treatment fails, the decision to operate often comes easily in patients with chronic anterior knee pain. The great challenge is to choose the correct operative procedure. If there is objective tilt of the patella with minimal articular damage to the patella and trochlea, many surgeons proceed to open or arthroscopic lateral release. Unfortunately, many patients have distal articular lesions, and lateral release inadvertently may place more stress on this lesion or on a medial lesion related to prior dislocation. Consequently, the decision to perform lateral retinacular release is much more difficult than simply considering it the proper alternative if there is tilting of the patella. Furthermore, lateral retinacular release fails to improve patellar subluxation consistently and even can make lateral subluxation worse if the proximal pull of the quadriceps is directed laterally. In its purest form, lateral retinacular release is indicated best if there is isolated patellar tilt with no subluxation and no articular disease. Furthermore, lateral release is most likely to bring benefit if there is tenderness in the lateral retinaculum (2). Many patients, therefore, have lateral retinacular release as a first attempt at relieving lateral overload and lateral retinacular stress, but shifting of load onto deficient articular cartilage can negate the benefit of the release.

Anteromedial tibial tubercle transfer is a much more major procedure but better addresses the problems of lateral patellar subluxation and distal or lateral articular disease related to malalignment. If these conditions exist and nonoperative treatment has failed, anteromedial tibial tubercle transfer offers a good alternative for relieving pressure on the distal central lesion and lateral facet lesion often present in the patient with chronic lateral tracking of the patella. In the majority of cases, surgeons perform lateral retinacular release also. The net result is transfer of loading onto the more proximal medial facet earlier in knee flexion, with a slight reduction of contact stress and release of restricting or painful lateral retinaculum.

Lateral Release   The author strongly recommends open lateral release. Visualization of the patella articular surface is better, hemostasis is easier and more complete, morbidity is less frequent, and the potential for consistently complete lateral release is greater.

Technique of Lateral Release   After anesthesia and tourniquet, the surgeon makes a short incision measuring about 3 cm long immediately adjacent to the lateral patella, extending from the midpatella level distally towards the tibial tubercle. The lateral retinaculum including both superficial and deep layers may be incised together, going directly into the joint sharply at a level of the incision about 1 cm behind the skin incision. Army–Navy retractors provide visualization of the entire lateral retinacula, after spreading the subcutaneous tissues immediately over the retinaculum itself. The surgeon should palpate the vastus lateralis tendon and visualize the vastus lateralis oblique muscle, so that there is no risk of cutting into the tendon itself.

The retinacular release is completed proximally by sliding Mayo scissors along the lateral patellofemoral joint line, about 1 to 2 cm lateral to the vastus lateralis tendon itself. Once the vastus lateralis oblique muscle is reached, the remainder of the proximal lateral release may be completed by spreading. There is no reason to cut the oblique fibers of the muscle.

Attention then should move to the distal end of the release. After spreading subcutaneous tissues to the distal pole of the patella and the tibial tubercle, the surgeon should palpate the patellar tendon and the tubercle itself. One must be certain to identify and localize these structures before extending the lateral release. Mayo scissors again may be used to extend the release distally, staying well lateral of the lateral joint line itself. The lateral release should continue well past the lateral tibiofemoral joint line, proceeding about midway between Gerdy's tubercle and the patellar tendon. The incision should be in retinaculum only, well lateral to the meniscus.

At this point, the patella is taken by the lateral edge and elevated away from the trochlea. In most cases, there are some tight bands of dense tissue extending into the fat pad behind the patellar tendon. The surgeon extends the lateral release into the retropatellar tendon fat pad, using Mayo scissors and releasing only those tight bands in the fat pad and elevating the lateral edge of the patella away from the trochlea. This release should continue until the lateral edge of the patella can be raised easily to a vertical position from the trochlea itself. There is no need to deepen the lateral release at the tibial femoral joint line, and the fat pad release permits most of the lateral facet elevation. In fact, it is likely that some patients with lateral retinacular tightness also have a secondary miniature infrapatellar contracture. This is apparent by the amount of patellar elevation that is possible on releasing a tethered fat pad in some patients undergoing lateral release.

Once the release itself is completed, cautery is used on the retinacular edges and any apparent bleeding points in the fat pad. After releasing the tourniquet, complete hemostasis is possible in most cases. Obtaining this hemostasis often takes as long as the release itself, if not longer. It is impressive how many bleeding points may be found, particularly in the fat pad area, and open hemostasis often yields knee without hemarthrosis or effusion postoperatively. This, of course, is very important in the optimal rehabilitation of every patient.

After achieving hemostasis, the surgeon should secure the subcutaneous tissues to be watertight and then close the skin securely, using full-length steristrips if a subcuticular closure is elected.

A light compressive wrap permits the surgeon to apply a cooling and compressive device. The patient starts weight bearing as tolerated with crutches initially and progresses off crutches once a full supportive quadriceps contracture permits single-leg knee bend with weight bearing. Patients start range-of-motion exercises immediately and return for the first postoperative visits at 10 to 14 days in most cases.

Technique of Anteromedial Tibial Tubercle Transfer   After anesthesia, the incision is made extending from the midpatella level, immediately adjacent to the patella, and proceeding distally to a point 5 to 7 cm distal to the tibial tubercle at the midline. Sharp dissection down to the retinaculum should be used, and incision made directly into the patellofemoral joint. A lateral release is completed as noted previously. The anterior compartment of the lower leg is exposed sharply, and the proximal anterior fibers of the tibialis anterior muscle are released using cautery. The electrocautering and a large Cobb elevator complete the reflection of the tibialis anterior from the lateral side of the tibia all the way to the posterolateral corner of the tibia. Retraction permits full visualization of the lateral tibia with protection of the tibialis anterior muscle (Fig. 11-1) (1).

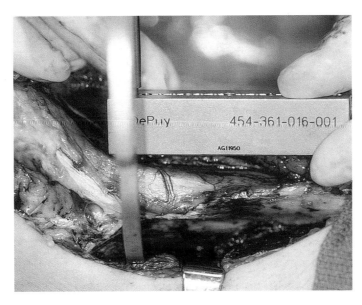

Cutting block positioned to create the desired osteotomy angle, using the "slope selector" of the Tracker guide.

Next, the patellar tendon insertion into the tibial tubercle should be identified, as well as the entire extent of the patellar tendon itself. A Kelly clamp is placed behind the patellar tendon, and the periosteum is incised along the medial crest of the tibia from the insertion of the patellar tendon distally. This line generally should be as far anterior as possible, starting immediately adjacent to the patellar tendon insertion. This should extend approximately 7 cm distal to the tibial tubercle and taper anteriorly to a point at the anterior crest of the tibia.

The Tracker guide block (Depuy, Warsaw, Indiana) is placed along the line defined along the medial tibia. The slope selector of the Tracker guide permits the surgeon to define the angle of the osteotomy (Fig. 11-2). Using the guide block alone, with the slope selector

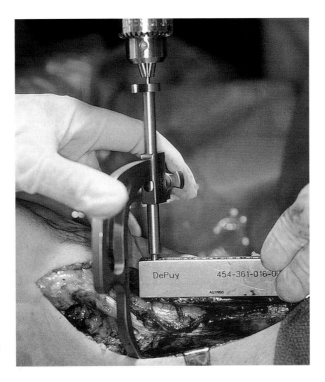

Only one cortex is drilled for fixation of the block proximally.

■ FIGURE 11-2

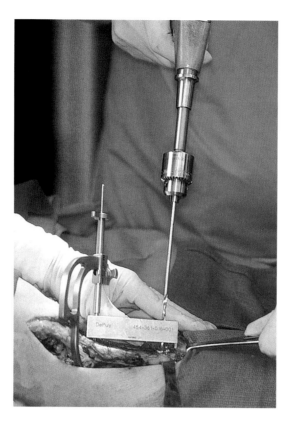

FIGURE 11-3

The distal fixation hole is well anterior and completely in cortical bone.

braced in the proximal pole of the guide block, the surgeon defines an oblique cutting plane extending from the anteromedial tibia to the posterolateral side of the tibia. A single drill hole through the slope-selector cannula then permits the surgeon to put a holding pin or drill bit in place to hold the guide at the selected slope through the proximal pole of the cutting block.

Next, the slope selector is placed in the most distal pole of the cutting block and a fixation point chosen, well anterior on the tibia so that the pin barely penetrates the anterior cortex, with the chosen osteotomy line tapering anteriorly. A second drill hole through the slope selector cannula permits a second pin to secure the cutting block in place (Fig. 11-3).

With the tibialis anterior retractor in place, preferably hooked behind the posterolateral corner of the tibia, an oscillating saw creates the osteotomy through the cutting block (Fig. 11-4). Great care should be taken to avoid entering the tibialis anterior muscle. Using the cutting block, with direct observation on the lateral side, the osteotomy should come out exactly where the slope selector had been placed. Once the lateral cortex has been cut, this cutting block may be removed and the remainder of the osteotomy completed under direct visualization proximally and distally. The surgeon should use a large Lambotte osteotome to create an osteotomy from a point just above (proximal to) the patellar tendon insertion to a point at the proximal lateral extent of the osteotomy towards the posterolateral tibia and tapered in a distal posterior direction (Fig. 11-5). This prevents the osteotomy from entering the metaphysis of the tibia. Additionally, the surgeon should use a 1/4-inch osteotome to cut the cortical bone proximal to the patellar tendon insertion into the tibia, connecting the lateral osteotomy with the medial osteotomy, which has been cut through the Tracker cutting block.

By greenstick fracture of the thin cortical bone at the distal point of the anteromedial tibial tubercle transfer osteotomy, the fragment of bone is displaced anteromedially along the precise osteotomy plane and secured with two cortical screws into the posterior cortex of the tibia (Fig. 11-6). The surgeon should use a lag principal, overdrilling the hole in the os-

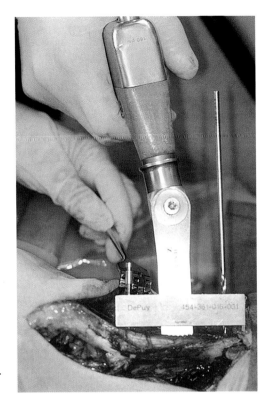

Once the cutting block is fixed in place, the os-
teotomy is cut with an oscillating saw.   ■ FIGURE 11-4

teotomy fragment and placing two screws securely into the posterior and posteromedial
cortex of the tibia. Of course, it is important to take great care not to penetrate beyond the
posterior cortex, because the popliteal artery is not far away. It is most desirable to place
one of the holding screws perpendicular to the osteotomy and the other in the anteroposterior plane.

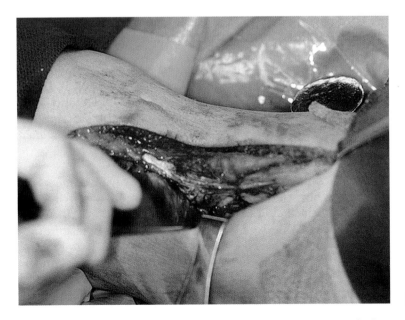

■ FIGURE 11-5

To free the osteotomy fragment, one makes a "back cut" on the lateral tibia, extending to a point just
proximal to the patellar tendon insertion.

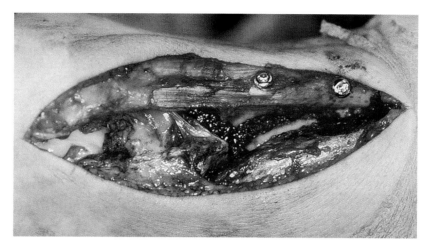

■ FIGURE 11-6

The displaced tibial tubercle is fixed securely with two cortical screws.

The surgeon chooses the amount of anterior and medial displacement depending on the needs of the specific patient. As a rule of thumb, if there is distal articular breakdown on the patella, the surgeon should try to achieve enough anteriorization to shift the load off of the distal patella. The more the distal articular breakdown on the patella extends proximally, the steeper the osteotomy, thereby permitting more anteriorization. The maximum anteriorization, using the steepest osteotomy possible without going out the back of the tibia, is no more than 2 cm.

If there has been significant patella instability with subluxation or dislocation, the surgeon wants more medialization; therefore the osteotomy is flatter with less anteriorization.

If there is both substantial instability and extensive articular breakdown on the distal patella extending towards the midpatella level, the surgeon needs to make a choice. Our approach has been to assure stability first. Therefore, the surgeon should create an osteotomy that permits enough medialization to make the patella stable. The surgeon may need to consider a standard Maquet procedure, fracturing the distal pedicle, taking an anterior iliac crest bone graft, and creating substantial medialization and anteriorization. This has not been necessary, however, in the author's experience.

■ TECHNICAL ALTERNATIVES AND PITFALLS

The most common pitfalls after lateral release are incomplete release, excessive release, inappropriate release, inadequate hemostasis, and releasing a patella to track onto deficient cartilage. These problems can be avoided by adhering closely to the defined guidelines for doing a lateral release, preserving the vastus lateralis tendon, obtaining complete hemostasis after tourniquet release, and assuring that distal medial patella cartilage is intact before doing a lateral release.

■ REHABILITATION

Patients use cryotherapy for 3 to 5 days following surgery. A knee immobilizer is used for 6 weeks but removed daily for range-of-motion exercises. By 2 weeks after the operation, the patient should have 90 to 120 degrees of knee flexion. Patients should remain on toe-touch ambulation for 6 weeks and then gradually resume full weight bearing. Most patients can ride an exercise bicycle by the sixth postoperative week, and at 4 months after the operation some patients can resume running short distances.

■ OUTCOMES AND FUTURE DIRECTIONS

Unfortunately, lateral release does not always produce a perfect result, even if indications are appropriate. There are a few patients who have some subtle cartilage lesion medially or postoperative medial subluxation, which can cause postoperative symptoms. It is imperative therefore to be very vigorous about indications and avoid being overzealous.

Nonetheless, lateral release can be useful, if done skillfully, in alleviating pain in 70 to 80% of patients with isolated tilt and tightness of the lateral retinaculum.

The future should bring further refinement of indications, particularly focusing on specific articular lesions and tailoring the release to minimizing load on areas of chondromalacia and assuring balance of the patella in the trochlea. As in most surgery, precision is most important.

References

1. Fulkerson JP. *Disorders of the patellofemoral joint.* Baltimore: Williams and Wilkins, 1996.
2. Fu FH, Maday MG. Arthroscopic lateral release and the lateral patellar compression syndrome. *Orthop Clin North Am* 1992; 23:601–612.

JOSEPH ABATE
RICHARD D. PARKER
GARY CALABRESE

12

Patellar Instability: Proximal and Distal Realignment

■ HISTORY OF THE TECHNIQUE

Surgical treatment of patellofemoral instability has evolved over the past 110 years. Roux in 1888 (1) described the three main components of patellar realignment procedures, namely, 1) release of the lateral retinaculum, 2) transposition of the patellar tendon insertion, and 3) medial reefing. In 1899, Goldthwait (2) described a modification of Roux's technique in which only the medial half of the patellar tendon insertion was transposed laterally. This technique was coined the *Roux–Goldthwait procedure* and is particularly useful in the skeletally immature patient, because it is purely a soft-tissue procedure. In 1938, Hauser (3) described his modification of Roux's procedure by distally, medially, and posteriorly transferring the patellar tendon insertion with a bone block (tibial tubercle). This procedure, though popular in the past, has fallen out of favor, because patellofemoral arthritis often developed as a result of increased pressure on the patellofemoral articular cartilage surfaces secondary to the posteriorization of the tibial tubercle.

Hughston in 1968 (4) reported excellent short-term results with proximal and distal realignment of the extensor mechanism. The results deteriorated over time, however. Hughston found that these procedures continued to eliminate or reduce patellar instability, but posttraumatic arthritis often occured. This may have been secondary to 1) preexisting chondral injury (posttraumatic arthritis) as a result of the patellar subluxations or dislocations, 2) postoperative immobilization, 3) postoperative rehabilitation, or 4) an increase in activity level once the patellar instability was eliminated.

Many other reconstructions have been described, but no one method is currently the procedure of choice. The two most popular reconstructions today are the Elmslie–Trillat and Fulkerson procedures. The Elmslie–Trillat procedure medializes without posteriorizing the tibial tubercle (5); the Fulkerson procedure medializes and anteriorizes the tibial tubercle and is indicated if patellofemoral arthritis is present at the time of surgery (6). Both procedures incorporate proximal realignment if indicated and utilize internal fixation of the tibial tubercle transfer, and their proponents recommend early motion and rehabilitation. We prefer a modified Elmslie–Trillat procedure in the patient without patellar posttraumatic arthritis (no chondrosis greater than grade II as described by Outerbridge [7]).

This chapter presents our preferred technique for patellar realignment of recurrent patellar subluxation or dislocation (patellofemoral instability) with or without patella alta and without significant patellar chondrosis (posttraumatic arthritis). In addition, we present indications, contraindications, technical alternatives, rehabilitation, pitfalls, complications, outcomes, and future directions.

■ INDICATIONS AND CONTRAINDICATIONS

Our indications for the modified Elmslie–Trillat procedure include current lateral patellar instability (subluxation or dislocation) that has failed nonoperative treatment (rehabilitation and bracing). The physical examination (8,9) may reveal patella malalignment consisting of any or all of the following:

1. Abnormal "Q" angle and femoral sulcus Q angle at 90 degrees flexion.
2. Laterally tilted or lateral subluxated patella.

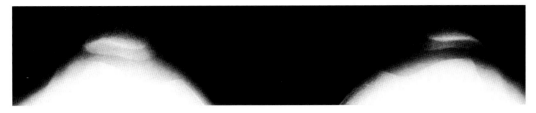

Mercer–Merchant patellar view at 45 degrees knee flexion revealing laterally subluxated and tilted patellae.

3. Lateral patellar glide into the third or fourth quadrant with apprehension with the knee flexed 30 degrees to allow for seating of the patella in the trochlear groove with or without patellar hypermobility.
4. Positive "J" sign (lateral pull test): lateral deviation of the patella in active terminal knee extension.
5. Normal patellar tendon length (patellar height) or patellar alta.
6. Normal trochlear morphology to moderate trochlear hypoplasia.
7. Vastus medialis obliquous atrophy or proximal insertion.

Radiographic evidence of patellar malalignment may include a Mercer–Merchant patellar view at 45 degrees revealing lateral tilt or lateral subluxated patella (Fig. 12-1). If the Mercer–Merchant view at 45 degrees is normal, additional views at 20 degrees (Laurin) and 55 degrees (Hughston) are obtained. If these are normal or equivical, then computed tomographic scans (tangential) of the patellae at 0 and 15 degrees with and without quadriceps contraction are obtained. Patellar tilt angle less than 13 degrees is considered abnormal and indicative of abnormal patellar tilt. In addition, the computed tomographic scan often reveals patellar subluxation, which is not seen easily on the plain radiographs.

Additional radiographs may include a lateral view of the knee at 30 degrees flexion to evaluate patellar height, patellar tendon length, and trochlear depth (gross); a 45-degree posteroanterior flexion weight-bearing view to function as a "tunnel view" and to aid evaluation for early arthritis of the lateral or medial compartments; and an extension weight-bearing view to evaluate the femorotibial axis anatomically and mechanically. These views, in addition to the Mercer–Merchant view at 45 degrees, often reveal an associated loose body if present.

Contraindications to the modified Elmslie–Trillat reconstruction include a history of voluntary habitual dislocations indicative of a psychological dysfunction requiring psychiatric treatment rather than surgical intervention. Though not as common in this setting as in shoulder instability, this does occur. Another contraindication is a history of pain primarily, rather than patellar subluxation or dislocation followed by pain for a short period. This pain is usually secondary to associated posttraumatic arthritis, in which case the Fulkerson procedure is indicated. On the other hand, the pain could be secondary to reflex sympathetic dystrophy, which is not as rare as previously believed. Finally a history of medial patellar subluxation or dislocation, active infection, and arthrofibrosis are contraindications.

We believe the success of any surgical procedure begins with preoperative counseling and teaching. It is much easier to teach a patient preoperatively than postoperatively, when he or she is in pain, taking narcotic medications, and often nauseated. It is extremely important that the patient and his or her family have the same expectations of the outcome as the surgeon. Therefore the expected outcome, risks, benefits, and potential complications should be explained completely to the patient by the surgeon. After the patient consents to surgery, a registered nurse who works with the surgeon in the office and operating room reviews the previous discussions, answers any remaining questions, and alerts the surgeon to any questions or issues that have been left unanawered or unresolved. In addition, a

■   SURGICAL
TECHNIQUES

physical therapist or athletic trainer teaches the patient the initial postoperative exercises consisting of straight leg raises, quadriceps sets, and active range of motion exercises (0–30 degrees flexion), as well as how to operate the postoperative brace and cryotherapy unit. Finally, the patient receives a set of handouts that reviews the preoperative teachings, as well as important information such as what to bring, what to wear, and where to report on the day of surgery; a reminder to stop all nonsteroidal antiinflamatory medications at least 5 days prior to surgery; responses to common postoperative scenarios (fever, nausea, pain); dressing care; and emergency phone numbers. The first postoperative visit is arranged, and the postoperative narcotic analgesic prescription is issued, allowing for an easier transition to home.

The surgery is performed on an outpatient basis. At our institution outpatient surgery encompasses both same-day discharges and those patients who are discharged within 23 hours. The majority of our patients fall into the latter group and therefore stay overnight. The patient meets with a representative from the anesthesia department as part of the preoperative visit, and the type of anesthesia is determined. We routinely perform the surgery under general anesthesia; however, spinal or epidural anesthesia is not unusual. After arriving in the preoperative area a peripheral intravenous line is placed, and prior to departing to the operating room the patient is given a broad-spectrum cephalosporin such as cephasolin (Ancef), or Vancomycin if the patient is allergic to penicillin or cephalosporins, as antibiotic prophylaxis. After the patient is anesthetized, he or she is positioned supine on the operating table, and both knees are examined and compared with the office examination. Often the affected patella (and sometimes the unaffected patella) can be dislocated with the lateral patellar glide, so care must be taken to not cause further injury. After satisfactory examination of both knees, a tourniquet is placed and preset to 250 to 300 mm Hg, depending on the patient's size and systolic blood pressure. A bolster is placed under the buttock of the operative leg to diminish its external rotation, allowing for easier leg control and visualization. Prior to surgical prepping, the operative knee is injected intraarticularily under sterile conditions with a 60-mL mixture of 0.025% bupivicaine, 1 : 400,000 epinephrine, and 2 mg preservative-free morphine as a form of preemptive analgesia. The operative leg then is prepped with Hibiclens (Zeneca Pharmaceuticals, Wilmington, DE) from the tourniquet to the tip of the toes. The leg then is draped free to allow for easy manipulation and positioning. All incisions and portals are marked and injected with the preemptive analgesia mixture. A diagnostic or operative arthroscopy is performed without the use of a tourniquet or leg holder. Careful attention is made to the patellofemoral articulation with respect to tracking and chondrosis (degree and location). If significant articular cartilage disease is found (grade III or IV), then the modified Elmslie–Trillat procedure is contraindicated and the Fulkerson procedure is performed. Patellar tracking via the superolateral portal can be assessed in various degrees of knee flexion to determine the amount of subluxation and patellar tilt. After thorough evaluation of the patellofemoral articulation, all other intraarticular pathology found is treated appropriately.

On completion of diagnostic or operative arthroscopy, the leg is exsanguinated with a Esmarck bandage, and the tourniquet is inflated to 250 to 300 mm Hg. A vertical incision is made from 1 cm lateral to the patellar tendon and inferior to the inferior pole of the patella to 2 cm below the tibial tubercle (Fig. 12-2). The skin is undermined subcutaneously superior to the vastus lateralis, and medially to the patella, patellar tendon, and tibial tubercle. The lateral release is performed by incising the lateral retinaculum and synovium from the vastus lateralis to the superior border of the lateral meniscus (anterior horn), taking care to protect the inferior lateral geniculate artery, which courses inferior to the lateral meniscus. The lateral release is performed with electrocautery to ensure cauterization of the superior lateral geniculate artery. Passive patellar tilt is measured and should be positive 70 to 90 degrees. If the passive patellar tilt is less than 70 degrees, further release can be done proximally along the vastus lateralis if an adequate release has been performed distally along the patellar tendon. Care should be taken not to perform an excessive lateral release in patients with hypermobile patellae.

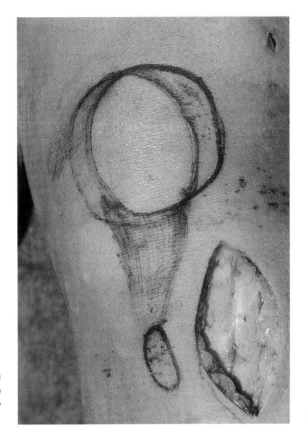

A vertical incision has been made from 1 cm lateral to the patellar tendon and inferior to the inferior pole of the patella to 2 cm below the tibial tubercle.

■   FIGURE 12-2

Once an adequate open lateral release has been performed, a decision is made between a distal tibial tubercle medial transfer and a medial reefing as the next step. Because a lateral release only addresses patellar tilt and not the Q angle or tubercle–sulcus Q angle, a distal tubercle medial transfer is the most frequent next step. The rationale for this decision is that a medial reefing increases both Q angles, whereas a distal tibial tubercle medial transfer decreases both Q angles, and an indication for the Elmslie–Trillat procedure is increased Q angles. The distal one third of the patellar tendon and its insertion on the tibial tubercle is demarcated both medially and laterally. An Army–Navy retractor is placed behind the patellar tendon, and the periosteum along its distal attachment is exposed. The periosteum is incised along both sides of the tibial tubercle, and laterally 2 cm of the anterior compartment musculature is elevated from the anterolateral tibia. Further release of the anterior compartment fascial is performed subcutaneously distally with blunt scissors as far as posible. Osteotomy of the tibial tubercle then is performed with an oscillating saw in a medial to lateral direction. The osteotomy is performed parallel or angled slightly posterior to the posterior cortex of the tibia. The osteotomy is initiated 2 cm posterior to the anterior cortex of the tibial tubercle, to increase the surface area of cancellous bone to enhance bone healing and to increase the posterior base for medial transfer of the tibial tubercle. The osteomy is extended distally 4 cm and angled anteriorly over the last centimeter and exits the cortex subperiosteally at the distal point. The knee is flexed to 90 degrees (in neutral rotation), and the tibial tubercle is medialized until the tubercle–sulcus Q angle is 0 degrees (usually 1–2 cm). The tibial tubercle is secured with a K wire, and the knee is extended and flexed throughout a full range of motion to ensure proper patellofemoral tracking (Fig. 12-3). The arthroscope can be placed superiorly laterally to verify proper tracking. The medialized tibial tubercle is fixed in position by two anterior-to-posterior 4.5-mm cortical screws that engage the posterior cortex of the tibia. The screws are placed in a lag fashion by overdrilling the tubercle, and the screw heads are countersunk to the surface of the cortex to prevent prominence under the skin (Fig. 12-4). Two screws are used to control rota-

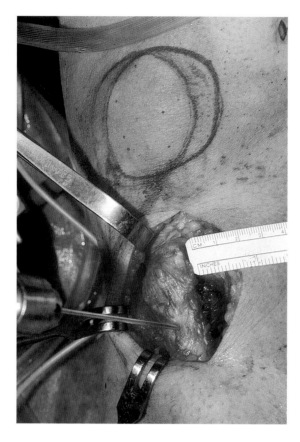

■   FIGURE 12-3

After medialization of the tibial tubercle to the desired position, a K wire is utilized to fixate the tibial tubercle temporarily, to allow for evaluation of patellofemoral tracking.

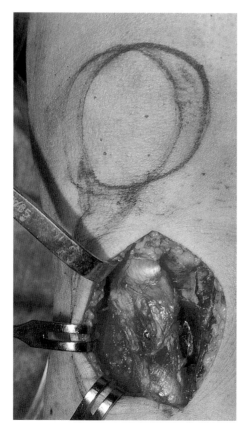

■   FIGURE 12-4

Once satisfactory medialization has been determined, the tibial tubercle is secured by placing two anterior-to-posterior 4.5-mm cortical screws in a lag fashion, which engage the posterior cortex of the tibia.

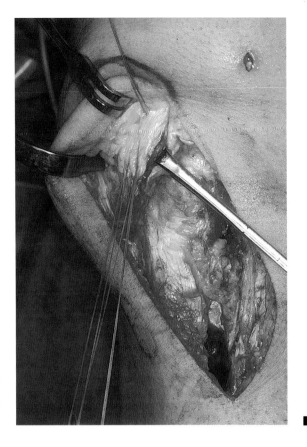

The vastus medialis oblique muscle and the medial retinaculum are transferred distally and laterally under the raised periosteum of the superior medial patella.

■ FIGURE 12-5

tion, although one screw is often sufficient. The knee again is flexed and extended through a full range of motion, to ensure adequate fixation of the tibial tubercle and proper patella tracking.

Once the lateral release and distal tibial tubercle medial transfer have been completed, a decision is made regarding the need for a medial reefing. Rarely is a medial reefing necessary; we feel it is indicated if lateral patellar subluxation still exists after the lateral release and distal tibial tubercle medial transfer. If indicated, the medial retinaculum and distal attachment of the vastus medialis oblique (VMO) muscle are detached from the medial and superomedial patella through the same lateral incision by extending the incision proximally 1 to 2 cm and medially retracting the skin edges. The periosteum is raised over the medial and superomedial patella, and the exposed patellar cortex is decorticated partially by a rongeour to create bleeding bone. The medial retinaculum and VMO muscle are transferred laterally and distally and imbricated under the raised periosteum and secured with multiple no. 2 nonabsorbable sutures (Fig. 12.5). The knots are tied in extension, and the knee is flexed fully after each knot is tied to ensure that the medial reefing does not decrease the range of motion. The raised periosteum then is sutured over the transposed tissue and nonabsorbable knots with no. 1 absorbable sutures.

Prior to wound closure, the tourniquet is deflated and hemostasis is achieved, with particular attention to potential geniculate artery bleeding. A 1/4-inch closed suction drain is placed intraarticularly and subcutaneously, and a two-layered wound closure is performed. The subcutaneous layer is closed with multiple interrupted no. 2-0 absorbable sutures and the skin is closed with a running no. 3-0 nonabsorbable monofilament suture. Steristrips (without tension on the skin) and a thin dry nonadherant sterile dressing are applied. Next a sterile cryotherapy pad (Donjoy Iceman) followed by a compression stocking are applied. Finally, an Extension Lock Splint (ELS) (Donjoy Inc., Vista, CA) brace is applied to the leg and locked in full extension.

As stated previously, the procedure is performed as outpatient surgery (23-hour stay in the hospital), and the suction drain is removed the morning after surgery prior to discharge. At this time the patient is permitted to bear partial weight on the operated leg with the use of crutches and begins quadricep sets, straight leg raises (with the ELS brace locked), and unlocks the brace to actively flex and extend the knee as tolerated. The patient returns to the office within the first week for a dressing change and removal of arthroscopic portal sutures. The subcuticular nonabsorbable monofilament suture is removed approximately 10 days postoperatively, and formal rehabilitation begun with a physical therapist and certified athletic trainer.

■ TECHNICAL ALTERNATIVES AND PITFALLS

Five main alternatives to the modified Elmslie–Trillat procedure are available to the surgeon treating patellar instability. The first alternative is the Roux–Goldthwait procedure, which is a medial transfer of the lateral half of the patellar tendon. Because this is a soft-tissue transfer, it is indicated primarily in the skeletally immature patient if further proximal tibial growth is expected. The second alternative is the proximal tube realignment as described by Insall (10). This procedure is indicated in the skeletally immature patient in whom the Roux–Goldthwait procedure is not sufficient or in the rare patient who has patellar instability without an elevated tubercle–sulcus Q angle (usually secondary to patellar hypermobility or trochlear hypoplasia). The third alternative is a distalization of the medially transferred tibial tubercle and is indicated in the skeletally mature patient with patella alta and patellar instability. Distalization is performed by extending the distal cut by 1 to 1.5 cm and then removing an amount of bone from the distal detached tibial tubercle equal to the amount of distalization desired. The desired distalization is determined by either gross visualization of the relationship between the trochlea and the inferior pole of the patella in full extension, because the inferior pole should be at the level of the superior trochlea; a lateral radiograph of the knee at 30 degrees flexion after trial distalization is fixated temporarily; or both. The fourth alternative is a deepening of the trochlear groove, which is known as the Albee procedure and is indicated in severe trochlear hypoplasia as a salvage procedure. The final alternative, the Fulkerson procedure, is employed most commonly and is indicated if grade III or IV chondrosis of the patella is discovered with associated patellar instability.

The potential for failure in the surgical treatment of patients with patellar instabiliy is present through every phase from patient selection through postoperative rehabilitation. Throughout this chapter the authors have identified several pitfalls and discussed them individually. A few major pitfalls, however, deserve repeating. Perhaps the major pitfall is ignoring the presence of patellar chondrosis with patellar instability. Failure to recognize the significance of this finding and not choosing the Fulkerson procedure instead of the modified Elmslie–Trillat procedure would result most likely in correction of the patellar instability but worsening of the associated patellofemoral arthritis symptoms. Another pitfall is the failure to recognize medial patellar subluxation or dislocation that is an iatrogenic condition, usually secondary to a generous lateral release in a patient with a hypermobile patella without tilt. Another pitfall is too superficial a cut through the tibial tubercle, resulting in little cancellous and mostly cortical bone left to transfer (Fig. 12-6). This often results in a delayed union and increases the potential for nonunion.

Postoperative Complications   Of all the surgeries that are performed around the knee, patellofemoral surgery is second only to tibial osteotomy in potential complications. Intraoperative complications include nerve or vascular injury. Postoperative complications include infection (deep or superficial), compartmental sydrome, neurovascular injury, deep venous thrombosis, pulmonary embolism, and even death. Luckily, these complications are rare and their liklihood diminished further by prophylactic antibiotics, attention to surgical detail, and early mobilization of the operative leg and patient. The most common complication is a hemarthrosis or subcutaneous hematoma, which can occur despite postoperative wound drainage. If the hemarthrosis or subcutaneous hematoma causes severe pain, jeopardizes rehabilitation, or begins to drain (potentially increasing the chance of in-

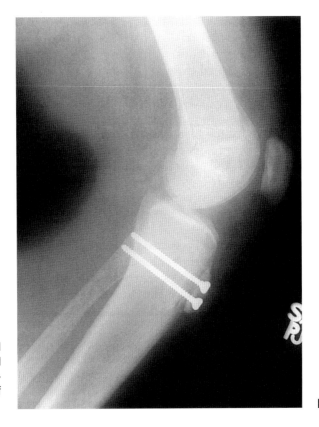

Too superficial an osteotomy of the tibial tubercle resulting in little cancellous and mostly cortical bone increases the possibility of a delayed union or nonunion of the medialized tibial tubercle.

■   FIGURE 12-6

fection) then the surgeon should perform an evacuation of the blood, lavaging of the wound or joint followed by complete hemostasis in the operating room under sterile conditions.

Other potential complications related to this surgery include loss of patellar tendon fixation, delayed union or nonunion of the tibial tuberosity, or fracture of bony osteotomy fragment and prominent hardware postoperatively. Recurrent extensor mechanism malalignment both medially and laterally also can occur postoperatively, and patients must be informed of this possibility preoperatively. Arthrofibrosis, patella baja and infrapatellar contracture syndrome, and reflex sympathetic dystrophy also can occur after this procedure.

Rehabilitation following a modified Elmslie–Trillat procedure should not be focused narrowly on strengthening exercises for the quadriceps musculature. Common postsurgical conditions seen in rehabilitation associated with this procedure are pain, intraarticular effusion, soft-tissue swelling, decreased patellar mobility, decreased active and passive ranges of motion, reduced muscular strength, and imbalance. Individualized postoperative progression and management should be based on clinical assessment and incorporate individualized goals that are established and discussed completely with each patient.

Initial postoperative rehabilitation focuses on promoting wound healing and decreasing pain and swelling. Early active range-of-motion exercises with the Donjoy ELS brace unlocked are initiated. A desired motion of 0 to 30 degrees of knee flexion is encouraged and progressed slowly as tolerated, to avoid excessive effusion and hemarthrosis. The use of a commercially available cryotherapy unit is encouraged for all nonambulating periods, to decrease pain and effusion. Partial weight-bearing ambulation with crutches and a locked brace is permitted, with emphasis on normalizing stride length in a heel–toe pattern. Patellar mobilization assessment and instruction is reviewed with the patient immediately after the operation. Superior, inferior, and lateral tilt of the patella is performed two times each day. With the quadriceps relaxed, the medial lateral borders of the patella are secured be-

■   REHABILITATION

tween the thumb and forefinger, which then can elevate the lateral border into a lateral tilt position. Superior patellar mobilization is necessary for normalized extensor mechanism biomechanics; inferior mobility is required for knee flexion. Quadriceps-strengthening exercises are started early to counteract the natural course of postsurgical muscle atrophy. Open kinetic chain exercises, such as quadriceps sets, hamstring sets, seated hip flexion, and straight leg raises, provide isolated muscle strengthening. Seated and assisted descending straight leg raises often are helpful with patients having difficulty initiating a good quadriceps contraction. Because the VMO muscle originates near the adductor magnus, the use of hip-adduction exercises follows for selective VMO training. Utilization of biofeedback and neuromuscular electrical stimulation has been shown to aid in early postoperative quadriceps reactivation and strengthening. Closed kinetic chain exercises with a locked brace, used to normalize gait such as weight shifting from side-to-side and in the anteroposterior directions, and calf raises, can facilitate muscular strengthening in functional patterns.

Active and active-assisted range of motion is progressed as tolerated to 90 degrees by 3 weeks. Once the straight leg raises can be performed easily, weights are added for progressive resistanc. The weight initially is placed proximal to the knee joint and is moved progressively distally as the patient regains strength. Only after the original weight is advanced to the ankle is additional weight added for resistance. Improving quadriceps strength with special consideration of the VMO aids in maintaining the patellar alignment. Balance and proprioception are enhanced with the use of balance-board training. The improved kinesthetic awareness can ease the transition into pure functional activities. Functional exercises are progressed to a walk stance with VMO contraction, wall-supported minisquats to 60 degrees of knee flexion, bilateral leg press with light weight and increased repetitions, box stepup, and eccentric stepdown. Exercises are progressed based on symptomatic response to the previous level of therapeutic activity. Exercises are not progressed if increased pain or effusion are noted after rehabilitation sessions. The ELS locking brace is discontinued if the patient demonstrates good active control of the knee during exercise and ambulation and after adequate bone healing has occurred (usually between postoperative weeks 4 and 6). A neoprene Donjoy "J" brace is ultilized at this time for lateral patellar support and reassurance. Crutches may be utilized for a short period of time to acclimate the lower extremity to ambulation without the brace support. Crutches can be discontinued at 6 weeks if the patient demonstrates a normal gait pattern without a limp. Biking is begun with a high seat position and low resistance in order to decrease the potential patellofemoral joint compressive forces. Rehabilitation should progress to functionally oriented activities, with resistance and repetition adjustments that meet the patient's functional status.

Functional training has been described as the process of motor relearning. A linear walk–jog program begins in the advanced phase of rehabilitation. The patient starts with a walking program, which is progressed to a walk–jog session if there is no pain or swelling. Progression to lateral activities, such as cutting and twisting, must be approached with caution and monitored closely for exacerbation of painful symptoms. Vertical activities, such as jumping rope and plyometrics, are the final series of functional training exercises. Finally, sport-specific rehabilitation is implemented.

■ OUTCOMES AND FUTURE DIRECTIONS

The outcome expected by the surgeon from a modified Elmslie–Trillat procedure is patellofemoral stability, full range of motion of the knee, full strength, no progression of arthritis, and no pain. More importantly, the patient expects a knee with patellofemoral stability so that he or she has no pain and full function. Unfortunately, not all patients who undergo this type of surgery experience either the surgeon's or their own expected outcomes. It has been our experience, however, that 85% of the patients who fulfill our indications, undergo the modified Elmslie–Trillat procedure as we have described it, and rehabilitate completely are satisfied with their outcomes. Ten percent are not completely satisfied for many reasons, which frequently revolve around unreasonable expectations such as "running faster," "jumping higher," or having "no pain" even though mild preexisting arthritis was present. The remaining 5% either experience some type of complication or more commonly have an unexpected progression of patellofemoral arthritis and complain of pain and a less than favorable outcome.

Future directions in the surgical treatment of patellofemoral instability recalcitrant to nonoperative rehabilitation should be focused on the patellofemoral ligament and laser medial contracture. In the future, the patellofemoral ligament's origin, insertion, and function will be understood and hence will be the focus of either repair or reconstruction as part of the surgical treatment of patellofemoral instability. Also, one should not underestimate the potential value of the laser. Perhaps the correct frequency will be discovered so that the laser can replace the open medial reefing currently employed. With lasers the medial retinaculum and VMO muscle theoretically could be contracted so that the VMO muscle would be distallized and lateralized, there would not be any tissue disruption that would require healing, and thus rehabilitation could be accelerated.

References

 1. Roux C. Luxation habituelle de la rotule: Traitemente operatoire. *Rev Chir* 1888; 8:682.
 2. Goldthwait JE. Permanent dislocation of the patella. *Ann Surg* 1899; 29:62.
 3. Hauser ED. Total tendon transplant for slipping patella. *Surg Gynecol Obstet* 1938; 66:199.
 4. Hughston JC. Subluxation of the patella. *J Bone Joint Surg* 1968; 50A:1003–1026.
 5. Cox JS. An evaluation of the Elmsie-Trillat procedure for management of patellar dislocations and subluxations: A preliminary report. *Am J Sports Med* 1976; 4:72–77.
 6. Fulkerson JP. Anteromedialization of the tibial tuberosity for patellofemoral malalignment. *Clin Orthop* 1983; 177:176–181.
 7. Outerbridge RE. The aetiology of chondromalacia patellae. *J Bone Joint Surg* 1961; 43B:752.
 8. Parker RD, Calabrese GJ. Anterior knee pain. In: Fu FH, Harner CD, Vince KG, eds. *Knee surgery*, volume 1. Baltimore: Williams & Wilkins, 1994; 929–951.
 9. Cox JS, Cooper PS. Patellofemoral instability. In: Fu FH, Harner CD, Vince KG, eds. *Knee surgery*, volume 1. Baltimore: Williams & Wilkins, 1994; 953–993.
10. Insall J, Bullough PG, Burnstein AH. Proximal-tube realignment of the patella for chondromalacia patella. *Clin Orthop* 1979; 144:63–69.

RUSSELL S. PETRIE
JOHN J.
KLIMKIEWICZ
CHRISOPHER D.
HARNER

13

Surgical Management of Chondral and Osteochondral Lesions of the Knee

■ HISTORY OF THE TECHNIQUE

In 1743 Hunter recognized that articular cartilage had limited ability to heal; he wrote that "ulcerated cartilage is a troublesome thing . . . that, once destroyed, is not repaired" (1). Articular cartilage injury remains a problem, especially in younger patients (2). An effective means of resurfacing the joint with a biologic solution would be ideal, because use of prostheses in young patients is inherently undesirable, because of the need for later revision (3). Numerous methods of treatment have been employed to this end. In 1959 Pridie (4) first reported on subchondral drilling of articular cartilage injuries. Steadman (5–7) improved on this technique with the use of small arthroscopic awls. Little progress was made in biologic resurfacing until the mid-1980s, when O'Driscoll et al. (3) reported on the use of periosteal autografts to treat articular cartilage injuries. Grande et al. (8,9) initially described autologous chondrocyte transplantation. More recently Brittberg et al. (10) reported on the use of autologous chondrocyte transplantation in 1994, which perhaps holds the most promise for hyaline cartilage regeneration. The advent of more precise instrumentation has improved autograft osteochondral transplantation. This technique in reality is an adaption of an technique described by Outerbridge (11) and popularized by Hangody et al. (12,13) and Bobic (14,15). The recent introduction of bioabsorbable screws and pins has made open and arthroscopic reduction and internal fixation of chondral and osteochondral fractures much easier, because the fixation device does not require removal. Initial fixation, however, may be an issue. Despite all these advances, there is little standardization in reporting on these injuries. Therefore, no technique has been established as the procedure of choice.

Techniques to address articular cartilage injuries can be broadly classified as resurfacing techniques that promote fibrocartilage formation (microfracture, abrasion chondroplasty), resurfacing techniques that promote hyaline-like cartilage formation (periosteal transplantation, autologous chondrocyte transplantation), osteochondral transplantation techniques (autograft "mosaicplasty" or core grafting, allograft osteochondral transplantation), and open or closed (arthroscopic) reduction and internal fixation of chondral and osteochondral fragments with bioabsorbable fixation if possible. This chapter focuses on the technical aspects of treating osteochondral and chondral injuries and presents the approach used at the University of Pittsburgh.

■ BASIC SCIENCE

Articular cartilage is the term used to describe normal joint cartilage macro- and microscopically. *Hyaline cartilage*, meaning "ground glass," is the term applied to the gross morphologic appearance (16). Articular cartilage ultrastructure can be divided into four zones (17,18), and it is composed primarily of type II collagen. The structure is highly organized. The first layer, the superficial zone, is a thin gliding surface. The second, transitional zone, has a higher proteoglycan content and larger collagen fibrils. The deep zone has the lowest water content and highest collagen content. The fourth zone is a calcified cartilage, formed from a mineralized matrix, and separates articular cartilage from subchondral bone. This ultrastructure makes articular cartilage particularly well adapted to withstand and distribute physiologic loads.

It is important to distinguish between repair and regeneration in discussing articular cartilage injury. Repair is the process of fibrocartlilage scar formation, whereas regeneration is the process of duplicating the original tissue. Once mature, articular cartilage loses its propensity to regenerate itself by cell division (17). Full-thickness articular cartilage injuries heal by fibercartilage formation. This type of cartilage is predominantly loosely organized type III collagen and does not have the same biomechanical characteristics as articular cartilage (16), making it an undesirable replacement for injured articular cartilage.

It is important to distinguish between pure chondral lesions and osteochondral lesions, which have both injured bone and cartilage, because treatment options may differ between these two entities. Injury to the subchondral bone in osteochondral lesions may need to be addressed, depending on the size of the lesion. In pure chondral injuries, the surgeon may "take advantage" of the intact subchondral bone in the treatment, as described in the surgical techniques section.

There are two classification schemes used commonly to describe chondral injury (11,19). The Outerbridge classification is perhaps the most widely used scheme for classifying articular cartilage lesions (11). This scheme has four gradations of injury. Grade I demonstrates softening or "bubbling" of the articular surface without fissuring. Grade II injury demonstrates superficial fissuring, grade III lesions have fissuring down to subchondral bone, and grade IV lesions exhibit exposed subchondral bone. This classification was developed to assess patellar lesions but is used for other articular cartilage injuries as well (16).

Bauer and Jackson (19) also have described a classification scheme, based on six gradations of injury. Grade I demonstrates a line crack; grade II, a stellate fracture; grade III, flap formation; grade IV, crater formation; grade V, fibrillation; and grade VI, degrading articular cartilage (19).

There are many other variables that need to be considered in classifying and treating these injuries. Etiology is often ignored in the literature. The presence or absence of trauma has treatment and outcome implications (20). The chronicity of the lesion is important; acute traumatic lesions fare better with treatment than chronic lesions (20). Size and precise location of the lesion is of critical importance. The distinction between weight-bearing and non–weight bearing zones needs to be made. Furthermore, meniscal and nonmeniscal weight-bearing zones and patellar and trochlear lesions should be differentiated.

Whether a lesion is on one (unipolar) or both (bipolar) sides of the joint has implications for ultimate outcome; bipolar lesions do not do as well as unipolar (20).

Focal versus diffuse and unicompartmental and bicompartmental distinctions need to be made also. Focal unicompartmental lesions are much more amenable to surgical treatment (21). Limb alignment is very important, because failing to correct limb alignment may lead to failure (20,21). Associated injuries such as anterior cruciate ligament and meniscal tears may have an effect on outcome (6).

The primary indication for addressing articular cartilage injuries surgically is a symptomatic chondral or osteochondral lesion of the knee. Symptoms typically include pain and swelling. Pain is usually focal, corresponding to the area of the lesion. Swelling may be large or small. Additionally, loose chondral flaps may cause catching, and intraarticular loose bodies may cause locking. Of particular interest is a change in symptoms. Osteochondral lesions consist of traumatic osteochondral fractures and osteochondritis dissecans (OCD). Osteochondral fractures are often loose and unlikely to heal. For this reason they require surgery. OCD in the skeletally immature patient, however, may heal if stable. If a previously asymptomatic lesion becomes symptomatic, surgical intervention is considered.

Stability of the lesion is also critically important. A lesion is considered unstable if joint fluid can be seen between the lesion and bone on a magnetic resonance image. This suggests communication with the joint (see Fig. 13-10). Asymptomatic unstable lesions are followed closely, and if symptoms develop surgical intervention is considered.

■ CLASSIFICATION

■ INDICATIONS AND CONTRAINDICATIONS

Choice of the procedure depends on the type, size, depth, location and grade of the lesion. One should distinguish between chondral lesions and osteochondral lesions; they differ in that the subchondral bone is intact with chondral injuries but not osteochondral lesions. Some lesions are amenable to internal fixation, in which case this is the preferred technique. Use of bioabsorbable fixation has aided this approach. Although adequate compression with these devices has been raised as a potential problem, this has not been the case in our experience. In lesions with inadequate or poor articular cartilage (e.g., comminuted osteochondral fractures, fragmented OCD), some techniques to regenerate or replace the cartilage must be considered. The degree to which subchondral bone is involved is also critically important, because the bone provides support for the cartilage. If subchondral bone is damaged, the reconstructive technique may or may not need to take this into account. Furthermore, the degree to which the cartilage cap is damaged, using the Outerbridge classification (11), dictates which reconstructive technique is employed.

■ SURGICAL
TECHNIQUES

Choice of Technique

Chondral Lesions   Pure chondral lesions are distinguished by undamaged subchondral bone. For grade III and IV lesions, we employ a microfracture technique in lesions up to 2 cm^2. If this is not possible, however, we consider autologous chondrocyte transplantation or allograft osteocondral transplantation. Figure 13-1 summarizes the approach used for chondral lesions at the University of Pittsburgh.

Because of the added complexity, cost, and concern for infection with autogenous chondrocyte transplantation, we have elected to use this technique sparingly. Abrasion chondroplasty and periosteal transplantation do not play a significant role in our current treatment regimen.

Osteochondral Lesions   The approach to osteochondral lesions used at the University of Pittsburgh is summarized in Figures 13-2 and 13-3. Figure 13-2 pertains to lesions amenable to open or arthroscopic reduction and internal fixation. These lesions can be divided into

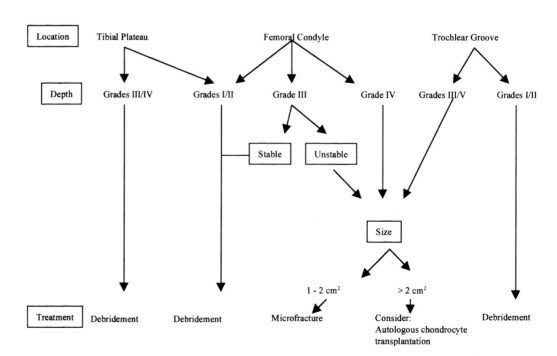

■ FIGURE 13-1

Treatment algorithm used for treating chondral lesions of the knee.

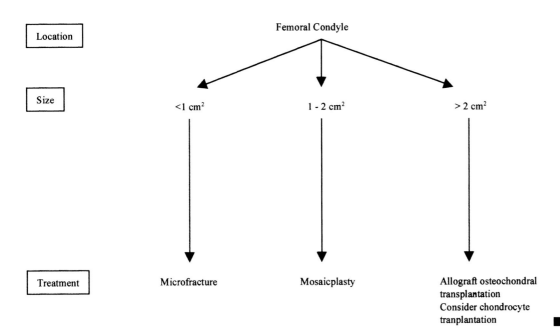

FIGURE 13-2

Treatment algorithm used for osteochondral lesions of the knee amenable to open or arthroscopic reduction and internal fixation, including osteochondritis dissecans lesions and acute and chronic osteochondral fractures.

OCD lesions, which by definition are chronic, and traumatic osteochondral fractures, which may be acute or chronic. OCD lesions can be subdivided further according to the integrity of the overlying cartilage. *In situ*, lesions have an intact articular cartilage surface, and they probably are treated best with *in situ* pinning. Some lesions have partially broken articular cartilage and are known as *"in situ* detached." In this case, the lesion remains in its bed but

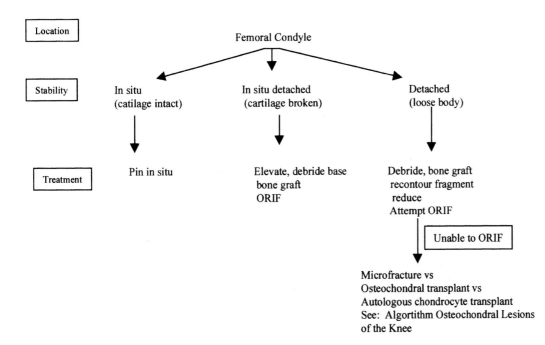

FIGURE 13-3

Treatment algorithm used for osteochondral lesions of the knee not amenable to open or arthroscopic reduction and internal fixation.

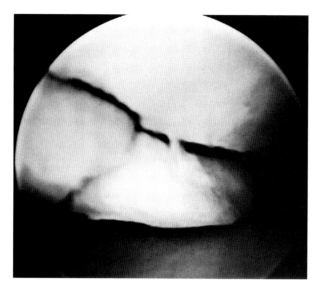

■ FIGURE 13-4

Comminuted chondral fracture of the
medial femoral condyle.

communicates with the joint by means of a break in the overlying cartilage. Treatment consists of hinging the fragment open, debriding fibrous tissue, bone grafting (if necessary), and internal fixation. Finally, detached lesions (i.e., osteochondral loose bodies) require debriding the bed, tailoring of the fragment, bone grafting (if necessary), and internal fixation. Traumatic osteochondral fractures are treated in the same fashion as detached OCD lesions.

Figure 13-2 pertains to lesions that either have failed reduction and fixation or are not considered amenable to internal fixation. Lesions occurring on the tibial plateau and the patella amenable to the techniques discussed in this chapter are rare; therefore this discussion focuses on femoral lesions. Location, grade, stability, size, and depth of the lesion dictate the procedure used. Grade I and II lesions, in general, are debrided irrespective of location. Grade III and IV lesions on the tibial plateau are debrided, as are diffuse lesions. For most lesions smaller than 1 cm^2, our initial procedure is a microfracture technique (Figs. 13-4 to 13-8). The calcified cartilage layer must be removed prior to performing microfracture. Lesions smaller than 1 cm^2 that fail microfracture are candidates for osteochondral autograft transplantation. For lesions between 1 and 2 cm^2, a single or multiple osteochondral plugs are preferred (i.e., mosaicplasty or COR grafting) (see Figs. 13-23 to 13-25). For those larger than 2 cm^2, an osteochondral allograft can be considered.

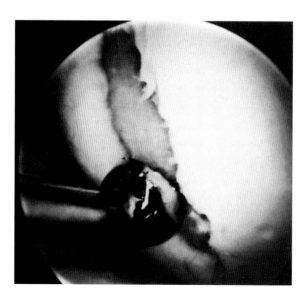

■ FIGURE 13-5

Debridement of loose chondral flaps back
to stable cartilage, and removal of the calcified cartilage layer.

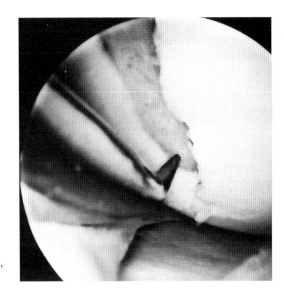

Thirty-degree microfracture awl (Linvatec, Largo, FL).

■ FIGURE 13-6

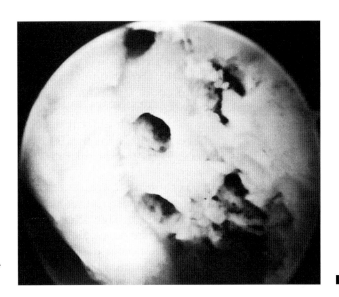

Lesion following microfracture, prior to releasing tourniquet.

■ FIGURE 13-7

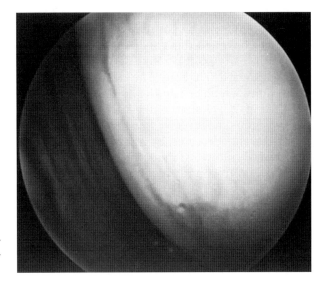

Repeat arthroscopy 1 year after microfracture, demonstrating the fibrocartilagenous cap.

■ FIGURE 13-8

Marrow-stimulating Techniques   Resurfacing techniques are designed to resurface denuded but intact subchondral bone. These techniques include subchondral drilling, microfracture, abrasion arthroplasty, periosteal transplantation, and autogenous chondrocyte transplantation. Certain techniques may be able to augment the subchondral bone, but the potential for this is somewhat limited. Recent reports have begun to challenge this doctrine (22).

Marrow-stimulating techniques are designed to allow marrow stem cells access to the exposed subchondral bone. This creates a fibrocartilagenous cap over the defect that does not have the same biomechanical characteristics as normal articular cartilage (16) and eventually breaks down, because of an inability to dissipate the ambient stresses.

Subchondral drilling first was reported by Pridie in 1959 (4). This technique employs drilling through the lesion into marrow bone to create vascular access channels. The subsequent clot over the subchondral bone establishes a new fibrocartlilage cap. Use of a drill generates heat and therefore can damage surrounding cells. Additionally, certain lesions (e.g., patellar lesions) are inaccessible with the drill. To avoid these problems, the microfracture technique was developed (5,7), which uses 30-, 60-, and 90-degree awls to create tunnels 2 mm round and 3 to 4 mm deep through subchondral bone into marrow bone (5,7). The lesion first must be debrided of loose articular cartilage (Fig. 13-4). A stable articular circumference must be established, and the calcified cartilage removed. The microfracture awl then is used to create small holes or "fractures" in the subchondral bone approximately 3 to 4 mm (i.e., three holes per square centimeter) apart so as not to fracture the subchondral bone between the holes (Figs. 13-6 and 13-7). The repair tissue is fibrocartilage and can be distinguished from articular cartilage at follow-up arthroscopy (Figs. 13-9). Six to eight hours per day of continuous passive motion treatment is required for 8 weeks following this procedure, for optimal results (5,7).

Abrasion arthroplasty is essentially a technique to abrade subchondral bone to bleeding bone, with the intention creating a fibrocartilagenous cap. This is accomplished using a rasp or motorized shaver (22,23). It has the disadvantage of disrupting of the congruence of the subchondral plate. We prefer the microfracture technique for this reason.

Biologic Resurfacing Techniques   The difference between biologic resurfacing and microfracture and abrasion arthroplasty is that biologic resurfacing has more potential to regenerate hyaline-like articular cartilage. Perichondral transplantation was reported on by Homminga et al. (24). Due to late ossification of the graft this technique was abandoned in favor or periosteal transplantation as described by O'Driscoll (3) and Bouwmeester (25). This technique requires an arthrotomy to gain access to the lesion, which then is resected back to healthy cartilage. A periosteal graft is taken from the medial proximal tibia and sewn to the defect with the cambrium layer facing the joint (3). Continuous passive motion treatment has been shown to have a significant positive influence on graft integrity at 1 year (3). Formation of hyaline cartilage has beem demonstrated. Bone grafting under the periosteal graft can be performed to augment deficient subchondral bone. The periosteal graft must be recessed in the defect to prevent shearing and damage to the cambrium layer during the early postoperative period. The graft itself is secured with sutures brought out through nonarticular bone. The technique is technically demanding, and overgrowth of the transplant sometimes requires additional surgery. Recently, use of this technique has been reported in OCD lesions of the knee (26).

Autologous chondrocyte transplantation is a two-stage procedure that first requires harvesting of chondrocytes, by arthroscopy. It then requires 14 to 21 days of *in vitro* chondrocyte cell culture. At the second operation a periosteal graft is harvested form the proximal medial tibia and sewn over the defect in a watertight manner. The autogenous chondrocytes are injected under the periosteal graft (10). In this situation the periosteal graft is sewn with the cambrium layer facing subchondral bone.

Open or Arthroscopic Reduction and Internal Fixation   Arthroscopic or open reduction and internal fixation is reserved for those lesions that have chondral or osteochondral fragments that can accept some form of pin or screw fixation. In some cases these lesions may

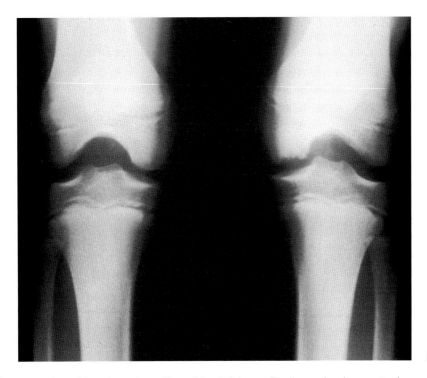

■ FIGURE 13-9

Fifteen-year-old male presenting with pain and swelling of the left knee. Radiographs demonstrating osteochondritis dissecans lesion.

be treated entirely arthroscopically. In other cases an arthrotomy may be required. Bioabsorbable fixation has made treatment of these injuries easier, because no additional surgical procedure is needed if healing occurs. In some lesions, such as OCD lesions, the subchondral bone has been violated and requires bone grafting. Figures 13-9 through 13-13 show an OCD lesion that required bone grafting for subchondral bone loss. The lesion was

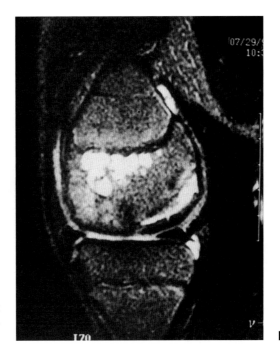

Magnetic resonance image demonstrating joint fluid beneath the fragment (i.e., "unstable" lesion), indicating communication with the joint.

■ FIGURE 13-10

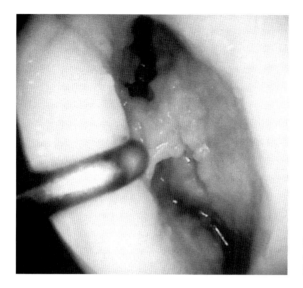

Fragment could be hinged on the intact medial border of the lesion (i.e., *in situ* detached).

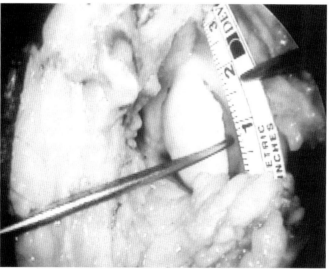

An arthrotomy was performed for improved access to the lesion. Debridement of fibrocartilage and bone grafting were performed.

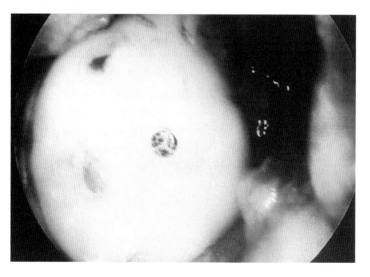

Final fixation obtained with bioabsorbable screws.

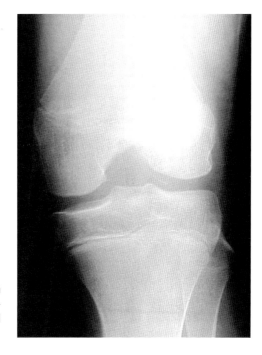

Fourteen-year-old boy presenting with an effusion and locking of the left knee. An osteochondral fracture fragment can be seen under the lateral femoral condyle.

■ FIGURE 13-14

hinged open to gain access to the subchondral bone. The bed was curretted of fibrous tissue and packed with bone graft taken from the ipsilateral Gerdy's tubercle. Definitive fixation was achieved with bioabsorbable screws. Alternatively, a 3.0-mm screw can be used for fixation and may provide better initial compression. A second operation is required 3 to 6 months later, however, to remove the screw.

It is important to note that if a chondral fragment has been loose inside a joint for a period of months it continues to receive nutrition from the synovial fluid and grow. Similarly, the edges of the defect grow to the center. The fragment then may appear too large for the defect; trimming of the fragment and defect allows a near anatomic fit. Figures 13-14 through 13-21 show the knee of a 14-year-old boy presenting with locking and swelling of the knee 6 months after trauma. Initial radiographs and magnetic resonance images demonstrated an osteochondral fracture of the lateral femoral condyle (Figs. 13-14 to 13-16). Diagnostic arthroscopy confirmed the presence of a large lesion of the lateral femoral condyle (Fig. 13-17). The fragment had become trapped behind the lateral femoral condyle (Fig. 13-18). A lateral arthrotomy was required to remove the fragment and debride the defect (Fig. 13-19). Tailoring of the fragment was required for optimal fit (Figs. 13-20 to 13-22).

Osteochondral Transplantation There is both auto- and allograft osteochondral transplantation. In each case injured cartilage and subchondral bone can be addressed. In the case of autograft osteochondral transplantation, cylinders of normal cartilage and bone are harvested from the intercondylar notch or the superior lateral femoral condyle. A cylinder similarly sized in diameter and depth is removed from the area of diseased cartilage and bone. The normal cylinder or "plug" is transplanted and press fitted into the osteochondral defect (Figs. 13-23 and 13-24). This technique can be done open or arthroscopically depending on the size, location of the defect and the preference of the surgeon. The technique is facilitated by the use of specially designed instrumentation. The number and size of the grafts that can be obtained from the knee limit this technique. The largest recommended graft is 8 to 10 mm, as larger grafts may result in significant donor-site morbidity. There have been numerous reports on this technique (12–15,27–30). A distinction can be made between mosaicplasty, in which multiple small 4- to 6-mm cylinders are used for a defect, and the technique in which one "large" 10-mm cylinder is used (Fig. 13-25). Proponents of mosaicplasty point out that the ability to recreate the curve of the femoral condyle is limited

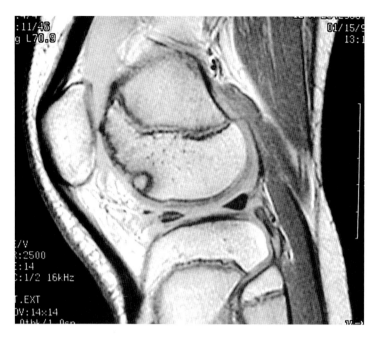

■ FIGURE 13-15

Magnetic resonance image showing the lateral femoral condyle osteochondral fracture site.

with large-plug techniques (12,13). The interface between graft and host cartilage fills with fibrocartilage. One single large plug minimizes the number of graft–host and graft–graft interfaces, which may be a potential advantage.

Allograft osteochondral transplantation and shell allograft transplantation have the advantage of no donor-site morbidity and the ability to cover lesions larger than 2 cm². The host cartilage is resected back to healthy stable cartilage. The subsequent defect often is irregular, requiring significant tailoring of the transplant for an optimum fit. Concern over disease transmission and immune reaction have limited the use of this technique.

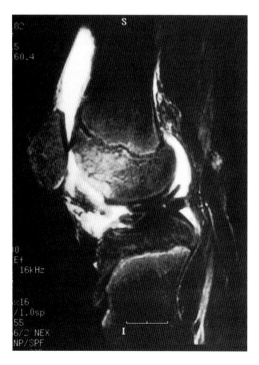

Magnetic resonance image showing that the fracture fragment is in the posterior aspect of the lateral compartment.

■ FIGURE 13-16

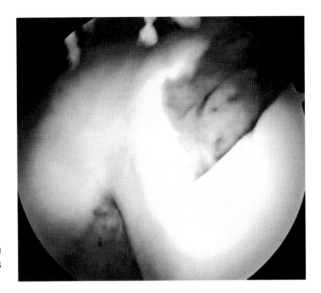

Arthroscopic view of the lesion seen on magnetic resonance imaging in Figures 13-15 and 13-16.

■ FIGURE 13-17

Subchondral drilling and microfracture techniques are both quick and very cost-effective (4,5). The repair tissue, however, is fibrocartilage (Fig. 13-7) and as such is considerably different from the hyaline cartilage it is meant to replace (31). Over time this fibrocartilage deteriorates (16). This technique also provides no means of reconstructing damaged subchondral bone and therefore is limited to use in pure chondral injuries or small (smaller than 1 cm) osteochondral injuries. The use of a drill limits the surgeon's ability to access many areas of the joint. The use of microfracture awls with varying angles at the tip solves this problem (Fig. 13-6) (5,7). Extensive use of continuous passive motion treatment following the operation can be very disruptive for some people, and optimal results may not be attained if there is noncompliance with this aspect of the treatment program. If insurance does not cover the continuous passive motion machine, patients must move the knee through a range of motion 1,500 times per day.

Periosteal transplantation has the potential for producing hyaline-like cartilage (3). This operation is technically demanding (32). Meticulous attention to detail is required, and the graft must be recessed into the subchondral bone to avoid excessive shearing of the cam-

■ TECHNICAL ALTERNATIVES AND PITFALLS

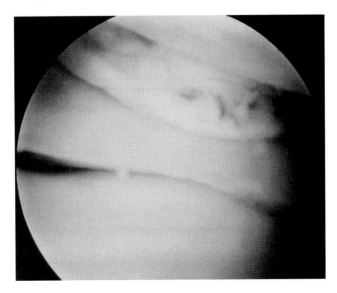

■ FIGURE 13-18

Diagnostic arthroscopy showing fragment trapped behind the lateral femoral condyle.

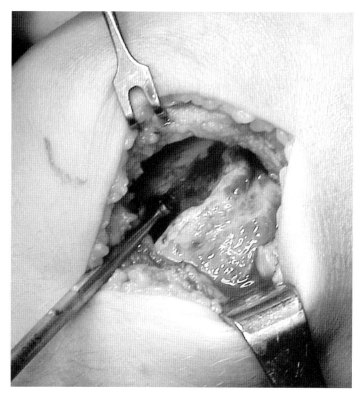

■ FIGURE 13-19

A lateral arthrotomy was performed to remove the fragment and debride the defect back to bleeding bone. The edges of the lesion also were trimmed back to healthy articular cartilage.

brium layer during the early postoperative period (33). Overgrowth of the transplanted tissue may require additional surgical procedures.

Autologous chondrocyte transplantation also holds potential for hyaline-like cartilage formation (10). This procedure is also technically demanding; furthermore, it is a two-stage procedure that requires a laboratory to grow the chondrocytes. In this procedure the periosteal graft is placed with the cambrium layer facing the subchondral bone. The amount of matrix synthesis has been shown to be related *in vitro* to the number of chondrocytes transplanted (34). This procedure is very expensive and may require 12 to 18 months for maturation of the lesional repair tissue and resolution of symptoms (10). There is some concern about *in vitro* culturing, because it has the potential for introducing an infection into the cultured chondrocytes and subsequently into the knee when transplanted.

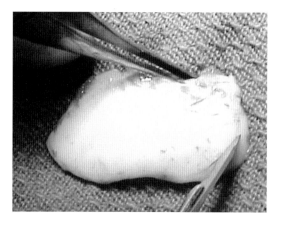

Macroscopic view of the fragment. It has grown and no longer fits in the defect. Tailoring of the fragment is required to achieve an optimal fit.

■ FIGURE 13-20

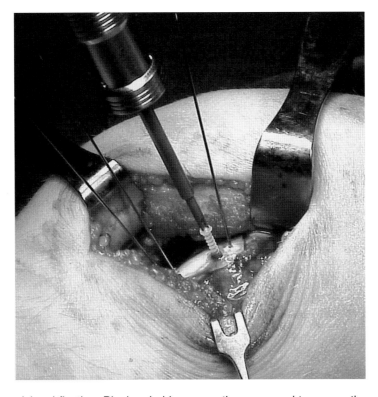

■ FIGURE 13-21

Kirchner wires are used for provisional fixation. Bioabsorbable screws then are used to secure the fragment to the lateral femoral condyle.

Open or arthroscopic reduction and internal fixation of chondral and osteochondral lesions is the preferred technique if possible. The advent of bioabsorbable fixation has aided this technique, because removal of the fixation device is no longer necessary. This technique is limited by the fact that many lesions cannot be treated in this manner because of

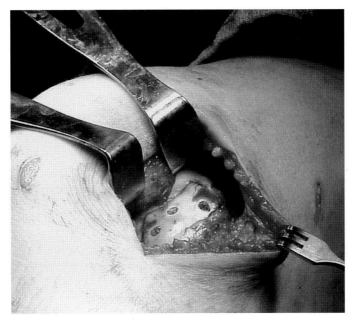

■ FIGURE 13-22

The graft after definitive fixation.

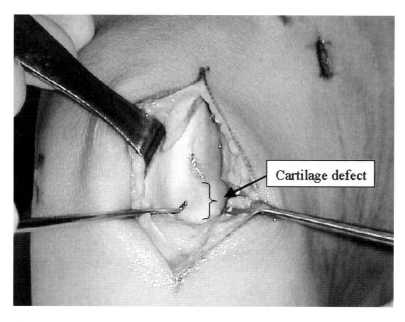

Cartilage defect seen in the lateral femoral condyle 2 years following an anterior cruciate tear with a large bone bruise in this area. Discolored and depressed articular cartilage can be seen on gross inspection.

comminution. Whether there is an ill effect of bioabsorbable fixation on articular cartilage and subchondral bone has not been determined fully yet.

Osteochondral autograft transplantation is the only technique that transplants true hyaline cartilage. This technique has numerous limitations, including the number of potential plugs that can be harvested from the knee (14,15). Although little has been written on in-

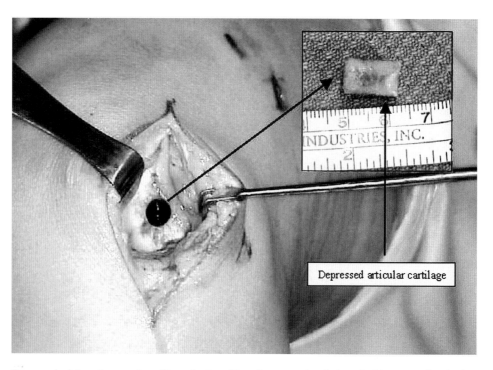

Removal of the diseased cartilage lesion. The depressed subchondral bone and articular cartilage can be seen (**inset**).

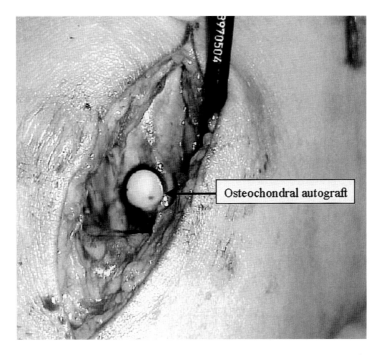

Autograft osteochondral plug, taken from the superolateral aspect of the knee (graft site not shown).

jury to the graft sites, it was shown recently that there are increased contact stresses at all of the currently used harvest sites (35). The long-term effect of these harvest sites on the knee is still unknown. This procedure has been improved with the use of better instrumentation. It is still challenging, however, to reconstitute the curvature of the femoral condyle with this technique (12). The graft–host and graft–graft interfaces fill in with fibrocartilage and not hyaline cartilage.

Osteochondral allografts have the advantage of potentially covering large areas, and there is no donor-site morbidity. This technique is limited by the fact that there is an added risk of infection. Furthermore, a significant amount of tailoring may be required to obtain an adequate fit.

Rehabilitation varies tremendously among techniques and authors. There are, however, some recurring themes. Resurfacing techniques such as subchondral drilling , microfracture, and periosteal and autologous chondrocyte transplantation probably require use of continuous passive motion treatment for an extended period of time following the procedure for optimal results. Six to eight hours a day for 8 weeks is recommended for microfracture (36). Patients should bear no or only touch weight during this period of time. Gillogly et al. (37) recently published an extensive rehabilitation protocol for autologous chondrocyte transplantation.

Osteochondral transplantation and internal fixation of chondral and osteochondral lesions do not require the use of continuous passive motion; rather the cartilage is mature at transplantation and the perioperative period focuses on allowing the repair to heal. Patients usually are held in extension for 1 to 2 weeks depending on the site, size, and stability of the repair, at which time range-of-motion exercises are instituted. Quadriceps straight leg exercises are encouraged immediately following surgery. Progressive weight bearing is begun 2 to 4 weeks postoperatively and progressed (38). Irrgang and Pezzulo (38) recently published the extensive protocol used at the University of Pittsburgh.

■   REHABILITATION

There are no long-term studies comparing microfracture to any of the other procedures used to treat articular cartilage defects. Furthermore, the studies reporting on microfrac-

■   OUTCOMES AND
FUTURE DIRECTIONS

ture fail to incorporate a control group (36). Long-term results recently were presented (39). Return to sports was evaluated by Blevins et al. (36), who found generally good results.

O'Driscoll has not published his results on periosteal transplantation yet; however, early results are encouraging (33). Brittberg et al. (10) reviewed 23 patients 66 months following autologous chondrocyte transplantation. Fourteen of 16 condylar defects and two of seven patellar defects had good or excellent results. Histologic evidence of hyaline-like cartilage was demonstrated by biopsy in 13 patients. Peterson (31) reported a series of 219 patients treated with autologous chondrocyte transplantation. Follow-up averaged 4 years (range 2–9 years). He reported 90% good or excellent results with isolated femoral condyle defects. Arthroscopic probing demonstrated similar stiffness between hyaline-like repair tissue and native articular cartilage. Areas of fibrocartilage formation, however, had significantly less stiffness. Outcome had been shown to correlate with formation of hyaline-like cartilage (40). Resolution of symptoms is time-dependent and correlates with maturation of the graft (10). Follow-up arthroscopy by Britteberg et al. (10) revealed a soft graft at 3 months, with slow complete incorporation over 12 to 18 months. Resolution of pain appears to mirror graft maturity, because it may require up to a year for symptoms to reach maximal improvement (21). This technique has been criticized for the significant cost involved and the potential for introducing an infection with *in vitro* cell culture. Also, it adds an additional surgical procedure.

Hangody et al. (12) have popularized the use of osteochondral autografts and recently published results in a series of 57 patients more than 3 years after surgery. They reported 91% good or excellent results. Outerbridge et al. (28) published a series of 10 patients in whom they used the lateral patellar facet for treating femoral condylar lesions. At 6.5 years after surgery, 6 of the 10 patients had no symptoms; four had mild symptoms.

Ghazavi et al. (21) reported on the use of osteochondral allografts for osteochodral lesions of the knee. Follow-up averaged 7.5 years. Survivorship analysis was 95% at 5 years, 71% at 10 years, and 66% at 20 years. The factors contributing to success include age younger than 50 years, unipolar defects, normal alignment, and an unloading osteotomy to improve alignment.

Studies often fail to report the chronicity, size, depth, and location of the lesions being treated. This makes it difficult to compare techniques and results. Good long-term data on all these techniques are lacking, because most studies are retrospective and lack control groups. As a result, this area is still very much in evolution, and the optimal technique has yet to be determined.

Attempts at producing artificial articular cartilage using a hydrogel of aqueous polyvinyl alcohol, chondrocyte-impregnated collagen bilayers, and mesenchymal cell transplantation have been reported (41,42). These types of technology may hold the most promise for the future.

In summary, over the past decade several techniques to manage chondral and osteochondral defects of the knee have been devised and used including fragment excision (43), arthroscopic debridement (23), abrasion chondroplasty (22,23), subchondral drilling (4), subchondral bone microfracture (5,7,36), periosteal transplantation (3), perichondral transplantation (24), autogenous osteochondral transplantation (12–15,27–30), allograft osteochondral transplantation (20,21), and autologous chondrocyte transplantation (10). Despite their promise, none has emerged as the clear method of choice. In treating these injuries, however, the surgeon should have some idea of the settings in which these techniques are used. Distinction between chondral and osteochondral lesions should be made. Our general approach is outlined in Figures 13-1 through 13-3. With respect to osteochondral lesions, we prefer to start with the least invasive technique, microfracture, and progress to more involved techniques if microfracture fails. With intermediately sized lesions the likelihood of success with microfracture is much less; thereofore we prefer to perform osteochondral transplantation as our initial procedure. Currently, we rarely perform autogenous chondrocyte transplantation, because this has significant cost and infectious concerns. Furthermore, there is no current evidence to indicate that it is superior to osteochondral transplantation techniques. Finally, the use of allograft osteochondral tissue typically is reserved for very large defects (larger than 2 cm^2) and patients in whom other techniques have failed. Investigation into chondrocyte-impregnated collagen and mesenchymal stem cell transfer may hold promise for the future (42).

References

1. Hunter W. On the structure and diseases of articulating cartilage. *Philo Trans R Soc Lond* 1743; 42B:514–521.
2. Johnson-Nurse C, Dandy D. Fracture-separation of articular cartilage in the adult knee. *J Bone Joint Surg Br* 1985; 57B:42–43.
3. O'Driscoll S, Keeley F, Salter R. Durability of regenerated articular cartilage produced by free autogenous periosteal grafts in major full-thickness defects in joint surfaces under the influence of continuous passive motion. *J Bone Joint Surg* 1988; 70A:595–606.
4. Pridie K. A method of resurfacing osteoarthritic knee joints. *J Bone Joint Surg Br* 1959; 41B:618–619.
5. Steadman J, Sterett W. The surgical treatment of knee injuries. *Med Sci Sports Exerc* 1995; 27:328–333.
6. Rodrigo JJ, Steadman RJ. Isolated chondral defects of the knee recover slower than defects combined with anterior cruciate ligament and/or meniscus pathology after debridement and microfracture. Presented at the American Academy of Orthopedic Sugeons annual meeting, New Orleans, LA, 1997.
7. Blevins FT, Steadman JR, Rodrigo JJ, et al. Treatment of articular cartilage defects in athletes: an analysis of functional outcome and lesion appearance. *Orthopedics* 1998; 21(7):761–767.
8. Grande D, Pitman MI, Peterson L, et al. The repair of experimentally produced defects in rabbit articular cartilage by autologous chondrocyte transplantation. *J Orthop Res* 1989; 7: 208–218.
9. Grande D, Singh I, Pugh J. Healing of experimentally produced lesions of articular cartilage following chondrocyte transplantation. *Anat Rec* 1987; 218:142–148.
10. Brittberg M, Lindahl A, Nilsson A, et al. Treatment of deep cartilage defects in the knee with autologous chondrocyte transplantation. *N Engl J Med* 1994; 331:889–894.
11. Outerbridge R. The etiology or chondromalacia patella. *J Bone Joint Surg* 1961; 43B:752–767.
12. Hangody L, Kish G, Karpati L, et al. Mosaicplasty for the treatment of articular cartilage defects: Application in clinical practice. *Orthopaedics* 1998; 21:751–756.
13. Hangody L, Kish G, Karpati L, et al. Arthroscopic autogenous osteochondral mosaicplasty for the treatment of femoral condylar articular defects. *Knee Surg Sports Traumatol Arthrosc* 1997; 5:262–267.
14. Bobic V. Autologous osteochondral graft in the management of articular cartilage lesions. *Orthopade* 1999; 28(1):19–25.
15. Bobic V. The utilization of osteochondal autografts in the treatment of artucular cartilage lesions. *Instr Course Lect* 1998; 146.4
16. Minas T, Nehrer S. Current concepts in the treatment of articular cartilage defects. *Orthopedics* 1997; 20:525–538.
17. Buckwalter J, Rosenberg K, Hunziker E. Articular cartilage: Composition, structure, response to injury and methods of facilitating repair. In: Ewing J, ed. *Articular cartilage and knee joint function: Basic science and arthroscopy.* Raven Press: New York, 1990:19–56.
18. Furakawa T, Eyre DR, Koide S, et al. Biochemial studies on repair cartilage resurfacing experimental defects on the rabbit knee. *J Bone Joint Surg* 1980; 62A:79–89.
19. Bauer M, Jackson R. Chondral lesions of the femoral condyles: A system of arthroscopic classification. *Arthroscopy* 1988; 4:97–102.
20. McDermott AG, Langer F, Pritzker KP, et al. Fresh small-fragment osteochondral allografts: Long term follow-up on first 100 case. *Clin Orthop Relat Res* 1985; 197:96–102.
21. Ghazavi M, Pritzker KP, Davis AM, et al. Fresh osteochondral allografts for post traumatic osteochndral defects of the knee. *J Bone Joint Surg* 1997; 79B:1008–1013.
22. Bert J, Maschka K. The arthroscopic treatment of unicompartmental gonarthorsis: A five-year follow-up study of abrasion arthroplasty plus debridement and arthroscopic debridement alone. *Arthroscopy* 1989; 5:25–32.
23. Freidman M, Berasi CC, Fox TM, et al. Abrasion arthroplasty in osteoarthritic knee. *Clin Orthop Relat Res* 1984; 182:200–205.
24. Homminga G, Bilstra SK, Bouwmeester PS, et al. Perichondral grafting for cartilage lesions of the knee. *J Bone Joint Surg Br* 1990; 72B:1003–1007.

25. Bouwmeester S, Beckers JM, Kuijer R, et al. Long term results of rib perichondrial grafts for repair of cartilage defects in the human knee. *Int Orthop* 1997; 21:313–317.
26. Angermann P, Riegels-Nielsen P, Pedersen H. Osteochondritis dissecans of the fermoral condyles treated with periosteal transplantation. Presented at the American Academy of Orthopedic Sugeons annual meeting, New Orleans, LA, March 1998.
27. Matsusue Y, Yamamuro T, Hama H. Arthroscopic multiple osteochondral transplantation to the chondral defect in the knee associated with anterior cruciate ligament disruption. *Arthroscopy* 1993; 9:318–321.
28. Outerbridge H, Outerbridge A, Outerbridge R. The use of a lateral patellar autologous graft for the repair of a large osteochondral defect in the knee. *J Bone Joint Surg* 1995; 77A:65–72.
29. Takahashi S, Oka M, Kotoura Y, et al. Autogenous callo-osseous grafts for the repair of osteochondral defects. *J Bone Joint Surg Br* 1995; 77B:194–204.
30. Yamashita F, Sakakida K, Suzu F, et al. The transplantation of an autogeneic osteochondral fragment for osteochondritits dissecans of the knee. *Clin Orthop Relat Res* 1985; 201:43–50.
31. Peterson L. Autologous chondrocyte transplantation articular cartilage regeneration and transplantation. Presented at the American Academy of Orthopedic Sugeons annual meeting, New Orleans, LA, 1998
32. Fitzsimmons J, O'Driscoll S. Technical experience is important in harvesting periosteum for chondrogenisis. *Trans Orthop Res Soc* 1998; 23:914.
33. O'Driscoll S. Current concepts review: The healing and regeneration of articular cartilage. *J Bone Joint Surg* 1998; 80A:1795–1812.
34. Chen AC, Nagrampa JP, Schinagl RM, et al. Chondrocyte transplantation to artucular cartilage explants in vitro. *J Orthop Res* 1997; 15:791–802.
35. Simonian P, Sussmann PS, Wickiewicz TL, et al. Contact pressures at osteochondral donor sites in the knee. *Am J Sports Med* 1998; 26:491–494.
36. Blevins FT, Steadman JR, Rodrigo JJ, et al. Treatment of articular cartilage defects in athletes: An analysis of functional outcome and lesion appearance. *Orthopaedics* 1998; 21:761–768.
37. Gillogly S, Voight M, Blackburn T. Treatment of articular cartilage defects of the knee with autologous chondrocyte implantation. *J Orthop Sport Phys Ther* 1998; 28:241–251.
38. Irrgang J, Pezzulo D. Rehabilitation following surgical procedures to address articular cartilage lesions in the knee. *J Orthop Sports Phys Ther* 1998; 28:232–240.
39. Steadmen J. Long-term result of full-thickness articular cartilage defects of the knee treated with debridement and microfracture. Presented at the Linvatec Sports Medicine Conference, Vail, CO, December, 1997.
40. Peterson L. Autologous chondrocyte transplantation: Articular cartilage regeneration: Chondrocyte transplantation and other technologies. Presented at the American Academy or Orthopedic Surgeons annual meeting, San Francisco, CA, February, 1997.
41. Gu Z, Xiao J, Zhang X. The develoment of artificial articular cartilage: PVA-hydorgel. *Biomed Mater Eng* 1998; 8:75–81.
42. Frenkel S. Evaluation of a novel two-layered collagen implant for articular cartilage repair in a rabbit model. Presented at the American Academy of Orthopedic Surgeions annual meeting, San Francisco, CA, February, 1997.
43. Ewing J, Voto S. Arthorscopic surgical management of osteochondritis dissecans of the knee. *Arthroscopy* 1988; 4:37–40.

14

ASHOK S. REDDY
RALPH A.
GAMBARDELLA

Arthroscopic Treatment of Degenerative Joint Disease of the Knee

The role of arthroscopy in the treatment of degenerative joint disease of the knee has been in a state of constant evolution. Although the first report of the use of arthroscopic lavage to treat patients with degenerative joint disease appeared in 1934 (1), significant advances in the development of arthroscopic techniques were not made until the 1970s. Since then, the equipment and techniques have improved and a plethora of clinical studies have been performed. Many investigators (2–4) have reported degenerative changes in the knee occurring after total and partial meniscectomy, similar to those first described by Fairbanks in 1948 (5). More recently, arthroscopic treatment of degenerative joint disease has been shown to be efficacious in certain situations. Burks, Metcalf, and Metcalf in 1997 (6) reported the results of arthroscopic partial meniscectomies at 15-year follow-up in 146 patients. Overall there were 88% good or excellent results in ligamentously stable knees, and age was not found to be a significant factor determining outcome. Several other authors also have described the benefits of arthroscopic meniscectomy in an older population, especially in the absence of significant articular cartilage damage and tibiofemoral malalignment (7–10). Similar success has been reported with arthroscopic lavage and debridement, but studies of abrasion arthroplasty have shown mixed results (11–14).

As with any open surgical procedure, selection of appropriate patients for arthroscopic treatment of degenerative joint disease is an important predictor of a successful outcome. Patients with pain of short duration (i.e., less than 3 months) respond better to treatment, especially those with a history of a specific twisting injury and ensuing mechanical symptoms. Mechanical symptoms also may suggest loose bodies or symptomatic osteophytes, both of which correlate well with good results postoperatively. Age alone should not be a factor in the selection process. Patients with pending litigation and work-related compensation claims tend to do poorly.

On physical examination, the recent appearance of an effusion, joint-line tenderness, and a positive McMurray's test usually correlate with a good result from arthroscopic treatment. Mechanical malalignment, with varus deformity greater than 10 degrees or valgus angulation greater than 15 degrees, correlates with poor results and is a relative contraindications to the procedure. Ligamentous instability also is associated with poor results.

The presence of loose bodies or osteophytes on radiographs that correspond with a patient's area of pain are associated with good results. Complete loss of joint space on standing films is associated with poor results. Because of a high incidence of incidental findings, results of magnetic resonance scans must be correlated with the area of the patients' symptoms and findings as noted on physical examination.

Excellent technique is necessary to treat patients with degenerative joint disease successfully, as these patients often have tight knee compartments that make access a challenge. Good visualization is mandatory and requires adequate fluid distension, high flow,

■ HISTORY OF THE TECHNIQUE

■ INDICATIONS AND CONTRAINDICATIONS

■ SURGICAL TECHNIQUES

159

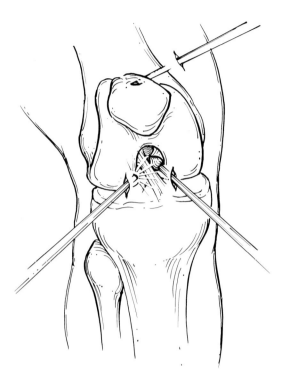

■ FIGURE 14-1   Schematic representation of portals used for
                                                            arthroscopic instrumentation.

and an adequate light source. Portal placement is extremely important, because correct placement not only enhances visualization but also facilitates instrumentation. We prefer vertical incisions with standard anteromedial, anterolateral, and superomedial portals (Fig. 14-1).

The anteromedial and anterolateral portals are made with the knee flexed 90 degrees. It is our preference to make the incision with a no. 11 scalpel blade, with the cutting edge facing proximally to avoid inadvertent incision into the meniscus. A straight Kelly clamp then is used to enlarge the portal, and the arthroscope is introduced using the blunt trochar and sheath, placing it into the suprapatellar pouch. The joint is distended with fluid, and a supramedial portal is established parallelling skin lines, using a large flow cannula. We prefer inflow through the arthroscope to keep debris away from the field of view.

It is important to perform the diagnostic arthroscopic examination systematically to ensure a complete evaluation regardless of the preoperative diagnosis. Failure to inspect each compartment in a standard order may result in areas being overlooked. We prefer a sequence of evaluation of the suprapatellar pouch followed by the patellofemoral joint medial to lateral. Next comes inspection of the medial gutter into the medial compartment, followed by visualization of the intercondylar notch area, inspection into the lateral compartments, and finally the lateral gutter. It also may be possible to visualize the posteromedial and posterolateral compartments through the intercondylar notch.

Accurate knowledge of the patient's specific preoperative complaints and the results of the physical examination can be extremely helpful in determining whether pathology viewed arthroscopically should be addressed. In general, unstable meniscal fragments and unstable tears should be removed and the remaining meniscal rims contoured to leave as much normal tissue as possible (Fig. 14-2A,B). We prefer, in performing chondroplasties, to remove only unstable tissue or chondral flaps, and to make specific effort not to be overzealous in the use of motorized instruments (Figs. 14-3A,B and 14-4). In general, abrasion arthroplasty should not be performed. Particularly in compartments of the knee in which preoperative symptoms have been minimal, every effort should be made to not traumatize the compartment.

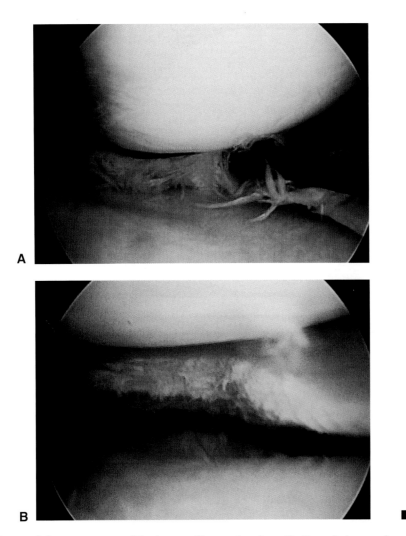

A

B

A: Arthroscopic view of the medial compartment of the knee, with a probe placed in the substance of a complex, degenerative meniscal tear. **B:** The same meniscus after removal of the torn tissue and contouring of the remaining meniscal rim.

There are several minor variations in technique that may be used, depending on the preference of the surgeon. The use of a leg holder is controversial in the older population. Particularly in men, it is not unusual to encounter a varus knee with a tight medial compartment, and in these instances a leg holder may help with visualization. In general, we prefer a single lateral post to provide valgus stress if needed, and the figure-four position for access to the lateral compartment.

The use of a tourniquet for arthroscopic surgery is also controversial. Bleeding may be minimized by the injection of both the portals and the joint with a combination of didocaine or bupivacaine with epinephrine. Sherman et al. (15) reported an increased complication rate with arthroscopic surgery associated with the use of a tourniquet for longer than 45 minutes. We prefer the tourniquet, however, as a means to enhance visualization and thereby decrease overall surgical time.

Some surgeons prefer to use only the two inferior portals, without using the superior portal for either inflow or outflow purposes. Their reasoning may be to avoid trauma to the quadriceps mechanism, which may impede postoperative rehabilitation. Because of the proven benefit of lavage in patients with degenerative joint disease, our preference is to use all three portals and enhance our ability to irrigate the joint thoroughly.

■ TECHNICAL ALTERNATIVES AND PITFALLS

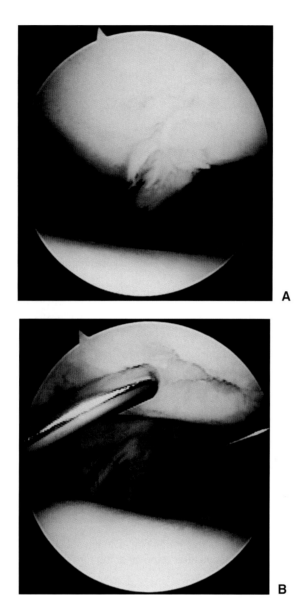

■ FIGURE 14-3

A: Arthroscopic view of the patellofemoral joint showing isolated chondromalacia of the patellar facet.
B: Removal of the loose, fibrillated tissue with a motorized shaver.

■ REHABILITATION

Rehabilitation after arthroscopic procedures must be tailored to the individual, in consideration of the findings at surgery. In general, patients who require only meniscectomies with minimal debridement are able to progress more quickly in a rehabilitation program than patients who have had extensive chondroplasties involving multiple compartments. Patients may present at the first visit after synovectomy with a large hematoma that requires aspiration or evacuation.

The patient should be encouraged to walk, but a cane or crutch may be necessary for a few days after surgery to assist with ambulation. It is important to emphasize early range-of-motion exercises, as well as an isometric quadriceps strengthening program, as soon as possible after arthroscopy. Many patients with degenerative arthritis do best with a supervised physical therapy program for 1 to 3 months. The use of a stationary bicycle and a walking program are encouraged in the first month. Most patients then can resume full activities gradually in the second or third month postoperatively.

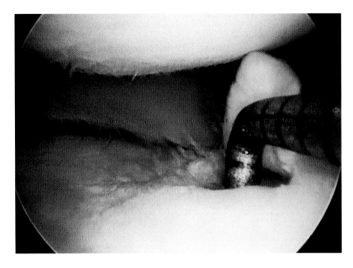

Arthroscopic view of the lateral compartment revealing a loose chondral flap on the tibial plateau.

■ OUTCOMES AND FUTURE DIRECTIONS

Arthroscopic treatment of degenerative joint disease is a very successful procedure, with a low incidence of morbidity if used in carefully selected patients. The treatment should be focused to address the areas corresponding to the patient's symptoms and physical findings.

Although abrasion arthroplasty and drilling of large chondral defects no longer are recommended, newer devices using thermal or radiofrequency energy to perform chondroplasties have been used. These instruments may be able to smooth the edges of the articular defects and help prevent fragmentation and ensuing synovitis, which can occur if the edges are left alone. One of these newer methods, called "coblation," involves a process of energy-mediated cold ablation in volumetric tissue removal, presumably with little or no collateral tissue damage. A preliminary anecdotal report of coblation in 130 patients with articular cartilage defects was encouraging, with improved postoperative recovery and less pain and swelling (16). More research is needed to define optimal parameters for the use of this technology, and more long-term clinical outcome studies must be done.

References

1. Burman MS, Finkelstein H, Mayer L. Arthroscopy of the knee. *J Bone Joint Surg Am* 1934; 16:255–268.
2. Tapper EM, Hoover NW. Late results after menisectomy. *J Bone Joint Surg Am* 1969; 51:517–526.
3. Jackson JP. Degenerative changes in the knee after menisectomy. *BMJ* 1968; 2:525–527.
4. Allen PR, Denham RA, Swan AV. Late degenerative changes after menisectomy. *J Bone Joint Surg Br* 1984; 66:666–671.
5. Fairbanks TJ. Knee joint changes after menisectomy. *J Bone Joint Surg Br* 1948; 30:664–670.
6. Burks RT, Metcalf MM, Metcalf RW. Fifteen year follow-up of arthroscopic partial menisectomy. *Arthroscopy* 1997;B6:673–679.
7. McBride GG, Constine RM, Hoffmann AA, et al. Arthroscopic partial medial menisectomy in the older patient. *J Bone Joint Surg Am* 1984; 66:547.
8. Bonamo JJ, Kessler KJ, Noah J. Arthroscopy menisectomy in patients over the age of 40. *Am J Sports Med* 1992; 20:422–429.
9. Covall DJ, Wasilewski SA. Roentgenographic changes after athroscopic menisectomy: five-year follow-up in patients more than 45 years of age. *Arthroscopy* 1992; 8:242–246.
10. Ogilvie-Harris DJ, Fitsialos DP. Arthroscopic management of the degenerative knee. *Arthroscopy* 1991; 7:151–157.
11. Livesley PJ, Doherty, Needoff M, et al. Arthroscopic lavage of osteoarthritic knees. *J Bone Joint Surg Br* 1991; 73:922–926.

12. Sprague NF III. Arthroscopic debridement for degenerative knee joint disease. *Clin Orthop* 1981; 160:118–123.

13. Shahriaree H, O'Connor RF, Nottage W. Seven years follow-up arthroscopic debridement of the degenerative knee. *Field of View* 1982; 1:1.

14. Rand JA. Role of arthroscopy in osteoarthritis of the knee. *Arthroscopy* 1991; 7:358–363.

15. Sherman OH, Fox JM, Snyder SJ, et al. Arthroscopy:"No-problem surgery." *J Bone Joint Surg Am* 1986; 68:256–265.

16. Kaplan L, Uribe JW, Sasken L, et al. The acute effects of radiofrequency energy in articular cartilage: an in vitro study. *Arthroscopy* 2000; 16(1):2–5.

F. DANIEL KHARRAZI
KELLY G. VINCE

15

Subvastus Surgical Approach for Total Knee Arthroplasty

The subvastus surgical approach provides an anatomic approach to the knee for arthroplasty surgery. It has been used for many decades in Europe, and Hofmann and associates revived interest in this approach with a study published in *Clinical Orthopedics* (1). Compared with the standard median parapatellar arthrotomy, its advantages are preservation of an intact extensor mechanism and the vascular supply to the patella and quadriceps expansion (2). An intact extensor mechanism may allow a more accurate assessment of patellar tracking during surgery. Although many investigators feel that the subvastus approach decreases the need for lateral patellar retinacular releases because the quadriceps tendon is not incised, this may not be the case. It is true, however, that the surgeon can make a more realistic evaluation of patellar tracking with an intact tendon and so is less likely to perform the release. A similar effect might be appreciated with standard approaches if the medial arthrotomy were closed with several sutures as the decision as to the necessity of a lateral patellar retinacular release was made (3). In a study comparing 40 total knee arthroplasties performed with the subvastus and 49 performed with a standard parapatellar approach, there was no statistically significant difference in patellar tracking between the two groups (4). Lateral patellar retinacular releases, however, were performed in almost twice as many cases with parapatellar arthrotomies. This strongly suggests that the standard approach overestimates the need for releases of the patellar retinaculum (5). Preservation of the vascular supply to the patella, quadriceps expansion, and soft tissues may decrease wound complications.

■ HISTORY OF THE TECHNIQUE

The subvastus approach is appealing in carefully selected patients undergoing primary total knee arthroplasty by a surgeon intimately familiar with knee anatomy. This approach for revision surgery, although feasible, is not the best choice, because a tibial tubercle osteotomy may be required to extend the approach.

Clearly, the obese, stiff, or muscular knee is better treated by standard arthrotomies for knee arthroplasty. It has been said that patients with badly deformed knees are poor candidates for the subvastus approach. It can be argued, however, that the bad valgus knee is usually quite supple, with a patella that everts easily. The bad varus knee yields to any approach more readily if a medial release is incorporated into the approach, allowing for external rotation of the tibia, which repositions the tibia and tubercle laterally and thus facilitates patellar eversion. Bad varus or valgus deformities do not constitute a contraindication to the subvastus approach.

Comparison of primary total knee arthroplasties performed through a subvastus approach with those performed through the standard median parapatellar approach has shown the former to have significantly greater strength after the 1-week and 1-month postoperative intervals. However, there is no significant strength difference at 3 months (2). Range-of-motion measurements comparing the two approaches have shown no difference (2,4). The lack of a clear long-term functional advantage of the subvastus approach makes the issue of approach in the appropriate patient more a matter of surgeon preference and style.

■ INDICATIONS AND CONTRAINDICATIONS

165

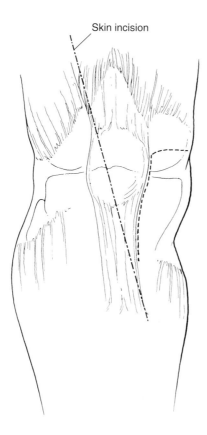

Skin incision

Skin incision and arthrotomy. The skin incision for a subvastus arthrotomy resembles standard approaches for
other arthrotomies (*solid line*). The distal incision should
stay off of the tibial tubercle, because healing is compromised over a boney prominence. It then angles parallel to
the quadriceps muscle, creating a smaller lateral flap that is
easier to evert. The arthrotomy is L-shaped, going all the
way to bone medial to the tubercle and proximal to the inferior third of the patella before turning posteriorly.

■   FIGURE 15-1

■   SURGICAL
    TECHNIQUES

Cutaneous Landmarks   The patella and the tibial tubercle must be identified to guide the
skin incision. Poorly placed incisions may stretch and compromise the skin and hamper exposure of the joint for the duration of the operation.

Incision   The incision spans the knee from a point proximal and lateral to the knee, over
the patella, ending approximately 1 cm medial to the tibial tubercle (Fig. 15-1). The lateral
origin of the incision facilitates patellar eversion and creates a smaller lateral skin and subcutaneous flap. The incision should be kept off of the tibial tubercle for three reasons: healing may be compromised over prominent subcutaneous bones, such as the tibial tubercle
and olecranon; incisions directly over the tubercle inevitably lie directly over and may
jeopardize the patellar tendon, essential to the arthroplasty; and incisions over the tubercle
may create discomfort druing kneeling.

Medial Skin Flap   A medial skin flap is created, establishing a plane deep to the light fascial layer. The fascial layer provides some of the skin vasculature. This medial flap is neither
everted nor stretched. Unlike lateral flaps, the medial flap is not susceptible to necrosis.

Elevation of the Vastus Medialis   The medial border of the vastus medialis is palpated.
With finger dissection (to protect the contents of Hunter's subsartorial canal) the vastus
medialis is elevated off of the medial femur, revealing the thin capsule and synovium on
the medial part of the suprapatellar pouch (Fig. 15-2). This sets the stage for the arthrotomy
itself.

Arthrotomy (Medial Limb)   An L-shaped arthrotomy is performed with an incision
made from posterior to anterior through the capsule, across the medial femoral condyle
and up to the edge of the patella. The arthrotomy leaves two well-defined edges of the capsule (used for a synovial closure at the completion of the arthroplasty; Fig. 15-3).

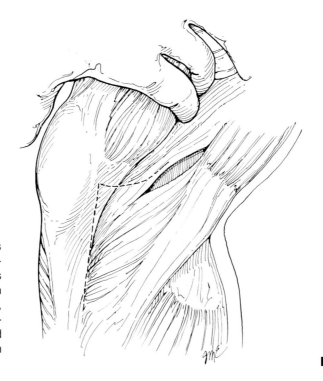

Blunt dissection and elevation of vastus medialis. The initial dissection on the medial side is performed best with scissors or scalpel. Because of the vasculature on the adductor side of the thigh, however, fingers are safer to drive under the muscle. The index finger is pushed deep and then driven medially until the femur can be palpated.

■ FIGURE 15-2

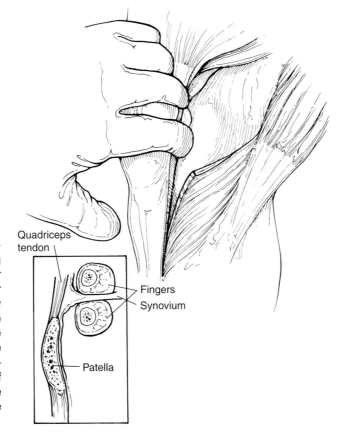

The synovium. Closure of the synovium can be facilitated by leaving a cuff of it attached to the extensor mechanism of the supra-patellar pouch. This is accomplished easily by inserting the index finger into the suprapatellar pouch near the patella, and the third digit on the other side of the synovium immediately superior (**inset**). A width of synovium corresponding to the thickness of the fingers is available for later closure.

Quadriceps tendon

Fingers

Synovium

Patella

■ FIGURE 15-3

Preserving the Capsule for Later Closure   The index finger is inserted into the suprapatellar pouch through the arthrotomy and the third finger is placed on the other side of the capsule (outside and above the knee joint) superiorly.

The edge of the capsule grasped between the fingers later is retrieved for capsular closure.

Division of the Capsule of the Suprapatellar Pouch   The capsule is cut to the midline of the femur, with a scalpel, just under the dorsum of the fingers. Unless the arthrotomy includes this capsular division, it is impossible to evert the patella.

Arthrotomy (Lower Limb)   The lower (vertical) limb of the L-shaped arthrotomy begins at the anterior end of the transverse incision. The lower incision proceeds along the medial border of the patella, within 1 cm of the medial border of the patellar tendon and down onto the anterior tibia. The medial capsule should be elevated sharply as one flap. Using the knife blade to create multiple ribbons of soft tissue, which ultimately cannot be closed, should be avoided.

Elevation of the Medial Capsule from the Tibia   A solid, intact flap of periosteum and overlying tissue is elevated sharply off of the tibia using a scalpel. This flap is initiated at its superior and lateral tip, using sharp dissection to develop a triangular flap. The flap is used for closure at the end of the case.

Separation of the Patellar Tendon from the Anterior Tibia   Several maneuvers may be used to facilitate patellar eversion without threatening the integrity of the extensor mechanism. To separate the fat pad from the anterior tibia, with the knee fully extended, one lifts the patella straight up off the anterior femur with two flexed fingers. Without pulling the extensor mechanism off to the lateral side, the scalpel blade is introduced against the anterior tibia, immediately proximal to the junction of the tendon and the tubercle. The blade should sweep proximally, away from the patellar tendon attachment.

Elevation of the Medial Capsule   To elevate the medial capsule and periosteum in one layer, a Key elevator is used with a small mallet to deliver discrete amounts of force to the tissue, without the risk of forcing, slipping, or plunging. The medial collateral ligament, situated further around the corner of the tibia, is a consolidation of the layers of the medial capsule, which at this location are neither as thick nor as strong as the "ligament" itself. The fibers of the ligament–capsule complex to be elevated are oriented vertically, free proximally, and attached distally. The Key elevator should be oriented to act as a wedge in the axilla of the tissue–bone interface, driven between the soft periosteum and bone.

Removal of Medial Osteophytes   The Key elevator can be used, if oriented proximally, to remove medial osteophytes around the medial edge of the tibia. The elevator can be used to elevate the most proximal attachment of the deep medial collateral ligament further from the tibia, irrespective of the deformity of the knee. This should continue medially to at least the midcoronal line. In exposing a varus knee, this elevation can be continued around the posteromedial corner of the knee, detaching the semimembranosis insertion. This medial release allows external rotation of the tibia at the moment of flexion and patellar eversion. External rotation of the tibia places the tibial tubercle more laterally and facilitates exposure. Except in severe varus deformities, the attachment of the pes anserinus should be spared.

Closure   The subvastus arthrotomy provides the opportunity for a near anatomic closure (Fig. 15-4). If the incision through the synovium was performed with care to leave a cuff on both sides, this too may be closed with a fine absorbable suture. The synovium is closed with running suture, and then the arthrotomy is reapproximated with heavier absorbable interrupted sutures. The extensor mechanism assumes its normal anatomic relationship very easily.

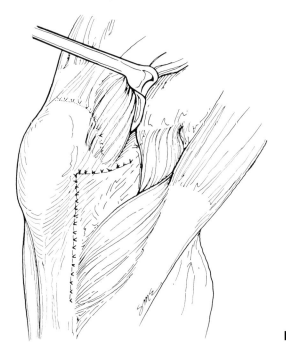

Closure. The synovium can be closed with a running absorbable suture (*lighter colored suture line superior to the patella*). Heavier (e.g., no. 1) absorbable suture works well in the arthrotomy. The extensor mechanism has not been disrupted by the arthrotomy, and the patient should enjoy rapid rehabilitation.

■ FIGURE 15-4

The standard approaches for knee arthroplasty continue to work well and are appropriate alternatives to the subvastus arthrotomy. In fact, many experienced knee surgeons feel that there is no particular advantage to this surgical approach.

If, however, the subvastus approach is used and there is difficulty with eversion of the patella, the surgeon must proceed slowly. Failure to do so can result in avulsion of the patellar tendon from the tubercle or rupture of the patellar tendon, both of which are regarded as catastrophic complications of knee arthroplasty. If exposure is difficult, the alternatives all require attention to detail. Small amounts of the patellar tendon insertion should be elevated from the tibial tubercle, extending more than 3 cm distally. In this way, if the forces are excessive, the tendon is more likely to peel off rather than tear. The tibia should be rotated maximally externally, so as to position the tubercle laterally, which facilitates eversion. The superior capsule, in the region of the suprapatellar pouch, must be divided up to its superior apex, and the vastus medialis must be free from the overlying skin and fascia. A large rongeur may be used to remove some of the cartilage, scar, and bone from the anterior aspect of the lateral femoral condyle. This makes it easier for the patella to be turned over the edge of the lateral femur, and the increased friction with the exposed cancellous bone prevents the patella from slipping back as the knee is flexed.

The surgeon needs help with eversion at this point. The assistant can aid by placing a hand behind the knee and helping to bend it. The surgeon uses one hand to externally rotate the tibia forcefully, and the thumb of the other to apply pressure on the articular surface of the patella to evert it. Persistent problems may require an extension of the arthrotomy into the tendon of the vastus medialis, converting the subvastus arthrotomy to a limited parapatellar approach. A full parapatellar approach still can be performed, although it rarely is required. The ultimate solution is a tibial tubercle osteotomy. Patience and attention to detail enable a successful subvastus arthrotomy to succeed in all but the most difficult cases.

Rehabilitation after subvastus arthrotomy if anything can be accelerated. There is anatomic, if not scientific, reason to believe that the forces on the repair of the extensor mechanism are less, given that the quadriceps tendon has been maintained intact. There should be minimal concern over disruption of the closure. Accordingly, the patients should

■ TECHNICAL ALTERNATIVES AND PITFALLS

■ REHABILITATION

experience less pain and be willing to proceed with an accelerated protocol. Anecdotes of straight leg raising in the recovery room following knee arthroplasty with the subvastus arthrotomy have been circulated but not substantiated with clinical studies.

■ OUTCOMES AND FUTURE DIRECTIONS

Future investigations may include larger numbers of cases and objective evaluation of strength testing, as well as electromyographic evaluation of knee function after various surgical approaches. Scintigraphic evaluation of circulation to the patella would be a welcome corroboration to the anatomic expectation that this approach spares the blood supply to the patella.

REFERENCES

1. Hofmann AA, Plaster RL, Murdock LE. Subvastus (Southern) approach for primary total knee arthroplasty. *Clin Orthop* 1991; 269:70–77.
2. Faure BT, Benjamin JB, Lindsey B, et al. Comparison of the subvastus and paramedian surgical approaches in bilateral knee arthroplasty. *J Arthroplasty* 1993; 8:511–516.
3. Ogata K, Ishinishi T, Hara M. Evaluation of patellar retinacular tension during total knee arthroplasty: Special emphasis on lateral retinacular release. *J Arthroplasty* 1997; 12:651–656.
4. Ritter MAK. Comparison of two anterior medial appraoches to total knee arthroplasty. *Am J Knee Surg* 1990; 3:168–171.
5. Bindelglass DF, Vince KG. Patellar tilt and subluxation following subvastus and parapatellar approach in total knee arthroplasty: Implication for surgical technique. *J Arthroplasty* 1996; 11:507–511.

16

Surgical Technique for Tibial Tuberosity Elevation

Adequate exposure of the knee in total knee arthroplasty, either primary or revision, can be difficult at times. There are various factors that come into play, including the adequacy of the skin and soft tissues, the number of prior surgical procedures, and the presence of infrapatellar contracture or patella baja. Although these factors are encountered most commonly in revision total knee arthroplasty, it is not unusual to encounter them in primary knee arthroplasty. In the case of primary arthroplasty, prior procedures may have included open meniscectomies or debridements, tibial osteotomy, or open reduction and internal fixation of tibial plateau fracture.

Soft-tissue procedures that have been described to enhance exposure include the rectus snip (1) and the quadriceps turndown (2,3). Although the rectus snip is useful in many situations, it does not always allow adequate exposure and knee joint mobilization in more difficult situations, particularly in the face of patella baja or infrapatellar contracture.

The quadriceps turndown allows for improved exposure but can result in an unacceptable quadriceps lag postoperatively (3). In addition, patella baja may result, particularly if a V-to-Y closure is used to improve the flexion range.

Tibial tuberosity osteotomy also has been reported to be a useful technique for exposure in difficult arthroplasty situations, both primary and revision (4–6). With this technique, proximal soft-tissue dissection is minimized, resulting in less disturbance to the quadriceps mechanism. Postoperative problems reported with this technique have included displacement of the osteotomized fragment (4), as well as tibial fractures (7).

The technique that is described in this chapter is one that involves the use of an extended tibial tuberosity osteotomy. Like other reported techniques, this technique allows for satisfactory exposure in most difficult knee arthroplasty situations. In addition, the described procedure can assist with enhancement of patellar tracking through medial or lateral translation of the tibial tuberosity. Proximal displacement of the patella can be achieved in a controlled manner in situations in which this is desirable to restore the relationship of the patella to the reconstructed tibial femoral joint line.

The approach to the difficult knee arthroplasty requires planned and controlled surgical aggression. Otherwise, inadequate exposure with the associated limitation of access to bone and soft tissue can compromise the surgeon's chances of achieving a satisfactory reconstruction.

■ HISTORY OF THE TECHNIQUE

Tibial tuberosity osteotomy is indicated if difficulty with exposure is anticipated in knee arthroplasty, either primary or revision. Specific indications may include the following clinical situations:

1. Multiple prior surgical procedures
2. Arthrofibrosis
3. Fusion take down
4. Patella baja
5. Severe patellar maltracking
6. Two-stage reconstruction for infection

■ INDICATIONS AND CONTRAINDICATIONS

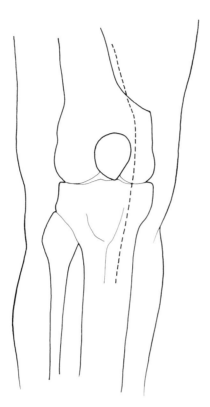

■ FIGURE 16-1   Extension of the skin incision medial to tibial tuberosity.

■ SURGICAL
TECHNIQUES

Step I   The skin incision should be distal to the tibial tuberosity approximately 8 cm (Fig. 16-1). One must stay off the tibial crest if possible and continue the incision either to the medial or lateral aspect of the crest, depending on the initial exposure. The skin incision may be determined by the presence of prior incisions, which may not be optimally located. If possible, the skin incision should be kept to the medial side of the tibial crest.

Step II: Delineation of Tibial Tuberosity Fragment To Be Elevated   The most superior insertion of the patellar tendon into the tibia should be identified (Fig. 16-2). With a right angle retractor, the patellar tendon is pulled anteriorly, and with sharp dissection the superior insertion can be identified clearly. The medial and lateral borders of the insertion are identified at the level of the tuberosity.

With either cautery or methylene blue, the distal extent of the osteotomy is measured and marked 6 to 7 cm from the superior margin of the patellar tendon insertion.

Step III: Elevation of Fragment   The dimensions of the fragment should be as follows: 6 to 7 cm long, 1.5 to 2.0 cm wide, and 1.0 to 1.5 cm thick at the upper end. The fragment should taper toward the distal end (Fig. 16-3).

Beginning medially, a sharp osteotome 2.0 cm wide is used. The planned position of the osteotomy along the medial tibial crest is marked, tapering the fragment distally. It is recommended that the osteotomy be performed with a sharp osteotome, but if the tibial bone is particularly hard, a thin-bladed oscillating saw can be used to cut the cortex. The cut plane is the coronal plane.

At the superior end (superior margin of the patellar tendon insertion), a transverse cut is made in the proximal tibia using an osteotome to create a platform at right angles to the longitudinal axis.

Inferiorly, the fragment should be tapered. The tapering can be to an apex, or a 45-degree bevel can be used. Again, if the tibial cortex is hard, a thin-bladed oscillating saw should be used to avoid splintering the tibial cortex.

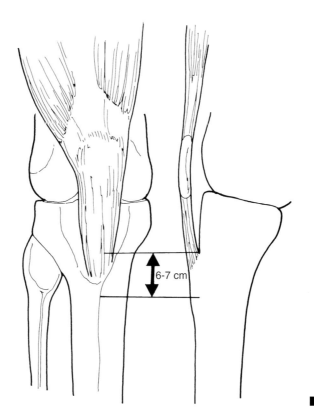

Definition of the extent of the osteotomy
fragment.

■ FIGURE 16-2

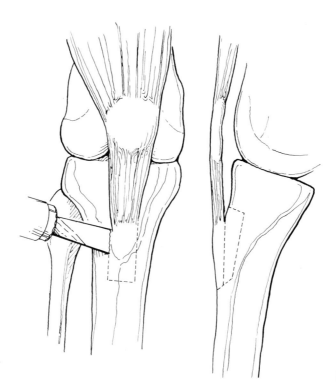

Osteotomy of the tuberosity fragment.

■ FIGURE 16-3

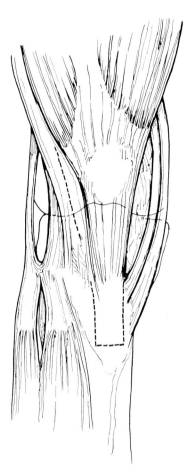

Elevation of the tuberosity.

With the superior, medial, and inferior cuts completed, the lateral cortex is broached using a sharp thin osteotome (Fig. 16-4).

The tibial tuberosity fragment then is reflected laterally.

No further elevation or dissection may be required in some circumstances. If satisfactory exposure still cannot be achieved, however, the lateral soft-tissue attachments of the tuberosity can be divided and the tuberosity elevated. The dissection can be carried laterally up to the level of the inferior margin of the vastus lateralis, preserving the superior lateral geniculate vessels.

Step IV: Reattachment of Fragment The tibial tuberosity fragment is reattached using a plate and screws (Fig. 16-5). The selection of plate and screw size is determined by the patient's size, bone size, and quality and adequacy of soft tissues.

In smaller patients or in those with thin skin coverage, a small-fragment semitubular plate with small-fragment screws can be used. In heavier patients and in those with more forgiving soft-tissue coverage, a large-fragment one-third tubular plate with large-fragment screws should be employed. The latter is optimal but is not always possible. A six- or seven-hole plate should be used. With the large-fragment plate, six holes usually are adequate; with the small-fragment plate, a seven-hole plate should be selected. The plate should be bent to match the contour of the tuberosity.

Depending on bone size and prosthesis dimensions, single-cortex screws may need to be used. If possible, however, bicortical fixation should be used.

The same situation applies if extension stems are used in a revision situation. If the stem is press-fit, then it is likely that single-cortex screws are required. In this case, it is recom-

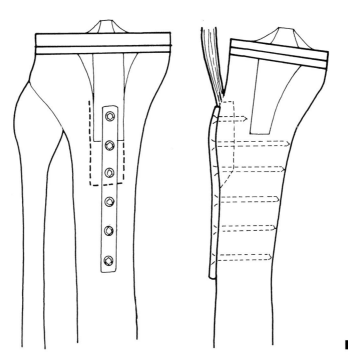

■ FIGURE 16-5

Reattachment of the osteotomy fragment.

mended that a seven-hole plate be used, so that four cortices can be engaged below the level of the osteotomy.

An osteotomy fragment 6 to 7 cm in length allows for the use of three screws in the osteotomy fragment.

Option: Alteration of Patellar Position Through Osteotomy This technique allows the patella to be shifted proximally, distally, medially, or laterally as necessary (Fig. 16-6).

To shift the osteotomy medially or laterally, one ascertains the optimal position for patellar tracking and fixes the osteotomy in this position.

Proximal shift of the patella may be desired in situations in which raising the tibiofemoral joint line is unavoidable to achieve satisfactory reconstruction and soft-tissue balance.

Superior elevation of the osteotomy fragment can be achieved as follows: With sharp dissection, the surgeon carefully separates the superior fibers of the patellar tendon insertion from the tibial tuberosity. The amount dissected should correspond to the desired amount of patellar elevation. The maximum that can be achieved through this technique is usually 1.0 cm, but if the tendon inserts over a longer distance, 1.5 cm of superior elevation can be achieved. Once the tendon has been dissected free from the tuberosity, a small rongeur or bone cutter is used to cut the osteotomy fragment at a right angle.

This allows abutment of the cut end of the tuberosity against the previously created platform of the proximal tibia. At times, particularly in the case of revision, the osteotomy fragment abuts up against the undersurface of the tibial component.

The tuberosity fragment then is reattached as described previously. Prior to plate application, the gap is bone-grafted at the inferior end of the tuberosity fragment.

Closure and Dressing Secure closure over the plate and screws and two layers is required. My preference is to use subcuticular suture at this level of the incision, and to reinforce this with interrupted 3-0 Prolene (or similar). The reinforcement sutures usually are removed after 5 to 7 days, once satisfactory wound healing has been achieved.

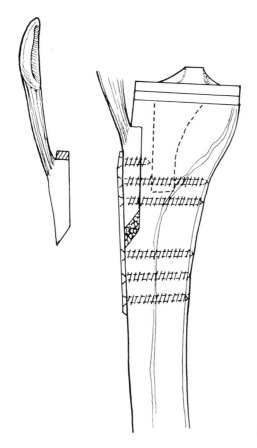

■   FIGURE 16-6   Proximal slide of the tuberosity and reattachment.

The dressing applied is a well-padded Jones bandage, with a knee immobilizer holding the knee in full extension.

■ TECHNICAL
ALTERNATIVES AND
PITFALLS

The following are to be avoided:

1. Too short an osteotomy fragment, which results in poor fixation with possible loss of control of the fragment
2. To thin an osteotomy fragment, which may result in vertical fracture of the fragment

In either of these situations, it is recommended that the fixation be supplemented with wires. It may be necessary to limit postoperative rehabilitation for the first 6 weeks, to allow healing to occur.

■ REHABILITATION

In general, it is possible to follow the rehabilitation guidelines generally used subsequent to an arthroplasty procedure.

If there is any concern about the integrity of the proximal tibia for weight bearing, then the patient should be kept to touch weight bearing with use of crutches for 6 weeks.

Range of movement can be achieved through the usual means, per the surgeon's preference. This may include passive movement, active assisted movement, or continuous passive motion.

Early quadriceps retraining is encouraged. Static quadriceps contractions are allowed, as well as active end-range extension, usually employed over a roll (30 degrees to maximum extension). Resisted quadriceps exercising is not allowed until 6 weeks after the operation to allow time for the osteotomy to unite.

■ DISCUSSION

This technique has been employed in both primary and revision total knee arthroplasty with success. Essential elements of the technique include use of a tuberosity fragment of appropriate size as described previously, as well as establishment of a superior platform if at all possible.

The advantage of this technique over other techniques is considered to be in the mechanics of the fixation achieved. The plate and screws act to stabilize the fragment in the direction of quadriceps pull and therefore reduce the risk of proximal migration of the fragment, which can be seen in methods tht employ fixation that is disadvantaged mechanically relative to the pull of the quadriceps.

The stress-riser effect of the osteotomy is reduced by application of the plate and screws. In addition, the length of the osteotomy usually brings it well below the level of tibial tray stems employed in primary arthroplasty. If extension stems are used, the osteotomy is located in the midportion of the device and therefore is protected through both intramedullary and extramedullary fixation.

This technique also allows for proximal shift of the patella of 1.0 to 1.5 cm in situations in which reconstruction of the knee has required elevation of the joint line. If this technique is employed in this situation, an early quadriceps lag is to be anticipated, with resolution of the lag generally seen by 3 months subsequent to the procedure.

Subcutaneous prominence of the plate and screws occurs occasionally. In these situations, it may be necessary to consider removal of the internal fixation subsequent to osteotomy union. It is recommended that the plate and screws be left *in situ* for 6 months, if possible.

References
1. Garvin KL, Scuderi G, Insall JD. Evolution of the quadriceps snip. *Clin Orthop* 1995; 321:131–137.
2. Coonse K, Adams JD. A new operative approach to the knee joint. *Surg Gynecol Obstet* 1943; 77:344–347.
3. Wolff AM, Hungerford DS, Krachow KA, et al. Osteotomy of the tibial tubercle during total knee replacement: A report of twenty-six cases. *J Bone Joint Surg Am* 1989; 71:848–852.
4. Whiteside LA, Ohl MD. Tibial tubercle osteotomy for exposure of the difficult total knee arthroplasty. *Clin Orthop* 1990; 260:6–9.
5. Whiteside LA. Exposure in difficult total knee arthroplasty using tibial tubercle osteotomy. *Clin Orthop* 1995; 321:32–35.
6. Trousdale RT, Hanssen AD, Rand JA, et al. V-Y quadricepsplasty in total knee arthroplasty. *Clin Orthop* 1993; 286:48–55.
7. Ritter MA, Carr K, Keating EM, et al. Tibial shaft fracture following tibial tubercle osteotomy. *J Arthroplasty* 1996; 11:117–119.

ROBERT W.
CHANDLER

17

High Tibial Osteotomy: Technique of Plate Fixation

■ HISTORY OF THE TECHNIQUE

High tibial osteotomy (HTO) as a treatment option for medial compartment arthritis of the knee was developed during the late 1960s (1–4). In the United States, Coventry (3,5–10) was an early and influential supporter of the method, promoting the use of a stepped staple as internal fixation. In the 30 years since its advent, the HTO has undergone many modifications. It has been combined with other procedures such as elevation of the tibial tubercle, anterior cruciate ligament reconstruction, and athroscopic joint debridement. External fixation has been explored with the Charnley clamp and later with a wide variety of external fixators. Internal fixation with staples, buttress plates, blade plates, and tension band devices has been explored. Finally, open wedge methods, using single-stage plates and iliac crest grafts or multistage techniques with osteotaxis, have gained some popularity.

In spite of these developments, the operation has retained its fundamental character from the early days. The angle of the leg is changed to a net valgus position to shift force into the healthy lateral compartment and away from the diseased medial compartment. The technique of lateral closing wedge HTO with preoperative planning and internal tension band fixation is described in this chapter.

■ INDICATIONS AND CONTRAINDICATIONS

Critical to the ultimate success of HTO is careful observance of the indications and contraindications for the operation. Pain should be localized predominantly to the medial compartment. If necessary as a confirmatory test, radionuclide imaging is used to identify increased uptake in the subchondral medial plateau cortex. Relative varus malalignment should be less than or equal to 12 degrees. Larger deformities are more difficult to correct with a lateral closing wedge technique and may be associated with instability. Bone quality must be adequate to hold fixation and not undergo collapse. If anterior cruciate instability is present, the surgeon must decide whether instability or arthritis dominates the clinical picture and perform the indicated procedure. HTO combined with anterior cruciate ligament reconstruction is technically demanding and typically best done by those experienced in the method. Finally, medial collateral ligament instability, if present, must be assessed with stress radiographs in order to avoid excess correction, because varus loading in single-limb stance shifts to valgus loading after osteotomy and therefore stresses the medial collateral ligament.

Contraindications to HTO include joint obliquity, lateral compartment pain, range of motion less than 90 degrees, and factors such as compromised healing, neurologic impairment, noncompliance, and inflammatory arthritis. Body weight greater than 30% above ideal has be cited as a relative contraindication for HTO (10).

■ SURGICAL TECHNIQUES

Preoperative Planning The goal of HTO is to direct the weight-bearing line into the lateral from the medial compartment. Ideally, the weight-bearing line intersects the line of the joint on the anteroposterior radiograph, at a point at one quarter of the distance measured from the center of the knee to the edge of the lateral plateau. The mechanical axis measures 5 to 7 degrees, and the anatomic or femoral tibial angle measures 8 to 10 degrees after correction.

These measurements can be made as follows: Full-length standing radiographs are obtained to plan the operation. The weight-bearing line is draw from the center of the hip to the center of the ankle, intersecting the joint line in the medial compartment in varus knees. HTO should shift the weight-bearing line into the lateral compartment, as long as excessive valgus does not result. The correction angle can be obtained on full-length films using the mechanical axis, which is the angle formed by the intersection of lines drawn from the center of the hip and the center of the ankle to the center of the knee (Fig. 17-1A).

Commonly, full-length views are not available. In such cases, radiographs should be obtained on the longest cassettes available. Lines drawn through the centers of the lengths of the femur and tibia intersect, forming the femoral tibial angle or anatomic axis. The femoral tibial angle is used to define the amount of deformity, assuming 7 degrees valgus to be the approximate population mean. The deformity angle is calculated by subtracting the measured angle from 7 degrees valgus. The difference plus up to an additional 3 degrees is the size of the wedge that must be removed in order to achieve the end result of a valgus of 8 to 10 degrees (Fig. 17-1B).

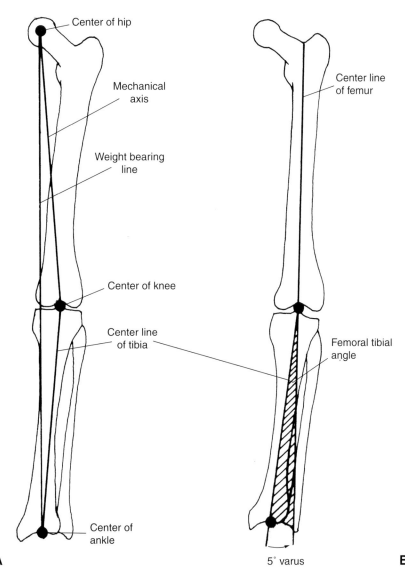

A   5° varus   B ■ FIGURE 17-1

A: The weight-bearing line indicates the line of force as it passes through the knee joint and requires radiographs extending from the hip to the ankle on a single film. Similarly, the mechanical axis must be drawn on long films. **B:** The anatomic axis, in contrast, can be measured on films including enough of the femur shaft and tibia shaft to find the center of the medullary canals.

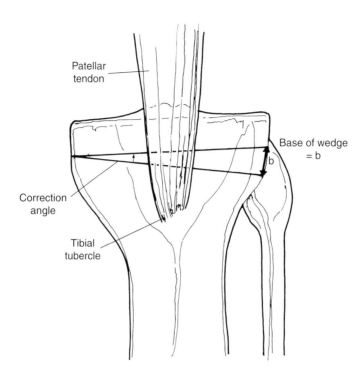

Patellar
tendon

Base of wedge
= b

b

Correction
angle

Tibial
tubercle

Using the more available anatomic axis, the correction angle is calculated by adding the measured relative varus deformity (equivalent negative valgus) angle from the ideal valgus angle of 8 to 10 degrees. For example, 5 degrees of relative varus deformity added to the ideal of 8 to 10 degrees gives a 13- to 15-degree correction angle. The correction angle then is drawn on an overlay of the proximal tibia, slightly oblique in the coronal plane and based as far distally as possible, yet still above the tibial tubercle. The base of the wedge is measured; this measurement is used intraoperatively to check the angle guide. The measured base of the wedge to be removed should correspond to within 15 to 20% of the base defined by the separation between angle pins (#1, #2), as defined by the angle guide.

The osteotomy lies between the tibial tubercle and the knee joint. The more proximal cut of the osteotomy should be situated distal to the joint by 5 mm. An additional few millimeters of bone should be retained in the proximal fragment to anchor the blade above the more proximal cut. The distal cut is planned as close to the level of the tibial tubercle as possible. Angling slightly obliquely from distal to proximal, the more distal cut can be started distal to the level of the tibial tubercle. The two osteotomy lines should intersect medial to the actual tibial cortex. The base of the triangle described is the lateral cortex of the tibia, which should approximate the linear distance of the actual wedge to be removed. Typically, this distance ranges from 10 to 15 mm. Corrections in excess of 15 degrees with associated large resections should be approached with considerable caution (Fig. 17-2).

The correction angle must take medial collateral ligament laxity into consideration. Otherwise, excessive valgus is produced. Valgus stress radiographs are useful in understanding what can happen under valgus loading conditions. If the patient's resting position, for instance, is 5 degrees of varus, and there is correction to 2 degrees of valgus with valgus stress, then a 5- to 8-degree wedge should be adequate, rather than the 10- to 12-degree wedge indicated based on standing films. Otherwise, the final alignment will be in excessive valgus.

Operative Setup The image table and image intensifier help expedite the procedure. The patient is placed prone on the operating table, with a small bump under the ipsilateral buttock. A plastic intravenous solution container (bladder bag) can be taped to the table to act as a foot rest to hold the patient's knee flexed to protect the posterior soft-tissue structures during the ostotomies. Prophylactic antibiotics are administered prior to preparation and draping, and a tourniquet is used. Transfusion is not planned.

Operation

Step 1   The extremity is prepared in a sterile manner up to the level of the tourniquet on the upper thigh. The leg is exsanguinated and the tourniquet is inflated. An incision is initiated above the level of the tubercle and below the level of the joint, at approximately the halfway point between them, that extends from the patellar tendon posterior to the line of the fibular head; care is taken to avoid fibular collateral ligament and the biceps femoris, as well as the patellar tendon. Proximal and distal flaps are immobilized, and the anterior compartment fascia is exposed. Using a scalpel, the anterior compartment fascia is released and reflected distally and posteriorly, extending to the level of the proximal tibia fibula joint. The patellar tendon also is identified and protected during the procedure, and the space posterior to the tendon freed by sharp dissection to allow for later placement of a protective retractor. The iliotibial band is released from distal to proximal up to the level of the coronary ligament (Fig. 17-3).

Step 2   The proximal tibia fibula joint is exposed, and the medial third of the fibular head is excised with an osteotome (Fig. 17-4). Alternatively, the joint can be released with an osteotome and bone spreader. Curettes and rongeurs are used to free the proximal tibia from the fibula sufficiently to allow for cephalad migration of the fibular head with closure of the tibial osteotomy. The fibula is a posterolateral structure and has a component directly posterior to the tibia, which requires careful removal if the fibula is to migrate proximally during closure of the osteotomy.

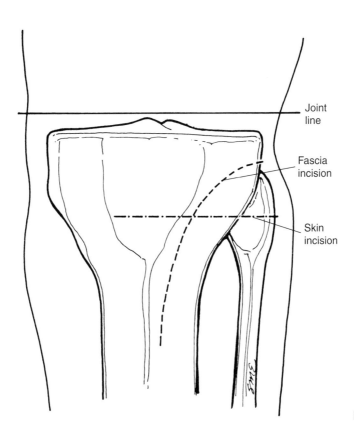

Joint
line

Fascia
incision

Skin
incision

■   FIGURE 17-3

The line of the skin incision extends from the tibial tubercle to the insertion of the fibular collateral on the proximal fibula. The fascial incision sweeps the fascia off the tibial crest and separates the iliotibial band from the anterior fascia of the leg. The anterior compartment musculature is reflected laterally to the proximal tibia fibula joint.

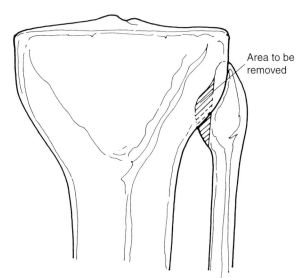

Area to be removed

The proximal fibula is freed from the proximal tibia by removal of the medial portion of the fibula with a small curved osteotome, with care taken to control the tip. Enough motion is necessary at this interface to allow placement of a posterior retractor during cutting of the wedge and cephalad migration of the fibula at the time at which the osteotomy is closed.

■ FIGURE 17-4

Step 3   The insertion of the patellar tendon on the tibial tubercle is carefully examined, because this is the time at which to plan the distal osteotomy cut. A guide pin is placed on the lateral cortex so that it crosses from lateral to medial and impales the medial cortex of the tibia, taking into consideration the level of the patellar tendon (Fig. 17-5). The ideal position is so that the entry point on the lateral cortex is actually at or below the tibial tubercle, but the cut crosses the sagittal plane of the tibial tubercle proximal to the insertion of the patellar tendon so that the patellar tendon is not injured. This tactic maximizes bone proximal to the inferior cut.

Step 4   The correction angle is identified on the angle guide. The distal pin is used as a mounting for the angle guide, and the proximal pin is placed. The lateral cortex between the two pins is measured and compared with the preoperative plan minus approximately 15% correction for radiograph magnification. A caliper is used to measure the closest points between the two pins, because the osteotomy follows the inferior surface of the proximal pin in the superior surface of the distal pin, so that the narrowest distance between the two pins constitutes the base of the resection wedge and should conform to preoperative estimates.

Step 5   The joint is identified using a thin spinal needle checking position under radiographic image intensification. A point 5 to 7 mm below and parallel to the joint is selected for placement of a guide pin, to help guide the placement of the plate. Ideally, 1 cm of bone should remain between the plate guide pin and the guide pin for the upper osteotomy cut. If this space is too small, less than 5 mm, then staples or buttress plating should be used. The seating chisel then is inserted on the guide pin and tapped into place, with proper rotation maintained in the coronal plane. The chisel should parallel the joint surface in both planes. The guide pin should be in the midlateral plane and should be placed from anterolateral to posteromedial to capture the thickest part of the tibia. The plate is designed to sit flush on the tibial cortex with this orientation. The seating chisel placed to depth of approximately 50 to 70 mm and then is withdrawn.

Step 6   Cutting blocks are slid on the two osteotomy guide pins and then anchored with a mallet (Fig. 17-6). A Z retractor is placed posterior to the tibia by sliding one end of the retractor along the posterior tibial cortex, and a second Z retractor is placed under the patellar tendon anteriorly. The knee is flexed to approximately 90 degrees, the foot is stabilized by the plastic water bottle. The oscillating saw is cooled by water during the cutting process. The shape of the upper tibia is triangular, with the apex anterior and the base lateral. The saw is directed with this in mind, with care taken to not advance the saw into the

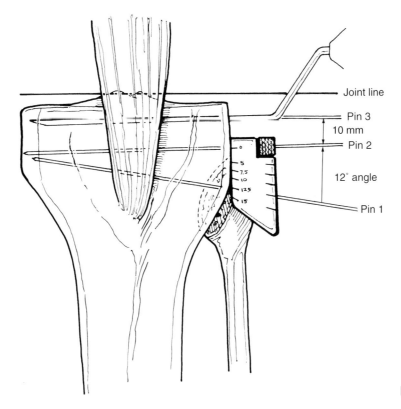

■ FIGURE 17-5

Pin #1 is placed obliquely cephalad, crossing the sagittal plane of the tibial tubercle at the level of the insertion of the infrapatellar ligament. Pin #2 is located with the angle guide at the appropriate angle. One centimeter above the top pin is the location for pin #3. The seating chisel must clear the joint by 5 to 7 mm.

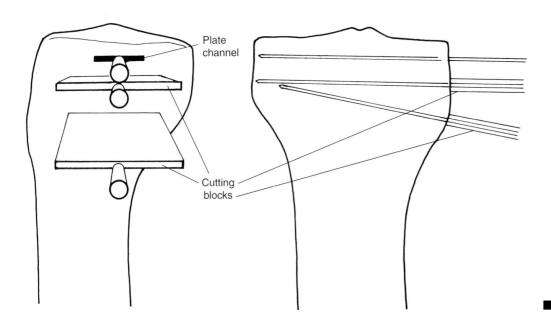

■ FIGURE 17-6

A seating chisel is placed over pin #3, driven to 50 to 70 mm, and then withdrawn. The pins are clipped and the cutting blocks placed over the pins.

soft tissue anteriorly or medially. Typically, the posteromedial cortex remains intact; it is best removed under direct vision with osteotomes and curettes. Additionally, the very back cortex of the tibia should be preserved, so that the saw is not advanced into the posterior compartment. The anterior cancellous portion of the resection wedge is removed, and the posterior cortex of the tibia is removed with 0.5 inches of osteotome under direct vision. A 3.2-mm drill is used to weaken the medial cortex.

Step 7   With the wedge removed, the blade plate is inserted onto the guide pin and seated with the cannulated impactor. The leg is brought into extension and the osteotomy gently closed. Ideally, there is a rubber-like consistency to the closure process, as the medial cortex gradually weakens to allow for closure of the osteotomy. The leg is held in extension with an applied valgus force. The guide pin is removed, and two cortical screws are placed after holes are drilled obliquely through the plate into the tibial cortex distal to the osteotomy (Fig. 17-7). The wound is irrigated, and the fascia of the anterior compartment is approximated loosely to the iliotibial band. A closed suction drain is placed in the subcutaneous space, the tourniquet is deflated, hemostasis is achieved, and the wound is closed.

■ TECHNICAL ALTERNATIVES AND PITFALLS

Staples offer ease of insertion and should be kept in mind for cases in which adequate bone stock laterally is not available. Aftercare must be modified in such cases to include protective support in the form of a cast for the first month following surgery. Alternative forms of internal fixation are available and may have compelling advantages in any given patient.

Technical problems fall into one of two categories: planning and execution. The most common planning error has to do with knees having an associated ligamentous instability, particularly of the medial collateral ligament. A valgus stress film should be obtained preoperatively in such cases to allow the surgeon to understand the effects of shifting the loading conditions from varus to valgus. On the other hand, cruciate ligament instability does not affect the outcome following HTO and requires no special consideration in planning of the osteotomy unless ligament reconstruction is to be undertaken at the same time as the HTO.

Over- and undercorrection constitute pitfalls of both the planning and execution phases of surgery. Ironically, overcorrection of modest proportion may provide a greater measure of relief than does a precise 7-to 10-degree valgus end result, which for most is the ideal fi-

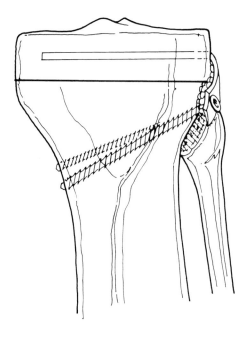

The plate is placed over pin #3, and lag screws are inserted. The wedge of bone removed is moralized and inserted under the overhanging proximal fragment.

■   FIGURE 17-7

nal position. Preparation of the patient prior to surgery helps postoperative adjustment to valgus.

Fracture of the lateral plateau, production of bony instability by improper location of the apex of the wedge resection, excessive bone resection, and improper location of the osteotomy are technical pitfalls in this procedure. Use of the image intensifier combined with preoperative planning helps reduce these problems.

■ REHABILITATION

The patient is placed in a continuous passive motion machine in the recovery room, and the drain is activated. A knee immobilizer is used when the patient gets up, until leg control returns as shown by the ability to do 10 sequential straight leg raises without pause. The patient begins touch weight bearing immediately and advances to full weight bearing at 6 weeks following surgery. Physiotherapy is useful for the first 6 weeks following wound healing to help the patient regain strength and motion.

■ OUTCOMES AND FUTURE DIRECTIONS

Despite widespread acceptance of total knee arthroplasty, HTO continues to play a role in the management of medial gonarthritis. Active young patients with localized disease and localized symptoms remain prime candidates for HTO. Long-term studies by Insall et al. (11) have shown 85% success at 5 years and 63% at 10 years. Rinonapoli et al. (12) reviewed a series of patients with 10- to 21-year follow-up and found that 53% had acceptable results. Coventry et al. (1) correlated results with residual angle of correction greater than 8 degrees valgus and body weight less than or equal to 1.32 times ideal. Preoperative planning combined with internal fixation should improve these results, with more reliable anatomic results and fewer complications. The future direction of HTO lies in improved operative techniques, which should reduce the incidence of technical errors and facilitate comfort and mobility of patients following surgery.

References

1. Wiley AM. Reconstruction of the osteoarthritic knee by high tibial osteotomy and joint clearance. *Can J Surg* 1967; 10:28–35.
2. Devas MB. High tibial osteotomy for arthritis of the knee: A method specially suitable for the elderly. *J Bone Joint Surg Br* 1969; 51:95–99.
3. Coventry MB. Stepped staple for upper tibial osteotomy. *J Bone Joint Surg Am* 1969; 51:1011.
4. Jackson JP, Waugh W, Green JP. High tibial osteotomy for osteoarthritis of the knee. *J Bone Joint Surg Br* 1969; 51:88–94.
5. Coventry MB. Upper tibial osteotomy for gonarthrosis: The evolution of the operation in the last 18 years and long term results. *Orthop Clin North Am* 1979; 10:191–210.
6. Coventry MB, Bowman PW. Long-term results of upper tibial osteotomy for degenerative arthritis of the knee. *Acta Orthop Belg* 1982; 48:139–156.
7. Coventry MB. Upper tibial osteotomy. *Clin Orthop* 1984; 182:46–52.
8. Coventry MB. Upper tibial osteotomy for osteoarthritis. *J Bone Joint Surg Am* 1985; 67:1136–1140.
9. Coventry MB. Proximal tibial osteotomy. *Orthop Rev* 1988; 17:456–458.
10. Coventry MB, Ilstrup DM, Wallrichs SL. Proximal tibial osteotomy: A critical long-term study of eighty-seven cases. *J Bone Joint Surg Am* 1993; 75:196–201.
11. Insall JN, Joseph DM, Msika C. High tibial osteotomy for varus gonarthrosis: A long-term follow-up study. *J Bone Joint Surg Am* 1984; 66:1040–1048.
12. Rinonapoli E, Mancini GB, Corvaglia A, et al. Tibial osteotomy for varus gonarthrosis: A 10- to 21-year followup study. *Clin Orthop* 1998; 353:185–193.

PETER J. EVANS
ANTHONY MINIACI

18

Distal Femoral Osteotomy

■ HISTORY OF THE TECHNIQUE

Valgus knee deformities requiring corrective surgery are uncommon and difficult to manage. Surgical management for lateral compartment osteoarthrosis associated with genu valgum have included proximal tibial varus osteotomy (1), supracondylar femoral varus osteotomy (1–10), intracondylar femoral osteotomy (11), and unicompartmental or total knee arthroplasty.

Genu valgum deformities severe enough to require osteotomy often have femorotibial angles that exceed 12 to 15 degrees, and slopes of the joint that exceed 10 degrees, making tibial osteotomies less favourable (1); therefore, most surgeons choose to correct the deformity above the level of the knee joint.

■ INDICATIONS AND CONTRAINDICATIONS

Careful evaluation of the patient clinically and radiographically is required for successful outcome following osteotomy. Gait should be evaluated, noting any dynamic medial or lateral thrust, recurvatum, or a flexed knee gait. Skin should be inspected for scars or any evidence of breakdown. Any evidence of ligament instability, joint line tenderness, effusion, or intraarticular pathology should be noted.

Ideal candidates for distal femoral varus osteotomy are younger than 60 years of age, have flexion arcs of greater than 90 degrees, and have good bone stock. Relative contraindications are similar to those for high tibial osteotomy and include age older than 70 years, patellofemoral osteoarthritis, a flexion arc less than 90 degrees, a fixed flexion deformity greater than 15 degrees, and peripheral vascular disease. Absolute contraindications include greater than 1 cm of tibial bone loss, multicompartment osteoarthritis, inflammatory arthritis, and significant ligamentous laxity.

Routine standing posteroanterior, lateral, and patellofemoral radiographs of the knee are needed to assess the joint adequately. Full-length, hip-to-ankle, single-leg standing radiographs should be obtained to assess the femorotibial angle and the mechanical axis of the extremity (12,13).

The normal femorotibial angle is 5 to 7 degrees of valgus and is formed by the intersection of the lines drawn through the long axis of the femur and the tibia (Fig. 18-1). The mechanical axis is drawn from the center of the hip joint to the center of the ankle joint and normally should intersect the center of the knee in the well-aligned leg. The surgical goal of distal femoral osteotomy should be to create a femorotibial angle of 0 degrees and a mechanical axis that is just medial to the center of the knee, which represents an overcorrection of 5 to 7 degrees from normal.

Using tracing paper and cutouts, the degree of angular correction, the angle of insertion of the internal fixation device (blade plate or dynamic condylar screw), and the subsequent amount of bony resection can be ascertained. In addition, the lengths of the plate, blade (or screw), and offset of the internal fixation device can be determined from the tracings.

■ SURGICAL TECHNIQUES

Although several techniques have been described (2), the most frequently reported approach is via a medial exposure and plate fixation. A lateral approach and plate fixation to the distal femur, however, are familiar to most orthopedic surgeons and provide a more biomechanically sound method of fixation, by placing the plate on the tension side of the

186

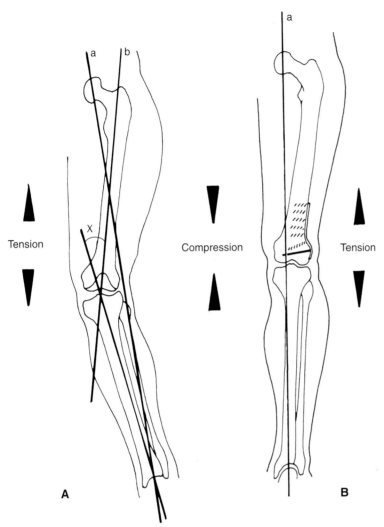

A: The mechanical axis (*a*) is measured by a line drawn from the center of the femoral head throught the center of the ankle mortise; the femorotibial axis (*b*) is subtended by the lines drawn down the center of the femur and tibia. A valgus knee shifts the normal mechanical axis from the center of the knee to the lateral compartment, causing compression and excessive wear. **B:** Distal femoral os-teotomy creates a femorotibial angle of 0 degrees (overcorrecting of 5 to 7 degrees), and a mechan-ical axis that is just medial of the center of the knee, which converts the lateral compartment from compression to tension.

■ FIGURE 18-1

femur. By creating an oblique osteotomy, mechanical compression can be applied via a screw through the third hole of the plate. The following techniques are described for the condylar blade plate but can be applied to the dynamic condylar screw, which is an easier device that we prefer to use because it does not have to be hammered into the distal femur, preventing possible comminution. In addition, because of the ability to rotate the plate about the screw, sagittal plane alignment of the side plate to the shaft is no longer critical.

Medial Plate Fixation The patient is placed supine on a radiolucent operating table, and the leg is draped to allow extensile exposure and allow the surgeon to flex and extend the knee to 90 degrees as needed. A tourniquet is placed. An arthroscopy is performed in the usual manner prior to performing the osteotomy, to rule out and treat any intraarticular mechanical pathology that might compromise the outcome of the osteotomy.

    Following arthroscopy a longitudinal medial incision is used that begins just distal to the joint and extends proximally 15 cm. If future arthroplasty is considered, a straight midline incision can be used, but it must be greater in length to allow equal exposure. Dissection is carried down to the joint capsule and the fascia of the vastus medialis muscle. The vastus medialis then is dissected from the septum and retracted anteriorly, exposing the medial femoral cortex and condyle. Blunt retractors maintain the exposure, with care taken to avoid injury of the femoral vessels. Bleeding from the posterior perforating arteries is common and should be controlled.

With the knee flexed 90 degrees, a guide wire is passed from medial to lateral through the joint and should rest on the most distal aspect of the medial and lateral condyle (Fig. 18-2). A small medial arthrotomy may be done to confirm placement if preferred. A second guide wire is placed 2.0 to 2.5 cm proximal to the articular surface and parallel to the first wire and the sagittal plane of the femur. The accuracy of these guide wires should be checked by fluoroscopy, because they guide the angle of insertion of the blade plate in the coronal plane and determine the subsequent angular correction. A third guide wire is inserted just proximal to the adductor tubercle and should be parallel to other two wires. This wire guides the osteotomy. A fourth guide wire is placed 3 cm proximal to the medial epicondyle and should be perpendicular to the long axis of the femur. A 90-degree pin guide may aid in its placement. This wire is proximal to and guides the proximal cut of the osteotomy. All guide wires should be parallel in the coronal plane to avoid rotational problems.

Once the guide wires are in proper position, the seating chisel is inserted just proximal to the second guide wire. Three 4.5-mm drill holes are made in the medial femoral cortex at the site at which the chisel is inserted, in order to prevent comminution. In order to ensure that the plate sits flush on the femoral shaft, the chisel should be placed in the anterior half of the femur, and the long arm of the plate holder should be attached to the chisel and kept parallel to the shaft during insertion (7). The chisel should be angled 10 to 15 degrees posterior to prevent the blade from cutting out of the anterior aspect of the lateral femoral condyle (2,4).

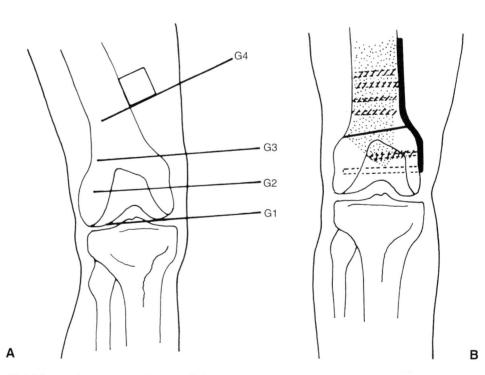

■ FIGURE 18-2   **A**   **B**

Distal femoral osteotomy via a medial approach. **A:** Intraoperative planning requires placement of three wires parallel to the joint line, the first (*G1*) intraarticular, the second (*G2*) 2.0 to 2.5 cm proximal representing the plate-insertion site, and the third (*G3*) proximal to the adductor tubercle representing the osteotomy site. **B:** An impaction of the proximal shift into the distal femur and 90-degree blade plate results in correction of alignment.

After placement of the chisel, the osteotomy can be performed with an oscillating saw. The distal cut should follow the third wire at least 2 cm above the chisel, to ensure good fixation and stability distally. The cut should be perpendicular to the anterior surface of the femoral shaft and should stop at the lateral cortex. The lateral cortex is perforated with a small osteotome to allow better control and prevent lateral translation proximally. The proximal cut then is made parallel and distal to fourth wire, approximately 1 cm above the distal cut. This distance depends on the size of the medial wedge determined from preoperative planning. Again, a small osteotome completes the cut on the lateral cortex. The wedge of bone removed is saved for bone graft.

The third wire can be removed and used to fix the osteotomy temporally until the condylar blade plate is inserted. The osteotomy is closed solidly, so that the second and fourth wires are parallel, assuring a femorotibial angle of 0 degrees. After the 90-degree condylar blade plate of the measured offset and length is selected and seated, provisional fixation can be removed and the femoral shaft secured. The first screw placed proximal to the osteotomy should be loaded according to the principles of dynamic compression plating, but the outrigger Association for Osteosynthesis (AO) compression device cannot be used because of the proximity to the femoral vessels. At least four bicortical screws should fix the proximal shaft. The knee should be moved through a full range of motion, and the osteotomy should be checked for stability.

An alternative and simpler method of medial plate fixation would be to remove only a small medial wedge, enough to allow impaction of the smaller-diameter proximal cortical fragment into the larger distal cancellous condylar fragment, thereby also improving stability and healing. Because the plate is angled at 90 degrees, the insertion of the blade parallel to the distal articular surface and the impaction of the osteotomy and the reduction of the medial femoral cortex to the side plate automatically eliminate the femoral valgus and ensure a femorotibial angle of 0 degrees.

The cancellous bone from the wedge is used to graft the osteotomy. The wound is closed in layers over suction drains. A sterile dressing, a full-leg elastic tube bandage, and a range-of-motion brace are applied.

Lateral Plate Fixation   The patient is placed supine on a radiolucent operating table with a sandbag under the ipsilateral buttock. The leg is draped to allow extensile exposure and allow the surgeon to flex and extend the knee to 90 degrees as needed. A tourniquet is placed. An arthroscopy is performed in the usual manner prior to performing the osteotomy.

A longitudinal lateral incision is made from just distal to the joint line for approximately 15 to 20 cm proximally. A straight midline incision can be used, but it needs to be slightly longer. The iliotibial band is exposed and incised just anterior to the intermuscular septum. The vastus lateralis muscle is identified, dissected from the intermuscular septum, and retracted anterior and medial with Homan retractors. The joint line and capsule are identified. The perforating vessels are exposed and cauterized.

With the knee flexed 90 degrees, a guide wire is inserted across the joint from lateral to medial at the distal articular surface (Fig. 18-3). A second wire is placed across the anterior aspect of the femoral condyles, pointing approximately 10 degrees posteromedial from the sagittal plane, indicating the plane of the patellofemoral joint. A third wire is inserted through the lateral femoral condyle 1.5 cm proximal and parallel to the joint in the coronal plane and the second guide wire in the sagittal plane. The wire should be placed at the midpoint of the anterior half of the lateral femoral condyle, which allows the plate to sit on the lateral aspect of the femur (10,14). The position of the wires should be checked with fluoroscopy. The amount of correction (in degrees and size of medial wedge) needed to achieve a femorotibial angle of 0 degrees is determined preoperatively. A fourth wire is placed proximal to the third wire and directed at the desired angle of correction relative to it, such that the two pins meet medial. Before beginning the osteotomy, the blade plate or screw and plate should be inserted partially. Because the angle of the insertion is not parallel to

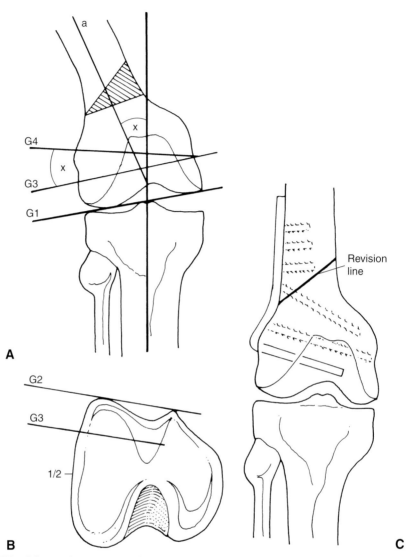

■ FIGURE 18-3

B

C

Distal femoral osteotomy via a lateral approach. **A:** Intraoperative planning requires placement of four guide wires, one (*G1*) intraarticular and parallel to the distal femoral joint line, one (*G3*) placed in the anterior quarter of the femur, 2.0 to 2.5 cm proximal and parallel to *G1* and *G2* (patellofemoral joint line). The final pin (*G4*) subtends the angle of correction required, meeting *G3* on the medial side. The osteotomy is performed 2 to 3 cm proximal to the supracondylar ridge, removing a wedge of bone corresponding to the desired angle of correction.

the joint, the 90-degree plate abuts the femur proximally and does not allow complete insertion yet.

The osteotomy is held laterally by a hinge of bone and should be performed just above the supracondylar ridge, approximately 2 to 3 cm proximal to the fourth wire. The osteotomy is oblique from proximal–medial to distal–lateral. An oblique osteotomy allows a compression screw to cross the site, allows the plate to act as a true buttress laterally, and increases the surface area of bone for better healing. Blunt Homan retractors retract the quadriceps, allowing good exposure medial and protecting the vascular structures. The medially based wedge of bone to be resected is marked. The femur should be cut with a reciprocating saw starting at the medial supracondylar area and proceeding laterally, not cutting but only perforating the lateral cortex. The wedge is removed and kept for bone graft, and the osteotomy is closed by using the plate as a handle. With the osteotomy closed, the plate should parallel the femur and be able to be fully seated. It is important to ensure that there has been no rotation. The third hole on the plate then is used to insert a compression screw across the osteotomy site. At least four bicortical screws should fix the proximal shaft. The knee should be moved through a full range of motion, and the osteotomy should be checked for stability. The wound is closed in layers over suction drains. A sterile dressing, a full-leg elastic tube bandage, and a range-of-motion brace are applied.

Combined Deformities   In addition to genu valgum, patients may present with significant flexion or recurvatum deformities, correction of which would benefit function. Preoperative assessment of gait, stability, and range of motion determines whether a corrective osteotomy is required and the degree of correction that is needed.

At the time of surgery an anterior-based closing wedge osteotomy can be combined with the previously determined medial-based closing wedge osteotomy in order to correct a combined valgus and flexion deformity. Similarly, a posterior- and medial-based closing wedge can be used to correct a combined valgus and recurvatum deformity. Like the osteotomies described previously, a wedge smaller than measured can be removed, and the remainder of the angular correction can be achieved by impaction of the proximal shaft into the distal femoral condyles as the plate is placed medial.

The angular correction can be performed accurately with placement of a guide wire perpendicular and into the anterior cortex of the femur, proximal to the site of the osteotomy. A second guide wire is placed just distal to the site of the osteotomy and at an angle from the first wire equal to the amount of correction. For an anterior-based osteotomy, the wire is directed posterior and proximal; for a posterior-based osteotomy it is directed posterior and distal. After closure of the osteotomy, both wires should be parallel and perpendicular to the anterior cortex.

■ REHABILITATION

Immediately postoperatively, analgesia and cold therapy are employed. Motion is started immediately, and continuous passive motion is optional. Patients walk with crutches, allowing feather-touch weight bearing for a period of 6 to 8 weeks. A physiotherapist is consulted for gait training and to initiate isometric exercises. Functional non–weight bearing exercises such as swimming and cycling are encouraged early in rehabilitation. A hinged range-of-motion brace is used for patient comfort but can be removed for exercises. Patients usually can be discharged on the first or second postoperative day. Serial radiographic evaluations of union and fixation are necessary to assess healing and allow full weight bearing and resisted exercises. The patient usually bears weight fully and is independent by 12 weeks postsurgery.

■ OUTCOMES AND FUTURE DIRECTIONS

Lateral joint pain and osteoarthritis associated with valgus deformity occur relatively infrequently, and the number of younger patients that are candidates for osteotomy rather than total knee replacement is small. For this reason a paucity exists in the literature of outcome data adequate to compare the available surgical techniques.

Although several early references to intercondylar and supracondylar osteotomies existed (5,6,8,9,11), it was not until 1988 that outcomes became available, when Healey et al. (4) and McDermott et al. (7) published their experiences with medial-plate, medial-closing wedge osteotomy. Healey et al. (4) reported good to excellent results in 14 of 15 patients with osteoarthritis, and complications in three patients in their series of 23, two of whom had nonunion. McDermott et al. (7) similarly found an improvement in 22 of 24 patients; one patient had hardware failure. Miniaci et al. (3) reviewed consecutive medial and then lateral plate fixation techniques for the treatment of osteoarthritis. They found good to excellent results in 6 of 10 patients treated with medial plate fixation (two had nonunion) and in 15 of 16 patients treated with lateral plate fixation.

Although the surgical approach for the lateral plate technique is simple and more familiar to most surgeons, and it has several biomechanical advantages, the medial plate technique is less demanding for preoperative planning and intraoperative execution. In the future, a supracondylar dome osteotomy performed via a lateral approach with a jig could simplify the intraoperative planning of the osteotomy.

References

1. Coventry MB. Osteotomy about the knee for degenerative and rheumatoid arthritis: Indications, operative technique, and results. *J Bone Joint Surg Am* 1973; 55:23–48.
2. Miniaci A, Watson LW. Distal femoral osteotomy. In: Fu FH, Harner CD, Vince KG, eds. *Knee surgery*, vol 2. Baltimore: Williams & Wilkins, 1994:1173–1180.
3. Miniaci A, Grossman SP, Jakob RP. Supracondylar femoral varus osteotomy in the treatment of valgus knee deformity. *Am J Knee Surg* 1990; 3:65–73.
4. Healey W, Anglen JO, Wasilewski SA, et al. Distal femoral varus osteotomy. *J Bone Joint Surg Am* 1988; 70:102–108.
5. Maquet PGJ. *Biomechanics of the knee*. New York, Springer-Verlag, 1976.
6. Maquet P. The treatment choice in osteoarthritis of the knee. *Clin Orthop Relat Res* 1985; 192:108–112.
7. McDermott AGP, Finklestein J, Farine I, et al. Distal femoral varus osteotomy for valgus deformity of the knee. *J Bone Joint Surg Am* 1988; 70:110–116.
8. Jackson PA. Ostotomy for osteoarthritis of the knee. *J Bone Joint Surg Br* 1958; 40:826.
9. Aglietti P, Stringa G, Buzzi R, et al. Correction of valgus knee deformity with a supracondylar V osteotomy. *Clin Orthop Relat Res* 1987; 217:214–220.
10. Muller ME, Allgower M, Schneider R, et al. *Manual of internal fixation*. Berlin: Springer-Verlag, 1979.
11. Debeyre J, Tomeno B. Treatment of axial deviations of the knee joint by means of intercondylar femoral osteotomies. *Clin Orthop Relat Res* 1973; 91:86–94.
12. Krackow KA. Approaches to planning lower extremity alignment for total knee arthroplasty and osteotomy about the knee. *Adv Orthop Surg* 1983; 1:69–88.
13. Moreland JR, Bassett LW, Hanker GJ. Radiographic analysis of the axial alignment of the lower extremity. *J Bone Joint Surg* 1987; 69:745–749.
14. Schatzker J, Tile M. *The rationale of operative fracture care*. Berlin: Springer-Verlag, 1987.

19

Fresh Osteochondral Allografts for Posttraumatic Knee Defects

In 1972, an Orthopaedic Transplant Program was established at the Mount Sinai Hospital, University of Toronto. The program has three major arms: revision arthroplasty of the hip and knee, orthopedic oncology, and reconstruction of posttraumatic articular defects. Deep-frozen irradiated bone is used for restoration of bone stock in revision arthroplasty of the hip and knee, and for tumor reconstructions, but fresh nonprocessed bone and cartilage is utilized to reconstruct traumatic joint defects. As of July 1, 1998, there had been 265 osteochondral allografts performed for posttraumatic articular defects, mostly around the knee. This program was initiated in order to reconstruct joints in patients who were too young for prosthetic joint replacement, and in whom arthrodesis or realignment by itself was not indicated. Today approximately 12 to 15 fresh osteochondral transplants are performed annually for posttraumatic articular defects, with the majority involving the knee.

■ HISTORY OF THE TECHNIQUE

Appropriate patient selection is tantamount to satisfactory outcome. The senior author and others have identified a number of patient characteristics that are predictive of success.

■ INDICATIONS AND CONTRADICTIONS

Diagnoses   McDermott et al. (1) reviewed 100 patients who received fresh, small-fragment osteochondral allografts for articular defects in and around the knee. The diagnoses included osteoarthritis, spontaneous osteonecrosis of the knee, steroid-induced avascular necrosis of the femoral condyles, osteochondritis dissecans, and trauma. Grafts done for posttraumatic changes in the joint had the best results. Those done for primary osteoarthritis had poor results. Meyers and coworkers also had poor results with fresh grafts placed into osteoarthritic knees (2,3). Garret (4) produced excellent results in patients treated for traumatic defects and osteochondritis dissecans. It is my opinion that posttraumatic defects and osteochondritis dissecans of the knee are the best indications for grafting (1,5–7).

Age   Beaver et al. (8), using Meier–Kaplan survivorship analysis, demonstrated that patients younger than 60 years of age in the posttraumatic group have grafts that survive longer than those in patients older than 60 years in the same group. Fortunately, the great majority of posttrauma patients are in their second and third decades.

Site   Unipolar or unicompartmental grafts are the most successful in considering the tibiofemoral articulation (1,5–9). Patients therefore should be referred for surgery before secondary charges occur on the nontraumatized side.

Deformity   If there is an associated deformity secondary to the joint defect, then an osteotomy is performed to decompress the compartment into which the graft is inserted. If the defect involves the medial femoral condyle and there is a secondary varus deformity, then a proximal tibial valgus osteotomy is performed. If the defect is in the lateral tibial plateau and there is a secondary valgus deformity, then a distal femoral varus osteotomy is performed. The osteotomy usually is done at the same time as the allograft.

It has been our experience that the best results with fresh osteochondral allografts are in patients with unipolar posttraumatic defects of the knee. We no longer perform this operation for osteoarthritis, spontaneous osteonecrosis, or steroid-induced osteonecrosis, or in patients with inflammatory arthroplasty. If the posttraumatic defect has been present for long enough to cause degenerative changes of a severe degree in the opposing articular surface, the graft is contraindicated. Also, the patient must be compliant and rehabilitable.

■ SURGICAL TECHNIQUES

Procurement   The local organ-procurement agency (in our case the Multiple Organ Retrieval and Exchange Program of Toronto) identifies potential donors. These donors must meet the criteria outlined by the American Association of Transplant Surgeons (AATS) (10). Also, donors are always younger than 30 years of age. This ensures that the grafts have healthy cartilage and strong bone.

The graft is harvested within 24 hours of the death of the donor, under strict aseptic conditions. The specimen consists of the entire knee joint, including an intact capsule. Aerobic, anaerobic, fungal, and tuberculosis cultures are obtained at the time of harvest. The specimen is stored in a sealed container in 1 L of Ringer's lactated solution with cefazolin (1 g) and bacitracin (10,000 U) added. The container is refrigerated at 4°C.

Operation   The transplantation usually is performed within 12 hours of harvest and always within 24 hours. The operation is performed in a clean-air room, with the surgeons wearing body exhaust suits. The patient receives preoperative antibiotics (cefazolin). Two surgical teams work simultaneously: one performs the arthrotomy, the other prepares the graft.

Ideally, the surgical approach is through an anterior, longitudinal incision over the affected knee. This may vary if old surgical scars are present about the knee. The incision is approximately 25 to 35 cm long and is centered over the patella. Proximally it overlies the quadriceps tendon; distally it overlies the tibial tubercle. Minor skin flaps are raised to fa-

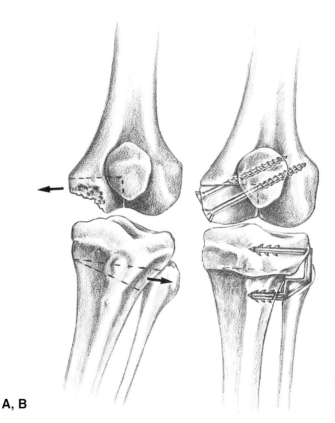

Medial femoral condylar allograft and high tibial osteotomy. **A:** Traumatic loss of medial femoral condyle with secondary varus deformity. *Dotted lines* show resection to healthy cancellous bone of femoral condyle and outline of tibial osteotomy. The allograft is fixed before osteotomy is performed. **B:** A medial femoral condylar allograft is inserted, with fixation by two 4.0-mm cancellous screws. A proximal tibial valgus osteotomy is performed to decompress the medial compartment.

■ FIGURE 19-1   **A, B**

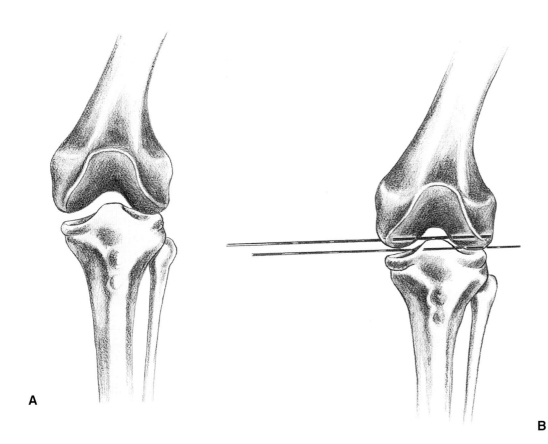

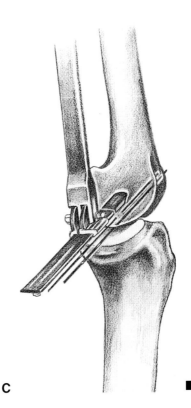

Lateral tibial plateau allograft and distal femoral varus osteotomy. **A:** Old fracture of lateral tibial plateau with secondary
valgus deformity. **B:** The plateau is resected to healthy cancellous bone, and lateral plateau osteochondral allograft inserted.
C: A lateral tibial plateau allograft is fixed by two 4.0-mm cancellous screws. A distal femoral varus osteotomy is made to decompress the lateral compartment, after the allograft is fixed.

C   ■ FIGURE 19-2

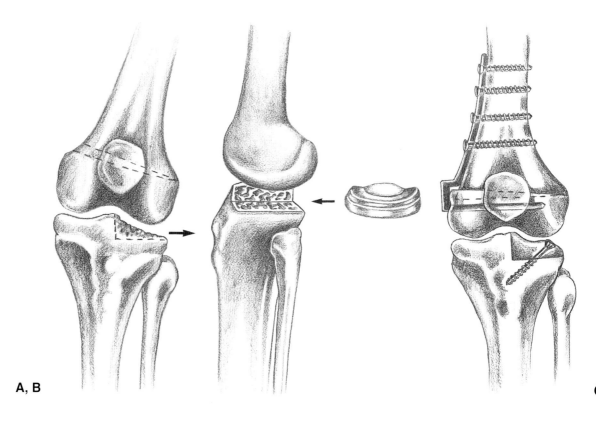

A, B

C

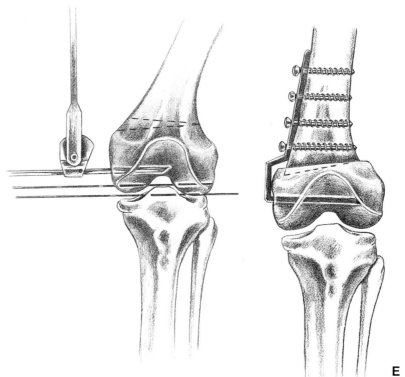

D

E

■ FIGURE 19-3   Technique of distal femoral varus osteotomy. **A:** Valgus knee. **B:** A guide wire is inserted parallel to the transcondylar axis of distal femur 1 cm from the joint line and confirmed on a radiograph. **C:** Seating chisel for the blade plate is inserted 2.5 to 3 cm from the joint line, parallel to the guide wire. **D:** Osteotomy is performed parallel to the chisel at least 1.5 cm proximal, and a 5-mm based wedge is removed. **E:** Osteotomy is held with a 90-degree offset blade plate.

cilitate later closure. A medial or lateral parapatellar arthrotomy is made, depending on the site of the defect. If a high tibial osteotomy is necessary, the skin incision is carried further distal to allow reflection of the anterior compartment off the proximal and lateral portion of the tibia. There is usually no difficulty doing a standard high tibial osteotomy through this approach. For the femoral osteotomy, the medial aspect of the distal femur is approached through the skin incision described above. The fascia over the vastus medialis is incised. The muscle then is dissected from the medial intermuscular septum and reflected anteriorly and laterally, exposing the medial portion of the distal femoral shaft and the medial femoral condyle.

Once exposure is obtained, the reconstruction is straightforward and quite conservative. The articular defect is "squared off," with the goal of removing as little bone as possible. The resection is down to bleeding cancellous bone. The graft is machined to fit the recipient bed accurately. As stated previously, the graft is orthotopic. The articular surface of the graft is made to lie flush with the surface of the host joint. The graft, whether tibial or femoral, is fixed with two 4.0-mm partially threaded cancellous screws. Enough bone must be retained on the graft to accommodate the two screws. In either scenario, fixation tends to be excellent.

The high tibial osteotomy that is done in concert with a medial femoral condyle graft is a lateral closing wedge osteotomy. The medial part of the proximal tibiofibular joint is excised, leaving the lateral proximal fibula intact and protecting the ligament and the nerve. The initial horizontal cut is made at the level of the insertion of the patellar ligament on the tibial tubercle and parallel to the tibial articular surface. The length of the wedge's base is determined by the amount of varus in which the limb is. I like to correct the limb to a tibiofemoral angle of approximately 10 degrees (valgus overcorrection). The osteotomy typically is fixed with two stepped staples (Figs. 19-1 and 19-4).

The distal femoral osteotomy that is done concurrently with a lateral plateau graft is well described by McDermott et al. (11). This is a medial closing wedge osteotomy. The first bone cut is made parallel to the transcondylar line of the distal femur. The transcondylar line connects the two distal most points on the femoral condyles. The base of the wedge is only 5 to 10 mm long. This conservative wedge allows the intercondylar line to become perpendicular to the medial cortex of the femur, producing the desired tibiofemoral angle of 0 degrees (varus overcorrection). If the wedge is too small, impaction of the proximal fragment into the distal fragment allows adequate correction. This construct is fixed with a 90-degree blade plate. The blade is placed parallel to the transcondylar line, and the plate is used to reduce the osteotomy as it is fixed to the femoral shaft. The plate forces the transcondylar line to be perpendicular to the medial femoral shaft (Figs. 19-2, 19-3, and 19-5).

The meniscus at the defect site is inspected and repaired by direct vision if damaged. If the meniscus is irreparable, however, a meniscal allograft is added to the reconstruction.

■ REHABILITATION

The patient receives postoperative antibiotics (cefazolin) for 2 days. The knee is mobilized immediately in the recovery room with a continuous passive motion machine designed to allow varus and valgus adjustments. Early motion facilitates cartilage nutrition and prevents stiffness (12). The patient is protected carefully. He or she is placed in a long-leg, ischial bearing caliper for 1 year. If an osteotomy is done, the patient does not bear weight until signs of radiographic healing are seen. The patient is allowed to bear full weight in the caliper if no osteotomy is done or after the osteotomy heals. Physiotherapy consists of active and active-assisted range-of-motion exercises and isometric strengthening exercises. No resistive work is done until the patient is out of the brace and the graft is healed.

■ OUTCOMES AND FUTURE DIRECTIONS

Materials   Between 1972 and 1992, 126 knees of 123 patients with osteochondral defects secondary to trauma (111 cases) or osteochondritis dissecans (15 cases) were reconstructed, using fresh small-fragment osteochondral allografts. The average age was 35 years (range 15–64); there were 81 males and 42 females.

A: Preoperative radiography of the left knee in a 33-year-old woman with traumatic loss of part of the weight-bearing area of medial femoral condyle. The screws are holding a patellar fracture. **B:** Postoperative standing radiograph in the same patient at 11 years. A fresh medial femoral condylar osteochondral allograft has been fixed with two screws. A high tibial valgus osteotomy was done in conjunction with the allograft. The knee is well corrected into valgus. The allograft is united, with no evidence of resorption or fragmentation, and the joint space is maintained.

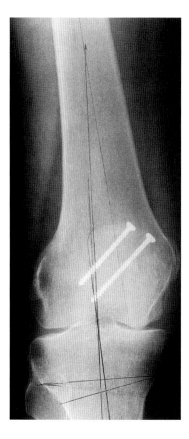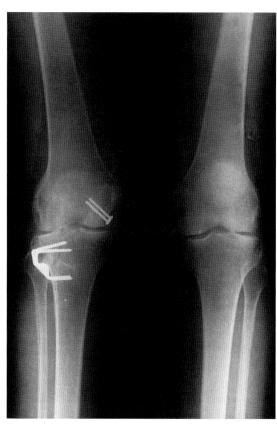

■ FIGURE 19-4

A, B

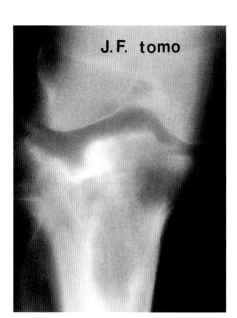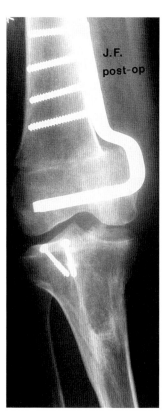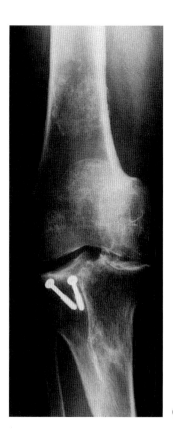

A, B

C

■ FIGURE 19-5   **A:** Preoperative anteroposterior computed tomographic scan of the right knee of a 32-year-old female, 2 years following fracture of the lateral tibial plateau. **B:** Postoperative radiograph 1 year following a lateral tibial plateau allograft done in conjunction with a distal femoral varus osteotomy. **C:** Postoperative radiograph at 11 years. The joint space is well maintained, with minor peripheral resorption of the graft.

The defects were located in the tibial plateau (55 lateral, six medial, and two combined medial and lateral), femoral condyle (27 medial and 23 lateral), bipolar tibial and femoral (seven lateral and ome medial compartment), and patellofemoral (1 in patellar groove of the femur and 1 in the patella).

The grafts, which were between 8 and 40 mm thick, were fixed to good bleeding cancellous bone after resecting the defect. In 47 cases the meniscus was included in the transplant. Sixty-eight knees underwent osteotomy to correct alignment (37 distal femoral, 31 upper tibial). Patients were assessed clinically pre and postoperatively, using a rating score based on subjective and objective criteria (Table 19-1). Radiographic assessment included alignment, graft union, fracture and resorption, joint-space narrowing, and osteoarthritis.

Results The average follow-up was 7.5 years (range 1–22). Failure was defined as a decrease in knee score or the need for further surgery.

Survivorship analysis (Kaplan–Meir life table) demonstrated 95% successful results at 5 years (95% confidence limits: 87–98), 71% at 10 years (95% confidence limits: 56–83), and 66% at 20 years (95% confidence limit: 50–81). Among 18 failures, one patient had an arthrodesis, eight had total knee replacement, the graft was removed in one, and eight experienced failure because of a decrease in score but still retain their grafts. The success rate was 85%.

Complications included three stiff knees, one wound hematoma, and one rupture of the patellar tendon. Log-rank analysis reveals a statistically significant relationship of failure with bipolar grafts ($P < 0.05$) and patients receiving workers' compensation ($P = 0.0396$),

TABLE 19-1. KNEE SCORING SYSTEM

Subjective Factors		Objective Factors	
Pain intensity		**Extension lack**	
None	35	No deformity	10
Mild	28	Less than 5 degrees	7
Moderate	21	5–10 degrees	4
(occasional analgesics)		10–20 degrees	2
Severe	14	More than 20 degrees	0
At rest	0	**Flexion**	
Instability		More than 120 degrees	20
None	10	90–120 degrees	15
Occasionally	7	45–90 degrees	8
Moderate	4	Less than 45 degrees	0
(with decreased activity)		**Effusion**	
Severe (using brace)	0	None	10
Walking aids		Moderate	5
None	5	Severe	0
Cane	3		
Crutches	1		
Walker	0		
Walking distance			
More than 1 mi	10		
1 to 5 blocks	6		
One block	3		
Inside house	1		
Confined to bed	0		

Adapted from Hospital for Special Surgery.

but no significant relationship with other factors such as osteotomy, meniscus transplant, sex, and medial or lateral side of the knee.

Also, analysis of variance in successful cases did not show any statistically significant effect of patient age or sex, postoperative complications, or preoperative scores. Radiographic assessment of 18 patients experiencing failures showed four collapsed grafts, seven patients with loss of joint space, and 10 with significant osteoarthritis.

Except for two instances of questionable union, all grafts solidly united to the host bone 6 to 12 months after surgery. Among clinically successful patients, we noted five instances of mild graft collapse (less than 3 mm), 11 of decreased joint space, and 18 of osteoarthritic changes. Among the patients who demonstrated negative radiographic changes, 11 were malaligned, with overstressing of the graft.

The rationale for fresh osteochondral allografts is clinical and experimental evidence of maintenance of viability and function of chondrocytes following fresh transplantation. There is also histologic evidence that the bony part of these grafts can be replaced by host bone in a uniform fashion in 2 to 3 years (7).

The survival rates for the allograft reconstructions in this study with long-term follow-up (95% survival at 5 years, 77% at 10 years, and 66% at 20 years) is very encouraging. The statistically significant relationships of failure with receipt of workers' compensation and bipolar grafts have provided guidelines for better selection of patients, and the suggestion that the procedure be performed in unipolar cases.

Although most patients experiencing failure showed radiographic changes of collapse (four), joint-space narrowing (seven) and osteoarthritis (10), similar changes were found in some patients in whom the procedure was successful.

Development of radiographic changes in 11 patients who were not properly aligned to shift the weight from the transplant indicates the importance of realignment osteotomy. Overall, the high success rate on long-term follow-up of this uncomplicated procedure, which not only does not compromise salvage surgery but facilitates it by restoring bone stock, makes it an appropriate procedure for unipolar osteochondral defects of the knee secondary to trauma, or for osteochondritis dissecans in properly selected patients.

Fresh osteochondral allografts also have been used for pure chondral defects, with precision instruments used to create a bony defect under the chondral defect. This allows the use of the bony part of the graft for fixation and anchorage of the cartilage (13). There has been recent interest in the use of autologous tissue for resurfacing joints. Both periosteum (14) and chondrocytes (15) are used. These techniques have the advantage of not exposing patients to the theoretic risk of an immune response, but even more importantly to bacteria or viruses carried by the donor. These autologous techniques are more appropriate for surface chondral defects, whereas the technique described in this chapter addresses the problem of major traumatic defects involving both cartilage and bone. Using proper screening protocols, the risk of transmitting HIV is 1 in 1,667,600 (16). The risk for hepatitis C has not been reported yet for bone and cartilage, but there have been case reports of transmission (17). The risk of transmitting hepatitis C in properly screened blood is 1 in 103,000; for hepatitis B it is 1 in 63,000; and for HTLV it is 1 in 641,000 (18). This same article states that the risk of transmitting HIV in properly screened blood is 1 in 493,000 (17). These figures represent the worst possible risks of disease transmission by allograft transplantation and should be used for unprocessed tissue (fresh or deep-frozen without irradiation or freeze-drying). In my opinion these risks are justified in patients with major bone or cartilage defects causing significant disability. In patients with pure chondral defects, the disability is not as great and the loss of tissue is not of the same magnitude. Autologous techniques may be more appropriate under these circumstances (15). If the antigen tests for viruses become precise enough to eliminate the window period for detection to less than 24 hours, then allograft tissue probably will become the tissue of choice for all of the aforementioned techniques, because there is no sacrifice of host tissue and it is less expensive.

References

1. McDermott AGP, Langer F, Pritzker KPH, et al. Fresh small osteochondral allografts. *Clin Orthop* 1985; 197:96.
2. Meyers MH, Akeson W, Convery FR. Resurfacing of the knee with fresh osteochondral allograft. *J Bone Joint Surg Am* 1989; 71:704–713.

3. Convery FR, Meyers MH, Akeson WH. Fresh osteochondral allografting of the femoral condyle. *Clin Orthop* 1991; 273:139–145.

4. Garret J. Osteochondral allografts for treatment of chondral defects of the femoral condyles: Early results. Proceedings of the Knee Society. *Am J Sports Med* 1987; 15:387.

5. Gross AE. Use of fresh osteochondral allografts to replace traumatic join defects. In: Czitrom AA, Gross AE, eds. *Allografts in orthopaedic practice*. Baltimore: William & Wilkins, 1992:78–82.

6. Zukor DJ, Paitich B, Oakshott RD, et al. Reconstruction of post traumatic articular surface defects using fresh small-fragment osteochondral allografts. In: Aebi M, Regazzoni P, eds. *Bone transplantation*. Berlin: Springer-Verlag, 1989:293–305.

7. Oakshott RD, Farine I, Pritzker KPH, et al. A clinical and histological analysis of failed fresh osteochondral allografts. *Clin Orthop* 1988; 233:283–294.

8. Beaver RJ, Mahomed M, Backstein D, et al. Fresh osteochondral allografts for post-traumatic defects in the knee, a survivorship analysis. *J Bone Joint Surg Br* 1992; 74:105–110.

9. Zukor DJ, Oakshott RD, Gross AE. Osteochondral allograft reconstruction of the knee: Part 2: Experience with successful and failed fresh osteochondral allografts. *Am J Knee Surg* 1980; 2:182–191.

10. Fawcett KJ, Barr HR, eds. Tissue banking. *In: American Association of Blood Banks*. American Association of Blood Banks: Arlington, VA, 1987:97–107.

11. McDermott AGP, Finklestein JA, Farine I, et al. Distal femoral varus osteotomy for valgus deformity of the knee. *J Bone Joint Surg Am* 1988; 70:110–116.

12. Salter RB, Simmonds DF, Malcolm BW, et al. The biological effect of continuous passive motion on the healing of full thickness defects in articular cartilage. *J Bone Joint Surg Am* 1980; 62:1232.

13. Garret JC. Treatment of osteochondral defects of the distal femur with fresh osteochondral allografts: A preliminary report. *Arthroplasty* 1986; 2:222–226.

14. O'Driscoll SW, Salter RB. The repair of major osteochondral defects in joint surfaces by neochondrogenesis with autogenous osteoperisoteal grafts stimulated by continuous passive motion: An experimental investigation in the rabbit. *Clin Orthop* 1986; 208:131–140.

15. Brittberg M, Lindahl A, Nilsson A, et al. Treatment of deep cartilage defects in the knee with autologous chondrocyte transplantation. *N Engl J Med* 1994; 331:889–895.

16. Buck BE, Malinin TI, Brown MD. Bone transplantation and human immunodeficiency virus: An estimated risk of acquired immunodeficiency syndrome. *Clin Orthop* 1989; 240:129–136.

17. Tomford WW. Transmission of disease through transplantation of musculoskeletal allografts. *J Bone Joint Surg Am* 1995; 77:1742–1754.

18. Schreiber GB, Busch MP, Kleinman SH, et al. The risk of transfusion-transmitted viral infections. *N Engl J Med* 1996; 334:1685–1689.

DOMENICK J. SISTO

20

Patellofemoral Replacement

■ HISTORY OF THE
TECHNIQUE

Isolated, severe patellofemoral degenerative disease is a rare but disabling disease of the knee. There are two groups of patients with advanced patellofemoral degenerative arthritis. The majority of patients have patellar malalignment with patellar tilt and compression, in addition to a history of subluxation and dislocation. These patients are younger (less than 55 years old) and have had previous surgery. The second group of patients is those who present with patellar pain later in life (50–70 years old) and have associated femorotibial arthrosis. This group includes only those patients with significant patellofemoral arthrosis with minimal femorotibial involvement. These patients do not have patellar malalignment and usually have not had previous surgery.

The nonoperative management includes quadriceps-strengthening exercises, nonsteroidal antiinflammatory drugs, weight loss if needed, and a modification of activities. These modalities rarely are beneficial in patients with severe patellofemoral degenerative disease, and surgical intervention frequently is necessary. The surgical treatment of advanced patellofemoral degenerative disease is controversial. There have been favorable reports following tibial tubercle elevation, but others have found this procedure unreliable (1–7). Some authors have advocated patellectomy, but these patients can complain of pain from residual disease in the femoral groove and can develop extensor-mechanism weakness (7–11).

The combination of unsatisfactory results in osteotomy and patellectomized patients and the excellent long-term results of total joint replacement initiated the development of patellofemoral replacement. Lubinus (12) introduced the patella glide replacement prosthesis in 1979 but did not report long-term results. Arciero and Toomey (13) and Cartier et al. (14) have reported good to excellent results in a significant number of patients, and all three of these investigators believe that patellofemoral surgery is indicated for patients with degenerative arthritis limited to the patellofemoral compartment (13,14).

Difficulties with femoral sizing and the necessity for removal of femoral bone stock initiated the deign of a custom patellofemoral replacement. A software program has been developed utilizing a computed tomographic scan of a patient's knee to construct a three-dimensional model of the patient's own femoral groove (15). This chapter presents the surgical technique and preliminary clinical results at a minimum of 2 years' follow-up.

■ INDICATIONS AND
CONTRAINDICATIONS

The indications for patellofemoral replacement are among the strictest for any orthopedic procedure. The patient must have intractable pain, palpable crepitus, and extreme retropatellar tenderness on examination, radiographic evidence of severe patellofemoral degenerative disease on both sides of the joint, and documented arthroscopic evidence of grade IV chondromalacia of the patella and femoral groove (Fig. 20-1). Most of the patients who eventually undergo patellofemoral replacement have failed previous surgical procedures, and the majority have undergone failed tibial tubercle elevations. It is difficult to determine whether a patient with moderately severe symptoms, radiographic changes on both sides of the patellofemoral joint, and documented grade IV lesions on both sides of the joint is best treated with a tibial tubercle elevation or a patellofemoral replacement. We usually recommend a tibial tubercle elevation in these patients and only recommend a patellofemoral replacement in those patients who have undergone failed tibial tubercle elevations or have severe symptoms and severe destruction of the patellofemoral joint. Age and weight certainly are factors, but the median age is younger among our patients un-

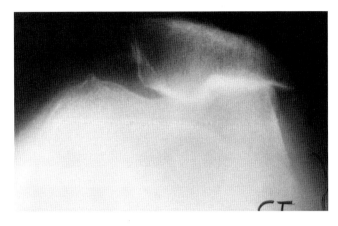

Severe patellofemoral degenerative arthritis in a 48-year-old woman.

dergoing patellofemoral replacement (44 years) compared with total knee replacement (69 years). The age disparity is secondary to the malalignment with significant patellar tilt and compression, which results in isolated patellofemoral degenerative disease at a younger age. These younger patients also have had numerous prior surgeries, and this may help account for the advanced degeneration. Our smaller group of patients with patellofemoral degenerative disease without malalignment who undergo patellofemoral replacement has a median age of 58 years, which is similar to those undergoing total knee replacement.

The final determination is between a patellofemoral replacement and a total knee replacement. Younger patients (less than 55 years old) with malalignment and isolated patellofemoral arthrosis are treated with patellofemoral replacement. A rare group is patients older than 55 years of age with isolated patellofemoral arthrosis. I recommend a patellofemoral replacement in this group but meticulously rule out the presence of femorotibial involvement, which would place these patients in a total knee replacement group. Younger patients (less than 55 years old) with tricompartmental degenerative disease are best treated with a total knee replacement if indicated.

An absolute contraindication is a past history of recent infection within the joint. The same precautions taken prior to total knee replacement are observed in indicating a patient for a patellofemoral replacement. Relative contraindications include age younger than 30 years, obesity, and age older than 55 years; these older patients are best treated with total knee replacement.

A software program utilizing a computed tomographic scan of a patient's knee has been designed that allows the construction of a three-dimensional model of the patient's own femoral groove (Fig. 20-2). A custom-fit cobalt–chrome femoral trial and a cobalt–chrome femoral groove prosthesis with fixation pegs are fabricated to be placed over the patient's own femoral groove. In essence, a custom resurfacing prosthesis is made. This eliminates the need to remove bone stock from the femur; impingement in flexion is eliminated, and revision to total knee is facilitated later, if necessary.

The patient is given epidural, spinal, or general anesthesia depending on the patient's and surgeon's choice. The leg is prepped and draped in the usual fashion. A midline incision is preferred, but frequently these patients have undergone previous patellofemoral stabilizing procedures or a tibial tubercle elevation through a lateral incision, and in these cases the original lateral incision is utilized. Minimal medial and lateral flaps are developed until the extensor mechanism is clearly visualized. The vastus medialis frequently is atrophied, and the quadriceps tendon is underdeveloped as well. A medial arthrotomy is preferred, but again, a lateral arthrotomy may be necessary if the patient has had a previous lateral incision, because a large medial flap should be avoided. The patella is everted and the knee flexed to 90 degrees. Patients who have had previous tibial tubercle elevations may require a quadriceps snip or an alternative quadriceps release in order to evert the patella.

■ SURGICAL TECHNIQUES

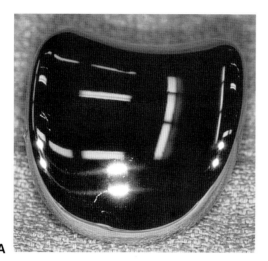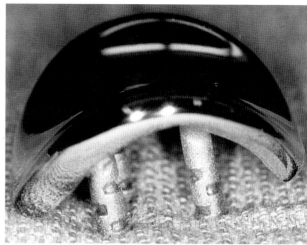

A   B

■ FIGURE 20-2   Custom cobalt–chrome femoral groove.

The entire knee is inspected, and the femoral groove is exposed completely by removing adherent synovium and osteophytes. The femoral template is placed on the femoral trochlear groove, and an outline is made with a marking pen to delineate the amount of groove to be decorticated (Fig 20-3).

The single most important technical consideration is to be certain that the prosthesis is not placed too far distally in the femoral groove, where it would impinge on the patella in flexion. The prosthesis must not overhang the intercondylar notch. The femoral groove is prepared for the implant by removing any remaining articular cartilage and decorticating the sclerotic degenerative surface with a curette or burr if needed. The fixation holes are prepared with a drill (Fig. 20-4), and the trial prosthesis is placed into position and evaluated for fit (Fig. 20-5).

Patella tracking and alignment are assessed closely at this time, with particular attention to poor tracking and patellar impingement on flexion. A lateral release is performed if the patella is subluxing laterally, and the femoral groove is shifted proximally if the patella is impinging in flexion.

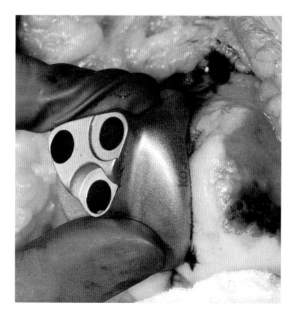

■ FIGURE 20-3   Femoral template in place outlining groove decortication.

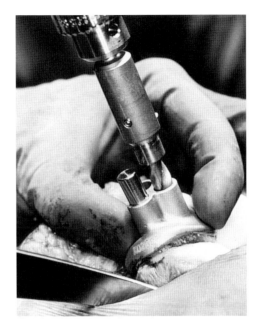

Femoral groove fixation hole being drilled.   ■ FIGURE 20-4

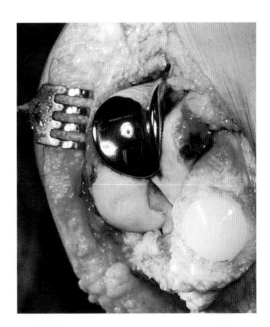

Femoral groove trial prothesis evaluated for fit.   ■ FIGURE 20-5

If patellar tracking is anatomic and there is no impingement in flexion, the femoral groove is irrigated and dried and the femoral implant is cemented into position and compressed until the cement is hardened (Fig. 20-6).

The patella is resurfaced in a standard fashion with a dome-shaped, nonanatomic implant and is cemented into position. Patella tracking and patellar impingement in flexion are assessed a final time, and a lateral release or revision of femoral groove position can be performed at this time.

A suction drain is placed, and the capsule is closed with a no. 2 nonabsorbable suture. The subcutaneous tissues and shin are closed, and a compression dressing and brace are

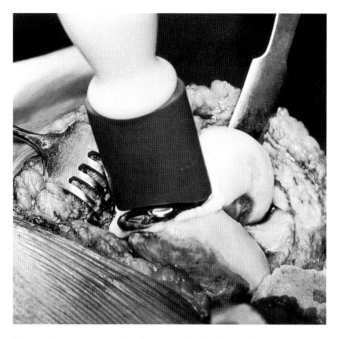

■ FIGURE 20-6

Femoral groove prosthesis cemented into position.

applied. The tourniquet is released, and the patient is brought to the postoperative recovery room. Radiographs are taken to observe position and cement fixation of the implants (Fig. 20-7A,B).

The immediate postoperative care is the same for any joint replacement of the lower extremity. Prophylactic antibiotics are given intravenously for 24 hours, and anticoagulation therapy is begun utilizing either warfarin or enoxaparin sodium. Continuous passive motion treatment is started immediately, with a full range of motion as tolerated.

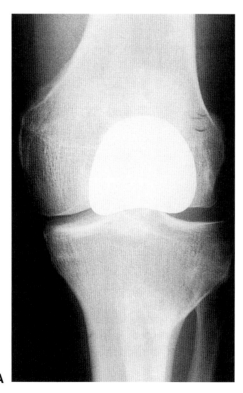 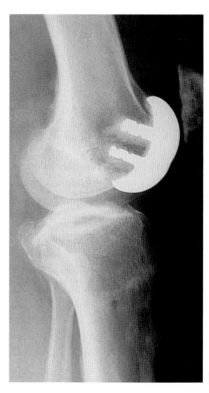

■ FIGURE 20-7   A   B

A,B: Anteroposterior and lateral radiographs of custom patellofemoral arthroplasty.

The surgical technique of patellofemoral replacement is standard, but alternative prostheses are available and can be utilized by the surgeon to reduce the costs of a custom patellofemoral replacement. Isolated patellar resurfacing is not a viable option, because of poor long-term results secondary to residual degenerative disease of the femoral groove. A constrained anatomic patella and a V-shaped femoral groove prosthesis are available, and long-term results have been favorable (13,14). There are two main disadvantages of this design: Patellar alignment must be precise, because the fit between the anatomic patella prosthesis and V-shaped femoral groove is constrained, and clicking and catching occur if patellar tracking is even slightly off-center; and the V-shaped femoral groove replaces significant femoral bone, which can make a revision to a total knee replacement difficult.

The custom patellofemoral replacement with a domed patella prosthesis allows for a wider range of patellar tracking, and catching of the prosthesis is avoided. The custom femoral groove removes very little femoral bone, and revision to a total knee replacement, if needed, is facilitated.

■ TECHNICAL ALTERNATIVES AND PITFALLS

The postoperative program includes immediate continuous passive motion treatment until a supervised physical therapy program is begun. Immediate full weight bearing is encouraged, and both closed- and open-chain kinetic exercises are utilized to develop quadriceps strength. Loss of motion is usually not a problem, and the majority of patients regain a full range in 3 to 6 months. A knee brace is recommended initially but should be discontinued when quadriceps function and strength return.

■ REHABILITATION

Twenty patients have undergone 23 custom patellofemoral replacements (three were bilateral). The average age at the time of replacement surgery was 44 years (range 31–70). Each of the knees had severe degenerative arthritis (grade IV chonromalacia) of the patellofemoral joint at the time of patellofemoral replacement. The average Hospital for Special Surgery knee score was 65 points (range 55–75) preoperatively and 85 points (range 65–95) postoperatively. The average follow-up was 46 months (range 24–134). There were excellent results in 10 patients, good in 10, and fair in two. One knee was revised to a total knee arthroplasty 6 years following the patellofemoral replacement and was considered a failure.

■ OUTCOMES AND FUTURE DIRECTIONS

Analysis of postoperative radiographs revealed no evidence of radiolucent lines in any of the femoral components. Radiolucent lines of less than 1 mm in thickness of the patella were seen in two knees, and radiolucent lines of 1 to 2 mm in thickness of the patella were seen in three knees. These lines were nonprogressive. No patient had radiographic evidence of loosening according to the criteria of the Knee Society or evidence of shifting or migration of any component. There were no infections, and there were no systemic complications.

References

1. Maquet P. Mechanics and osteoarthritis of the patellofemoral joint. *Clin Orthop* 1979; 144:70–73.
2. Ferguson AB, Brown TD, Fu FH, et al. Relief of patellofemoral contact stress by anterior displacement of the tibial tubercle. *J Bone Joint Surg Am* 1979; 61:159–166.
3. Radin E, Leach R. Anterior displacement of the tibial tubercle for patellofemoral arthrosis. *Orthop Trans* 1979; 3:291.
4. Silvello L, Scarponi R, Guazetti R, et al. Tibial tubercle advancement by the Maquet technique for patellofemoral arthritis or chondromalacia. *Ital J Orthop Traumatol* 1987; 13:37–44.
5. Friedman MJ. Modified Maquet tibial tubercle elevation. *Am J Knee Surg* 1990; 3:114–118.
6. Insall JN. Disorders of the patella. In: Insall JN, eds. *Surgery of the knee.* New York: Churchill Livingston, 1984:252.
7. Sisto DJ. Patellofemoral degenerative joint disease. In: Cooke D, Grayson TH, eds. *Knee surgery,* vol 2. Baltimore: Williams & Wilkins, 1994:1203–1221.
8. Boyd HB, Hawkins BL. Patellectomy: A simplified technique. *Surg Gynecol Obstet* 1948; 86:357–358.
9. Baker CL, Hughston JC. Miyakawa patellectomy. *J Bone Joint Surg Am* 1988; 70:1489–1494.
10. Lewis MM, Fitzgerald PF, Jacobs B, et al. Patellectomy: An analysis of one hundred cases. *J Bone Joint Surg Am* 1976; 58:736.

11. Kelly MA, Insall JN. Patellectomy. *Orthop Clin North Am* 1986; 17:289–290.
12. Lubinus HH. Patella glide bearing total replacement. *Orthopedics* 1979; 2:119.
13. Arciero RA, Toomey HE. Patellofemoral arthroplasty: A three-to nine-year follow-up study. *Clin Orthop* 1988; 236:60–71.
14. Cartier P, Sanouiller JL, Grelsamer R. Patellofemoral arthroplasty: Two-to twelve-year follow-up study. *J Arthroplasty* 1990; 5:49–55.
15. Blazina ME, Anderson LJ, Hirsh LC. Patellofemoral replacement: Utilizing a customized femoral groove replacement. *Tech Orthop* 1990; 5:53–55.

PETER J. THADANI
KELLY G. VINCE

21

Surgical Technique for Posterior Cruciate Retaining and Posterior Cruciate Substituting Total Knee Arthroplasties

Posterior Cruciate Ligament–retaining Arthroplasty Modern, condylar-type total knee arthroplasties probably began with the ideas of Townley in the late 1940s. His anatomic total knee arthroplasty, introduced in 1972, included retention of both cruciate ligaments and articulation of a condylar resurfacing metal femoral component with a high-density polyethylene tibial plate (1–4). Cloutier (5,6), another "biologically minded" surgeon, introduced his nonconstrained resurfacing prosthesis in 1975; this design also retained both cruciate ligaments. The concept of preserving both cruciate ligaments faded with the introduction of bicondylar arthroplasties, which were essentially the mechanical union of two unicompartmental arthroplasties. At this time emphasis was placed on larger tibial components that would be less likely to break or loosen (7).

The duocondylar prosthesis was introduced by Ranawat and Shine (8) at the Hospital for Special Surgery in 1973 as a posterior cruciate ligament (PCL)–retaining device. It later was modified to include patellofemoral resurfacing, which resulted in the duopatellar prosthesis (9). Further research dedicated to prosthetic design with PCL preservation led to the development of the linematic prosthesis (10), which subsequently evolved into a variety of modern PCL-retaining prostheses. Proponents of PCL retention argue for improved posterior tibial stability, potentially less transmission of forces through the prosthesis to the fixation interface, and a theoretically near normal gait (11).

Posterior Cruciate Ligament–substituting Arthroplasty The concept of kinematic conflict, whereby the articular geometry dictates a different motion of the femur on the tibia than does that of the cruciate ligament, brought to light the issue of PCL retention versus substitution (11,12). With a knee arthroplasty, if the PCL induces femoral rollback but a dished or conforming tibial articulation does not permit it, the knee impinges posteriorly and flexes poorly (11). The first modern type of arthroplasty to incorporate PCL resection was the Freeman–Swanson prosthesis, first implanted in March 1970 and described as a "roller in a trough" (13). One of the design criteria for this prosthesis was that it should not depend on the integrity of the cruciate ligaments for stability (14). The total condylar prosthesis, introduced in 1973 at the Hospital for Special Surgery, also was an early example of a PCL-sacrificing device (15–17). The total condylar prosthesis subsequently evolved into the posterior stabilized prosthesis, which incorporated a post and cam mechanism to address the issues of anteroposterior stability and simulation of femoral rollback to improve flexion. This has served as the basis for modern PCL-substituting prosthetic designs. Those in favor of cruciate excision believe that this concept is technically easier to execute and necessary to correct fixed deformities. Additionally, wear may be less than with PCL-retaining prostheses, because of the generally conforming surfaces that can be used (11).

■ HISTORY OF THE TECHNIQUE

209

Total knee arthroplasty is indicated for patients with end-stage degenerative and inflammatory arthritidies that have failed conservative treatment. In the straightforward case, cruciate retention or cruciate substitution is largely a matter of surgeon preference, with most arthroplasties being performed today using cruciate retention. If the reconstruction must include correction of a deformity, cruciate substitution may be a more sound choice (18–21).

Contraindications include active or subacute sepsis and the medical inability to withstand the surgical procedure. Relative contraindications include the diagnosis of neuropathic joint, extensor mechanism rupture, severe soft-tissue inadequacies with severe peripheral vascular disease, and the presence of a stable, painless arthrodesis.

Posterior Cruciate Ligament–retaining Arthroplasty   Certain principles should be applied to all total knee arthroplasties regardless of the design that is used. It is essential to produce a neutral mechanical axis from the center of the femoral head through the center of the knee to the center of the ankle by creating a valgus anatomic alignment of the femoral and tibial axes (22,23). This involves balancing the medial and lateral ligamentous structures, also required for knee stability. Knee flexion and extension gaps should be equalized, in order to maximize motion and retain stability. Failure to do so results in either a painful, stiff knee or one that is subject to instability in extension or dislocation in flexion (24).

Posterior cruciate ligament tension is decided by:

1. The thickness of the articular polyethylene.
2. The level of the tibial cut.
3. The slope of the tibial cut as viewed from the side.
4. The size of the femoral component and position of the femoral cuts.

All of these variables must be optimized to ensure that stability and mobility are preserved. Perhaps the most significant decision is the selection of femoral component size. The "overstuffed" knee joint, troubled by an overly large or posteriorly displaced femoral component, is problematic for all arthroplasties and especially with PCL retention. Furthermore, the positions of the femoral cuts are critical, in that the distance from the epicondyles (the attachment of the collateral ligaments) to the articular surface should be preserved.

Two types of femoral instrumentation prevail in knee arthroplasty surgery: those that reference from the anterior femoral cortex and those that reference from the posterior femoral condyles (25). The former facilitate avoidance of notching of the anterior femur, because the anterior cut is always made flush with the anterior cortex. The intervals between available sizes are reflected in differences in tension posteriorly. Surgeons who favor cruciate ligament retention often select instruments that reference from the posterior articular surface, arguing that it is this dimension that is essential to preserve if the collateral ligaments and the PCL are expected to function normally.

So-called classic alignment, which seems to be used more commonly in knee arthroplasty, involves resection of the proximal tibia at a right angle to the long axis of the tibia as viewed anteriorly. This is in contrast to the normal alignment of the articular surface of the tibia, which lies at approximately 3 degrees of varus with respect to the tibia's anatomic axis (26). The so-called anatomic instrument systems, introduced in 1982 with the Universal Total Knee Instrumentation System (Howmedica, Rutherford, NJ) (27,28), replicated normal anatomy if all of the cuts were made accurately. The pitfall of aiming for a 3-degree varus tibial cut, however, was that despite a reasonable margin of error, the actual cut resulted in an unacceptable degree of varus, which subsequently led to tibial component subsidence and failure of the arthroplasty (29–31).

The implication of classic alignment is that by performing a perpendicular tibial resection, more bone is removed from the lateral tibial plateau than from the medial plateau. Accordingly, a commensurably larger amount of bone would be resected from the medial posterior femoral condyle than the lateral, in order to create a symmetric, rectangular flexion space, which is essential for satisfactory collateral ligament function (Fig. 21-1) (32,33).

This rotational positioning concept has become known popularly as "external rotation of the femoral component." A more reliable and anatomic guide for proper femoral component rotation is the axis formed by the medial and lateral epicondyles, or the transepicondylar axis. These epicondylar prominences correspond to the origins of the collateral ligaments (34–37). If the femoral component rotation is parallel to the transepicondylar axis and is coupled with a classic resection of the tibia, it is critical to determine whether the PCL and collateral ligaments can be balanced.

Because tibial component loosening was of such concern a decade ago, surgeons were compelled to resect minimal amounts of tibial plateau, with the goal of preserving the maximally strong proximal tibia. This led to suboptimal reconstructions, with relatively little space between the femur and tibia and the implantation of thin polyethylene inserts. These arthroplasties were subject to catastrophic failure resulting from wear (38–42).

To accommodate thicker, more durable articular polyethylene inserts, one might consider resecting additional femoral bone. This is to be avoided, especially with PCL retention, because it elevates the joint line from its normal anatomic position and thus significantly alters normal cruciate function. The PCL in a knee with an elevated joint line becomes increasingly tight with further flexion and can cause excessive rollback and increased posterior stresses (43–45).

Of the three conflicting goals–preservation of proximal tibial bone, implantation of sufficient polyethylene thickness, and maintenance of the joint line—it seems that the first goal can be most safely compromised by additional resection of proximal tibial bone. Neither the material properties of the proximal tibia nor the kinematics of the knee should suffer from removal of a few additional millimeters of bone. (25). This, however, places the PCL at risk. As thicker pieces of proximal tibia are removed, the PCL attachment is jeopardized. A resection of 10 mm may result in complete detachment (46).

Creation of an island of bone in the posterior middle region of the proximal tibial articular surface (at the insertion of the cruciate ligament) ensures preservation of the PCL insertion. This is created most easily with two saggital saw cuts initiated from the front of the knee (Fig. 21-2A) to create a pie-shaped wedge whose apex is in the middle of the plateau.

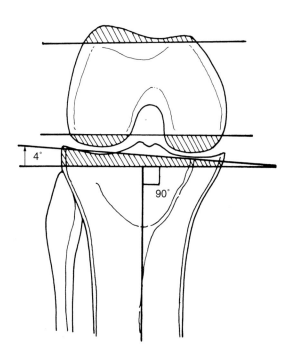

Bone resection with classic arthroplasty alignment. The ibial plateau is cut perpendicular to its anatomic axis, resulting in more bone resection from lateral plateau than medial. Correspondingly more bone is resected from the medial posterior femoral condyle than the lateral, to equalize medial and lateral flexion spaces.

■ FIGURE 21-1

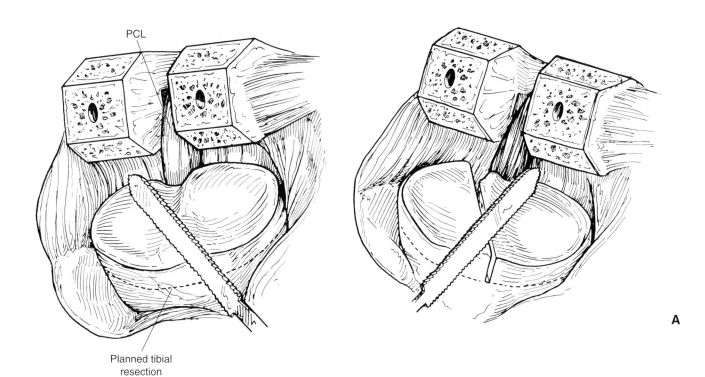

PCL

Planned tibial
resection

A

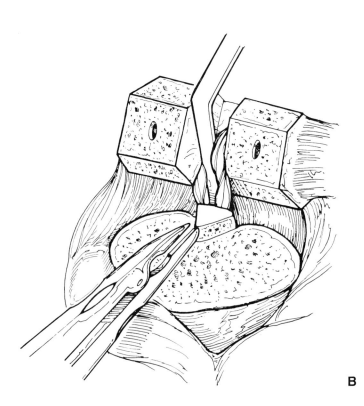

B

Posterior cruciate ligament preservation. **A:** Two sagittal saw cuts are made to resect the tibial
plateau, with preservation of an island of bone containing the ligament attachment. **B:** After the
plateau is resurfaced, a rongeur is used to trim the bone island carefully, to accommodate the tibial
component.

■ FIGURE 21-2

This ater can be reduced in size with a rongeur to accommodate the tibial component (Fig. 21-2B).

The insertion of spacer blocks was popularized with cruciate ligament–sacrificing and –substituting designs (32,33). Many knee arthroplasty systems intended for use with PCL preservation have not included these blocks as a formal step in the procedure but rather have relied on trial reduction to assess flexion–extension and varus–valgus balance. It is often useful, however, to insert blocks as a formal step, to demonstrate that flexion and extension gaps are indeed equal and of the appropriate tension. This step also can give early clues to the need for collateral ligament releases. If used in conjunction with an alignment rod, the spacer block is an accurate guide to the posterior slope of the tibial bone cut as viewed from the side.

Ultimately, trial components are inserted, and the knee is evaluated in flexion and extension. Three criteria must be met in extension (Fig. 21-3):

1. Absolutely full extension without recurvatum or residual flexion contracture.
2. Satisfactory valgus anatomic alignment (neutral mechanical axis).
3. Satisfactory varus–valgus stability.

In flexion, the knee should feel just slightly more lax than in extension, corresponding to the normal knee. Without this slight difference the patient will flex poorly. This difference in laxity, however, should not result in gross anteroposterior instability in flexion.

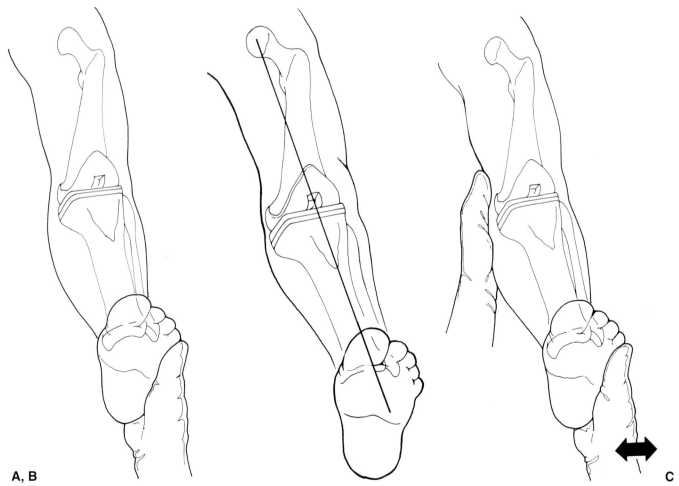

A, B

C

Evaluation of the knee in extension with trial components. **A:** The knee should achieve full extension without recurvatum. **B:** The mechanical axis should be neutral with trial components in place. This can be checked with an electrocautery cord. **C:** Satisfactory varus–valgus stability.

■ FIGURE 21-3

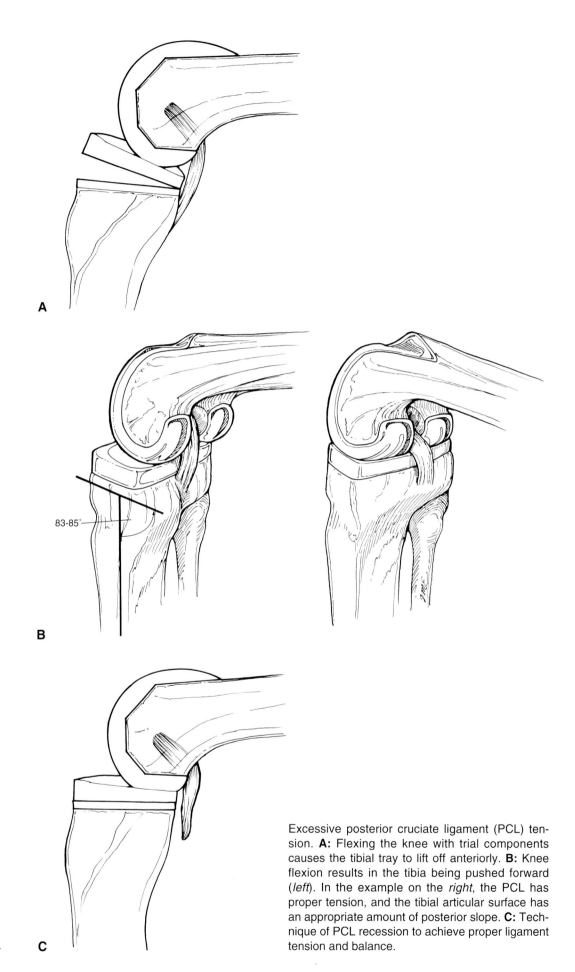

A

83-85°

B

C

■ FIGURE 21-4

Excessive posterior cruciate ligament (PCL) tension. **A:** Flexing the knee with trial components causes the tibial tray to lift off anteriorly. **B:** Knee flexion results in the tibia being pushed forward (*left*). In the example on the *right*, the PCL has proper tension, and the tibial articular surface has an appropriate amount of posterior slope. **C:** Technique of PCL recession to achieve proper ligament tension and balance.

It has become clear that the arthroplasty that is excessively tight in flexion will neither bend well nor feel comfortable for the patient. The knee that is moderately tight in flexion eventually succumbs to increased posterior polyethylene wear with osteolysis and consequently exhibits subluxation, instability, and ultimately dislocation (41,42,44,45). The culprit is the excessively tight PCL and the excessive femoral component rollback that accompanies it.

Several criteria have been developed to assess PCL tension and femoral rollback intraoperatively with trial components (45,47). Excessive PCL tightness is suggested if during flexion the tibial component lifts off anteriorly from the resected surface of the tibial plateau, or if the tibia is thrust forward more than a few millimeters (Fig. 21-4). The femoral component also may be pushed off the distal femur if the knee is too tight in flexion. If any of these signs are observed, the thickness of the tibial tray and the anteroposterior size of the femoral component must be checked to ensure that neither is too large. It is also important to verify that the posterior tibial slope is adequate, because insufficient or neutral slope results in a tight PCL. (48) The desired slope is usually between 5 and 7 degrees. If the PCL is excessively tight despite proper slope, adjustment of the tension by recession is required (Fig. 21-5).

Posterior Cruciate Ligament Recession   Just as collateral ligament tension sometimes is adjusted by releases in the correction of varus or valgus deformities, the PCL tension occasionally requires similar attention. This can be accomplished by releasing fibers of the PCL from either the femoral or tibial attachments (Fig. 21-6). Each technique has proponents (47,49–51). Release from the posterior femur can be regarded as somewhat selective: Release of some of the anterior fibers may produce the desired balance and leave the posterior fibers intact. Surgeons who favor release from the tibia argue that there is still an intact sleeve that theoretically can reattach itself to the posterior aspect of the tibia in its lengthened or recessed state.

Inability to sufficiently balance the PCL despite a complete ligament resection creates

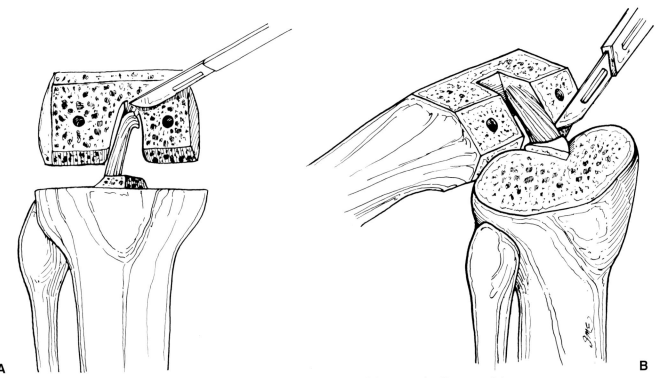

A

B

Technique of PCL release. **A:** Release of anterior fibers from femoral origin; posterior fibers are left intact. **B:** Release performed from tibial insertion.   ■ FIGURE 21-5

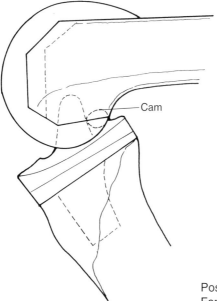

■ FIGURE 21-6   Posterior stabilization through spine and cam mechanism. Femoral rollback allows for improved flexion.

two choices for the surgeon: perform a cruciate ligament–sacrificing knee arthroplasty or a cruciate ligament–substituting arthroplasty. In straightforward cases, cruciate sacrificing arthroplasties have functioned extremely well with excellent stability and good motion (without risk of dislocation), provided the flexion and extension gaps have been carefully balanced (17,52). With complete PCL release, it is also important that the articular geometry of the implants have some conformity in order to provide additional stability.

The goal of cruciate ligament recession is to maintain femoral contact within the central portion of the tibial articular platform and not to recreate femoral rollback, as opposed to the original goals of cruciate ligament–retaining arthroplasties. In this manner posterior tibial component wear can be minimized.

Posterior Stabilized Arthroplasty   The PCL was excised during creation of some early total knee prostheses, because of the belief that it not only contributed to the pathology but also was difficult to integrate into the kinematics of the articular surface (7). Early designs such as the Geometric (Howmedica), which featured a highly conforming articular geometry as a means of enhancing stability, did not tolerate the preservation of the PCL because of a phenomenon known as "kinematic conflict" (53,54). In this situation, both the articular geometry and the PCL tried to engineer femoral rollback. These were not in agreement, and stiffness usually resulted, sometimes in conjunction with premature loosening (55–57).

Accordingly, more conforming (though not constrained) articular geometries were developed in prosthetic devices intended for implantation with resection of both cruciate ligaments. One of the earliest successful designs employing this concept was the total condylar knee arthroplasty, introduced in 1973 (15–17). Although the majority of implants worked very well despite the absence of the PCL, it became clear that a small percentage, especially those in patients with prior patellectomies, were susceptible to posterior dislocation in flexion (17). There was also concern that flexion, which averaged about 90 degrees, was poor because of lack of femoral rollback. Consequently, posterior stabilization was introduced through a spine and cam mechanism as a means of increasing femoral rollback in order to improve flexion (58). This concept was substantiated through various clinical reports describing increased flexion in posterior stabilized arthroplasties (59,60).

Excision of the PCL can be accomplished most efficiently by first removing it from the posterior femur with the knee in a flexed position. Bone resection on the tibia can proceed without regard for the PCL attachment. Accordingly, the bony resection can incorporate a slight degree of posterior slope to facilitate flexion. The thickness of bone removed from the proximal tibia can be duplicated easily by selection of an identical thickness of articular polyethylene.

Once all the bone cuts and appropriate collateral ligament releases have been performed, insertion of spacer blocks should demonstrate full extension with proper valgus alignment and good varus–valgus stability. Additionally, the flexion gap should be stable.

An alternative to total knee arthroplasty is unicompartmental replacement. The ideal candidate is in the same age group and has a similar demand level as the candidate for total knee arthroplasty but has disease limited to a single compartment. Additionally, angular deformities should be less than 15 degrees, flexion contractures less than 5 degrees, and the anterior cruciate ligament should be intact. Inflammatory arthridities represent a contraindication to the use of this technique. It has been theorized to be a bone-sparing operation, thereby making it appealing to the younger patient in whom later revision may be necessary, but this has not been the case in practice (61,62). Advantages include faster recovery and improved motion compared with tricompartmental arthroplasty, as well as preservation of both cruciate ligaments and bone stock in the uninvolved and patellofemoral compartments. Slight undercorrection of varus alignment and adequate tibial component polyethylene thickness are important contributors to long-term success (63). With proper patient selection, good long-term results can be achieved, although tricompartmental arthroplasties have demonstrated better results with statistical survivorship analysis (63,64).

Some surgeons mistakenly may select a prosthesis with varus–valgus constraint as an alternative to posterior stabilization. It is important to discriminate between the two, because a constrained device compromises long-term fixation of the arthroplasty and remains, if not essential, too high a price to pay for simple posterior stabilization (65). The indication for varus–valgus constraint is the inability to balance the collateral ligaments, as is the case with an absent or damaged collateral ligament. Other options for collateral ligament balance or reconstruction must be considered before resorting to the use of a constrained prosthesis.

Common pitfalls associated with cruciate ligament–retaining arthroplasties include the use of articular polyethylene that is too thin, and failure to recess the PCL that is too tight. The surgeon who correctly identifies a problem and its implications can readily address the dilemma using the strategies just described.

Attempting to use a cruciate ligament–retaining implant in the stiff knee, in the knee with considerable varus or valgus deformity, or in the face of a severe flexion contracture may produce a result inferior to that produced using the implant in which the PCL is resected (18–21). A posterior stabilized design also has been shown to be a better choice in the patient who has had a prior patellectomy (17,60,66,67).

■ TECHNICAL ALTERNATIVES AND PITFALLS

■ REHABILITATION

Postoperative rehabilitation after primary total knee arthroplasty is the same regardless of the manner in which the PCL is addressed. Full weight bearing and range-of-motion exercises may start in the immediate postoperative period for all cemented primary arthroplasties. As discussed in Chapter 25, this protocol also is used in cases requiring bone graft, because we feel that structural graft is mechanically strongest when initially implanted. This type of graft usually is protected by an intramedullary stem.

Preoperative exercise and strengthening programs have not changed any outcome measures (68), but preoperative teaching programs have been extremely valuable in educating patients and lessening fear and anxiety (69). It is also during the preoperative period that realistic goals and expectations for functional levels are established.

Postoperatively, some surgeons temporarily employ posterior splints or knee immobilizers until patients can demonstrate straight leg raising, but this is largely a matter of surgeon preference. Early rehabilitation should proceed with the goals of regaining full extension and maximal flexion. The surgeon must recognize that adequate analgesia and an optimal hemodynamic status are absolute requirements for patients to participate in a postoperative therapy program. The use of continuous passive motion treatment is controversial. Although it appears to result in faster return of motion and potentially earlier hospital discharge, long-term advantages have not been proven (70,71). With economic constraints resulting in earlier hospital discharge, the rehabilitation program must be coordinated to continue in the outpatient setting. After the initial recovery phase, endurance and strength become important to long-term success of the arthroplasty.

■ OUTCOMES AND FUTURE DIRECTIONS

Despite philosophic differences between surgeons, leading some to favor one style over another, both cruciate ligament–retaining and posterior stabilized knee arthroplasties have produced excellent long-term durability and functional results. More wear has been observed with cruciate ligament–retaining arthroplasties (42,72,73). This problem can be solved in the cruciate ligament–substituting design with thicker polyethylene, more conformity, and proper ligament balance. Finally, meniscal bearing knees may represent the next step in knee arthroplasty. These designs have been introduced as a means of permitting motion yet reducing polyethylene contact stresses (74,75). With this technology, however, comes the concern over backside polyethylene wear.

References

1. Townley CO. *The anatomic total knee.* Port Huron, MI: Acorn Press, 1973.
2. Townley CO. The anatomic total knee: Rationale, surgical technique, and long term results. *Orthop Trans* 1983; 7:531.
3. Townley CO. The anatomic total knee resurfacing arthroplasty. *Clin Orthop* 1985; 192:82–96.
4. Townley CO, Hill L. Total knee replacement. *Am J Nursing* 1974; 74:1612–1617.
5. Cloutier JM. Results of total knee arthroplasty with a non-constrained prosthesis. *J Bone Joint Surg Am* 1983; 65:7.
6. Cloutier JM. Long term results after nonconstrained total knee arthroplasty. *Clin Orthop* 1991; 273:63–65.
7. Vince KG. Evolution of total knee arthroplasty. In: Scott WN, ed. *The knee.* St. Louis: Mosby, 1994:1045–1078.
8. Ranawat CS, Shine J. Duocondylar total knee arthroplasty. *Clin Orthop* 1973; 94:185–195.
9. Ewald FC, Thomas R, Poss M, et al. Duopatellar total knee replacement in rheumatoid arthritis. *Orthop Trans* 1978; 2:202.
10. Ewald FC, Jacobs MA, Miegel RE, et al. Kinematic total knee replacement. *J Bone Joint Surg Am* 1984; 66:1032–1040.
11. Insall JN. Historical development, classification, and characteristics of knee prostheses. In: Insall JN, ed. *Surgery of the knee,* 2nd edition. New York: Churchill Livingstone, 1993:677–717.
12. Andriacchi TP, Stanwyck T, Galante JO. Knee biomechanics and total knee replacement. *J Arthroplasty* 1986; 1:211–219.
13. Freeman MAR, Swanson SAV, Zahin A. Total replacement of the knee using a metal-polyethylene two-part prosthesis. *Proc R Soc Med* 1972; 65:374.
14. Freeman MAR, Swanson SAV, Todd RC. Total replacement of the knee using the Freeman-Swanson knee prosthesis. *Clin Orthop* 1973; 94:153–170.
15. Insall JN, Ranawat CS, Aglietti P, et al. A comparison of four models of total knee replacement prosthesis. *J Bone Joint Surg Am* 1976; 58:754.
16. Insall JN, Ranawat CS, Scott WN, et al. Total condylar knee replacement: Preliminary report. *Clin Orthop* 1976; 120:149–154.
17. Vince KG, Insall JN, Kelly MA. The total condylar prosthesis: 10-12 year results of a cemented knee replacement. *J Bone Joint Surg Br* 1989; 71:793–797.
18. Laskin RS, O'Flynn HM. The Insall Award. Total knee replacement with posterior cruciate ligament retention in rheumatoid arthritis: Problems and complications. *Clin Orthop* 1997; 345:24–28.
19. Laskin RS. Total knee replacement with posterior cruciate ligament retention in patients with a fixed varus deformity. *Clin Orthop* 1996; 331:29–34.
20. Hood RW, Vanni M, Insall JN. The correction of knee alignment in 225 consecutive total condylar knee replacements. *Clin Orthop* 1981; 160:94.
21. Hungerford D, Krackow K, Kenna R. Management of fixed deformity at total knee arthroplasty. In: *Total knee arthroplasty: A comprehensive approach.* Baltimore: Williams & Wilkins, 1984:163–192.
22. Maquet PGJ. Mechanical stresses in the knee. In: Maquet PGJ, ed. *Biomechanics of the knee.* Heidelberg, Germany: Springer-Verlag, 1984:15–73.

23. Krackow KA. *The technique of total knee arthroplasty.* St. Louis: Mosby, 1990.
24. Pagnano MW, Hanssen AD, Lewallen DG. Flexion instability after primary posterior cruciate retaining total knee arthroplasty. *Clin Orthop* 1998; 356:39–46.
25. Insall JN. Surgical techniques and instrumentation in total knee arthroplasty. In: Insall JN, ed. *Surgery of the knee,* 2nd edition. New York: Churchill Livingstone, 1993:739–804.
26. Kapandji IA. *The physiology of the joints.* New York: Churchill Livingstone, 1976.
27. Hungerford DS, Kenna RV, Krackow KA. The porous-coated anatomic total knee. *Orthop Clin North Am* 1982; 13:103–122.
28. Greenberg RL, Kenna RV, Hungerford DS, et al. Instrumentation for total knee arthroplasty. In: Hungerford DS, Krackow KA, Kenna RV, eds. *Total knee arthroplasty: A comprehensive approach.* Baltimore: Williams & Wilkins, 1984:35–70.
29. Ewald FC, Jacobs MA, Miegal RE, et al. Kinematic total knee replacement. *J Bone Joint Surg Am* 1984; 66:1032–1040.
30. Tew M, Waugh W. Tibiofemoral alignment and the results of knee replacement. *J Bone Joint Surg Br* 1985; 67:551.
31. Jeffery RS, Morris RW, Denham RA. Coronal alignment after total knee replacement. *J Bone Joint Surg Br* 1991; 73:709.
32. Freeman MAR. *Arthritis of the knee: Clinical features and surgical management.* New York: Springer-Verlag, 1980.
33. Insall JN. Technique of total knee replacement: American Academy of Orthopaedic Surgeons. *Instr Course Lect* 1981; 30:324.
34. Berger RA, Rubash HE, Seel MJ, et al. Determining the rotational alignment of the femoral component in total knee arthroplasty using the epicondylar axis. *Clin Orthop* 1993; 286:40–47.
35. Poilvache PL, Insall JN, Scuderi GR, et al. Rotational landmarks and sizing of the distal femur in total knee arthroplasty. *Clin Orthop* 1996; 331:35–46.
36. Mantas JP, Bloebaum RD, Skedros JG, et al. Implications of references axes used for rotational alignment of the femoral component in primary and revison knee arthroplasty. *J Arthroplasty* 1992; 7:531–5.
37. Stiehl JB, Abbott BD. Morphology of the transepicondylar axis and its application in primary and revision total knee arthroplasty. *J Arthroplasty* 1995; 10:785–789.
38. Bartel DL, Bicknell VL, Wright TM. The effect of conformity, thickness, and material on stress in ultra-high molecular weight components for total joint replacement. *J Bone Joint Surg Am* 1986; 68:1041.
39. Collier J, Mayor MB, McNamara JL, et al. Analysis of the failure of 122 polyethylene inserts from uncemented tibial knee components. *Clin Orthop* 1991; 273:232.
40. Wright TM, Bartel DL. The problem of surface damage in polyethylene total knee components. *Clin Orthop* 1986; 205:67.
41. Tsao A, Mintz L, McRae CR, et al. Failure of the porous-coated anatomic prosthesis in total knee arthroplasty due to severe polyethylene wear. *J Bone Joint Surg Am* 1993; 75:19–26.
42. Wright TM, Rimnac CM, Stulberg SD, et al. Wear of polyethylene in total joint replacements: Observations from retrieved PCA knee implants. *Clin Orthop* 1992; 276:126–134.
43. Ryu J, Saito S, Yamamoto K, et al. Factors influencing the postoperative range of motion in total knee arthroplasty. *Bull Hosp Jt Dis* 1993; 53:35–40.
44. Corces A, Lotke PA, Williams JL. Strain characteristics of the posterior cruciate ligament in total knee replacement. *Orthop Trans* 1989; 13:527.
45. Swany MR, Scott RD. Posterior polyethylene wear in posterior cruciate ligament-retaining total knee arthroplasty: A case study. *J Arthroplasty* 1993; 8:439–46.
46. Girgis FG, Marshall JL, Al Monajem ARS. The cruciate ligaments of the knee joint: Anatomical, functional, and experimental analysis. *Clin Orthop* 1975; 106:216–231.
47. Ritter MA, Farris PM, Keating EM. Posterior cruciate ligament balancing during total knee arthroplasty. *J Arthroplasty* 1988; 3:323.
48. Singerman R, Dean JC, Pagan HD, et al. Decreased posterior tibial slope increases strain in the posterior cruciate ligament following total knee arthroplasty. *J Arthroplasty* 1996; 11:99–103.
49. Bertin KC. Instrumentation. In: Fu FH, Harner CD, Vince KG, eds. *Knee surgery.* Baltimore: Williams & Wilkins, 1994:1303–1312.
50. Arima J, Whiteside LA, Martin JW, et al. Effect of partial release of the posterior cruciate ligament in total knee arthroplasty. *Clin Orthop* 1998; 353:194–202.
51. Worland RL, Jessup DE, Johnson J. Posterior cruciate recession in total knee arthroplasty. *J Arthroplasty* 1997; 12:70–73.
52. Ranawat CS, Flynn WF Jr, Deshmukh RG. Impact of modern technique on long-term results of total condylar knee arthroplasty. *Clin Orthop* 1994; 309:131–135.

53. Coventry MB, Upshaw JE, Riley LH, et al. Geometric total knee arthroplasty: I. Conception, design, indications and surgical technique. *Clin Orthop* 1973; 94:171.
54. Coventry MB, Upshaw JE, Riley LH, et al. Geometric total knee arthroplasty: II. Patient data and complications. *Clin Orthop* 1973; 94:177.
55. Rand JA, Coventry MB. Ten-year evaluation of geometric total knee arthroplasty. *Clin Orthop* 1988; 232:168.
56. Riley D, Woodyard JE. Long-term results of geometric total knee replacement. *J Bone Joint Surg Br* 1985; 67:548
57. Skolnick MD, Coventry MB, Ilstrup DM. Geometric total knee arthroplasty: A two year follow-up study. *J Bone Joint Surg Am* 1976; 58:749.
58. Insall JN, Lachiewicz PF, Burstein AH. The posterior stabilized condylar prosthesis: A modification of the total condylar design. *J Bone Joint Surg Am* 1982; 64:1317.
59. Scott WN, Rubinstein M. Posterior stabilized knee arthroplasty: Six-year experience. *Clin Orthop* 1986; 205:138–145.
60. Vince KG. The posterior stabilized knee prosthesis. In: Laskin RS, ed. *Total knee replacement*. New York: Springer-Verlag, 1991.
61. Barrett WP, Scott RD. Revision of failed unicondylar unicompartmental knee arthroplasty. *J Bone Joint Surg Am* 1987; 69:1328.
62. Padgett DE, Stern SH, Insall JN. Revision total knee arthroplasty for failed unicompartmental replacement. *J Bone Joint Surg Am* 1991; 73:186.
63. Cartier P, Sanouiller JL, Grelsamer RP. Unicompartmental knee arthroplasty surgery: 10-year minimum follow-up period. *J Arthroplasty* 1996; 11:782–788.
64. Scott RD, Cobb AG, McQueary FG, et al. Unicompartmental knee arthroplasty: Eight-to 12-year follow-up evaluation with survivorship analysis. *Clin Orthop* 1991; 271:96–100.
65. Vince KG, Long W. Revision knee arthroplasty: The limits of press fit medullary fixation. *Clin Orthop* 1995; 317:172–177.
66. Bayne O, Cameron HU. Total knee arthroplasty following patellectomy. *Clin Orthop* 1984; 186:112–114.
67. Laskin RS, Palleta G. Total knee replacement in the post patellectomy patient. *J Arthroplasty* 1994; 9:109.
68. Colwell CW Jr. Rehabilitation following total knee arthroplasty. In Callaghan JJ, Dennis DA, Paprosky WG, Rosenberg AG, eds. *Orthopaedic knowledge update hip and knee reconstruction*. American Academy of Orthopaedic Surgeons, 1995:301–302.
69. Underhill MA. Nursing care of a patient having a total knee arthroplasty. In Scott WN, ed. *The knee*. St. Louis: Mosby, 1994:1229–1238.
70. Colwell CW Jr, Morris BA. The influence of continuous passive motion on the results of total knee arthroplasty. *Clin Orthop* 1992; 276:225–228.
71. Romness DW, Rand JA. The role of continuous passive motion following total knee arthroplasty. *Clin Orthop* 1988; 226:34–37.
72. Rose RM, Crugnola A, Ries M, et al. On origins of high in vivo wear rates in polyethylene components of total joint prostheses. *Clin Orthop* 1979; 145:277.
73. Wasielewski RC, Galante JO, Leighty RM, et al. Wear patterns on retrieved polyethylene tibial inserts and their relationship to technical considerations during total knee arthroplasty. *Clin Orthop* 1994; 299:31.
74. Buechel FF. Long-term outcomes and expectations: cementless meniscal bearing knee arthroplasty: 7- to 12-year outcome analysis. *Orthopedics* 1994; 17:833–836.
75. Jordan LR, Olivo JL, Voorhorst PE. Survivorship analysis of cementless meniscal bearing total knee arthroplasty. *Clin Orthop* 1997; 338:119–123.

PAOLO AGLIETTI
JOHN N. INSALL
FRANCESCO GIRON
PETER S. WALKER

22

The Meniscal Bearing Knee

The concept of the mobile bearing knee was developed in the late 1970s in an effort to mimic the normal anatomy of the knee. With this prosthetic design the developers intended to achieve better joint kinematics and reduced polyethylene wear. Other possible advantages included less stress on fixation and self-adjusting rotational tibial position.

The most widely known models of this prosthetic include the Oxford (Biomet, USA), the low contact stress (LCS) (De Puy, Warsaw, IN), and more recently the Rotaglide (Corin), the TACK (Link, Hamberg; Germany), and the SAL (Protek). Good mid- to long-term results have been published with the Oxford (1) and the LCS (2) knees. The results obtained with these two models therefore represent the baseline of comparison for other mobile bearing knees being introduced.

In 1992 a new prosthesis was developed called the *meniscal bearing knee* (Zimmer, Warsaw, IN). The concept underlying the design of this prosthesis is to have complete congruency between the femoral component and the polyethylene insert at all degrees of flexion and allow rotation between the polyethylene insert and tibial tray.

Rotation occurs at the knee during most activities, including walking. It has been calculated in walking volunteers that 5 degrees of internal tibial rotation takes place during the stance phase and 10 degrees of external rotation occurs during the swing phase (3). It is an accepted principle that some freedom of rotation in the knee is required for several everyday activities and certainly in sports. Rotation is decreased by weight bearing, and it is now recognized that at least 12 degrees of rotational freedom are required for total knee prosthesis (4).

During physiologic motion a certain amount of femoral rollback occurs in flexion. This is more evident in the lateral compartment (5,6). This causes a simultaneous internal tibial rotation in flexion, which occurs around a center located in the medial compartment. At the same time a few millimiters of anteroposterior motion take place, again more pronounced laterally. No interpretation of these events is accepted universally. Some investigators believe that the "rollback phenomenon" is an illusion and results from the shape of the femur. According to those authors, good kinematics can be reestablished simply by placing the axis of flexion permanently in a posterior position rather than by imposing femoral rollback with the action of the posterior cruciate ligament (PCL) (7).

Classic studies of femoral anatomy describe a decreasing radius for the posterior condyles, but more recent studies (8,9) have shown a costant posterior condylar radius on the order of magnitude of 21 to 33 mm for medial femoral condyle.

A complete congruency between the femoral component and the polyethylene insert at all degrees of flexion was desired in the prosthesis to reduce polyethylene wear. Wear is a long-term problem, which may become apparent only at 10 years after implantation. It involves three mechanisms: adhesion and abrasion (superficial wear) and fatigue (delamination or deep wear). The latter modality is predominant in knee prostheses; the first two predominate in hip replacements. Wear is also a multifactorial problem. Some factors are under industry control; others are under the surgeon's control. Manufacturers control the quality of polyethylene, including fusion defects, molecular weight, and the sterilization method. Oxidative degradation (which reduces molecular weight), the formation of crosslinks, and in general stiffness influence wear-resistance. The surgeon chooses the thickness of polyethylene, and above all prosthetic design. The most important design factors in this

221

respect are conformity of the prosthetic surfaces and the resultant contact stresses generated in the bearing area. Polyethylene wear in knee prostheses is related to the sliding motion between the metal femur and the tibial polyethylene, and to high contact stresses (10). Contact stresses increase significantly if the ratio between the radii of the prosthetic design surfaces becomes larger. An increasing potential for polyethylene damage occurs with increasing contact stresses. Ten megapascals or even better 5 MPa is considered the safe limit. For a load of 4.000 N, equivalent to approximately five times body weight, a contact surface of at least 400 mm^2 is required to stay within the 10-MPa limit.

Wear, bearing surfaces, and PCL function are interrelated. A flat tibial articular design with low conformity requires an intact PCL for stability. This increases the risk of wear caused by a sliding mechanism, if the PCL is lax, or by increased posterior compression forces, if the PCL is too tight. Clinical experience with PCL-preserving knee prostheses has shown that tension in the PCL is frequently either excessive or insufficient. PCL strain was measured at surgery and before and after implantation of a total knee prosthesis (11). Out of 10 knees the PCL was found to be lax in six and tight in three and to have normal tension in only one.

Proprioception, measured as the threshold of motion or reproduction of position, was found to be no different for PCL-saving or -substituting designs (12). PCL receptors were studied in osteoathritic knees and in a control group with gold chloride staining and a histomorphometric computerized method in 40 to 80 transverse sections (13). The neural component area was found to be significantly larger in normal knees.

Gait-analysis studies have showed the same degree of flexion up and down stairs with PCL-preserving and the -substituing types of protheses (14). Fluoroscopic analysis of PCL-retaining knee arthroplasties with a flat tibial component showed abnormal kinematics with erratic or even paradoxic motion of the femorotibial contact point (15). The femorotibial contact point was noted to be posterior to the midline with the knee near full extension, possibly because of the flat tibial design and the absence of the anterior cruciate ligament. An *in vivo* determination of condylar liftoff, using the inverse-perspective technique with fluoroscopy (16), showed lateral liftoff, again possibly resulting from the absence of the anterior cruciate ligament.

For the previously mentioned reasons, PCL preservation designs with flat tibial components without a functioning anterior cruciate ligament do not restore normal kinematics and increase the risk of wear. This risk is particularly high with a flat design, in which there is a higher potential for lateral translocation, instability, and "edge loading" if the prosthesis is malaligned.

We believe that in order to use a more conforming or curved design, which decreases contact stresses and wear, a reasonable solution might be PCL recession or release to adjust its tension. PCL release can be performed in various degrees.

INDICATIONS AND CONTRAINDICATIONS

The meniscal bearing knee prosthesis has complete femorotibial conformity throughout motion, owing to the fixed radius of the posterior femoral condyles. The ratio of the radii of the femoral to the tibial articular surface is 1:1 in both the sagittal and frontal planes. Axial rotation takes place between the tibial tray and the polyethylene insert, around a medial center of rotation, for a maximum total of about 25 degrees. Some anteroposterior motion (3–4 mm) is also possible between the polyethelene insert and tibial tray. The PCL is preserved but may be released.

The femoral component (Fig. 22-1) has separate patellar and tibial articular surfaces. The femorotibial articulations, the posterior femoral condyles, are separated from the patellar flange by two condylotrochlear grooves. The femoral condyles have a costant radius of curvature. Its magnitude changes with the prosthetic size. The patellar sulcus is deep and prolonged distally. It is slightly displaced laterally to improve patellar tracking. There are right and left femoral components. The profile of the patellar component is between the "dome" and the "Mexican hat" designs, in order to mantain a linear contact area in the arc of motion, and in deep flexion of the knee joint.

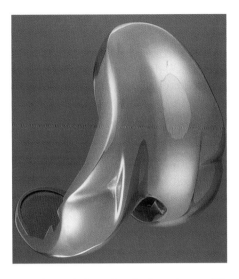

The femoral component of the meniscal bearing knee.

The tibial component has a metal tray and a single mobile polyethylene insert (Fig. 22-2). The guiding mechanism is shaped like a mushroom placed on the tibial tray; this fits into a slot on the undersurface of the polyethylene. The polyethylene insert can be implanted from the top, to enhance insertion or exchange of the insert at surgery. The tibial tray has an anterior stop to prevent anterior subluxation of the plastic insert. The polyethylene insert can rotate externally by 8 degrees and internally by 17 degrees. The articular surface of the polyethylene insert has two cupped surfaces for articulation with the femoral condyles, and a prominent intercondylar "saddle" eminence to prevent medial or lateral translocation. The prosthetic design allows 12 degrees of hyperexension. This is necessary, because the tibial component is implanted with 7 degrees of posterior tilt and the femoral component with 3 degrees of flexion.

Contact areas of various prostheses have been evaluated using either radiographs or computer-assisted methods. It has been found that the average "fixed bearing" prosthesis has only about 100 mm^2 per condyle; the LCS has approximately 200 mm^2; the Rotaglide 400 mm^2; the Oxford almost 600 mm^2; and the size E (available A through H) of the meniscal bearing knee 535 mm^2. Therefore, for the meniscal bearing knee prosthesis at a given load of 4,000 N, if contact occurs symmetrically in both condyles, contact stresses should be 3.6 MPa. If contact occurs in only one condyle, contact stresses should be no more than 7.0 MPa. Experimental studies in a knee simulator have shown limited scratching in the upper and lower surfaces of the plastic at up to 10 million cycles equivalent to 10 years of life. *In vivo* fluoroscopic studies have shown good meniscal motion with a near normal kinematic pattern.

Posterior cruciate ligament substitution has been, in our experience, a valuable option in the field of the total knee replacement. With the Insall–Burstein posterior stabilized total

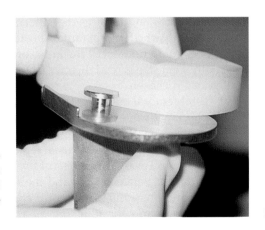

The tibial component has a metal tray and a single mobile polyethylene insert. The guiding mechanism is in the shape of a mushroom placed on the tibial tray, which fits into a slot of the undersurface of the polyethylene.

knee replacement, most deformities can be corrected, including severe ones. This procedure has proved valuable particularly in the treatment of stiff knees, knees with severe flexion contractures, patella dislocation, and knees with insufficient PCLs and in most revisions. The Insall–Burstein knee replacement has been used for many years, with minor design modifications from the original form. Good long-term results have been reported by many authors (17,18). Therefore we feel that the posterior stabilized knee will mantain its place in the field of total knee replacement as a "generic" knee used by most surgeons in most cases, with a standard technique and reliable results. There is a place, however, for a "high-tech" knee to be used by specialized surgeons in younger patients with increased demands. This implant should allow improved performance with reduced polyethylene wear. The initial results are promising and require long-term evaluation. The meniscal bearing knee design is based on sound principles and offers the advantages of full conformity throughout flexion and the possibility of keeping the PCL and releasing it. We prefer to use it in cases of mild to moderate deformity.

■ SURGICAL
TECHNIQUES

Under general or epidural anesthesia, the patient is placed in the supine position and a tourniquet is applied at the root of the limb.

The author's preferred surgical approach involves a straight longitudinal anterior skin incision. After the extensor mechanism is exposed, an anteromedial capsulotomy with a straight incision is made, beginning at the apex of the quadriceps tendon, proceeding distally in the substance of the tendon immediately adjacent to the vastus medialis, and extending distally over the medial border of the patella and then through the anterior capsule parallel to the patellar tendon and onto the anteromedial tibia. The quadriceps expansion usually is peeled from the anterior medial surface of the patella by sharp dissection. The distal extension of the incision on the tibia is continued through the periosteum 1 to 2 cm medial to the tibial tubercle. This leaves some tissue (periosteum) attached to the tubercle, with the advantage that, in case of accidental avulsion of the patellar tendon, the tendon remains in continuity with a sleeve of periosteum covering the tibia, which is helpful anchoring the tendon.

At the end of the exposure the patella is everted and the tibia is subluxed forward by releasing around the proximal tibia the medial meniscotibial ligaments and the deep medial collateral ligament. With the knee flexed, remnants of the anterior cruciate ligament are excised.

The operation includes the following steps: a distal femoral cut, anterior and posterior femoral cuts with selection of the rotational alignment, a proximal tibial cut, a check of extension and flexion gaps with spacer blocks, possible medial or lateral collateral ligament release, insertion of trial components, possible PCL release, and finally patellar resurfacing.

Before cutting the distal femur, a 12-mm hole is drilled in the femoral epiphisis above the PCL insertion. This allows the introduction of the 8-mm femoral intramedullary guide. The hole should be approximately 1 cm anterior to the origin of the PCL. The drill is a step drill and should be used to enlarge the entrance hole on the femur to 12 mm. This allows exit of the bone marrow and reduces the intramedullary pressure.

Subsequently, the femoral (anteroposterior) sizing instrument is inserted in the femoral canal. This guide references the anterior cortex and the posterior condyles of the femur. The component size is read directly from the guide. If the indicator is in between sizes, the smaller one is chosen.

The distal femoral cut is performed using an intramedullary instrument, but often we double check with an extramedullary rod. The distal 8 to 10 mm of bone is removed (from the normal condyle), and an alignment of 6 to 7 degrees of valgus in relationship to the anatomic axis is obtained. The distal femoral cut has 3 degrees of flexion in relationship to the distal femoral axis. This is useful to avoid notching of the anterior femur, particularly if the indicator is between sizes and the smaller size has been selected.

The preparation of the distal femur continues with exposure of the epicondyles, which are useful landmarks for adjusting the rotational position of the femoral component (19). We try to achieve a few (3 or 4) degrees of external rotation in relationship to the posterior condylar line; this is useful for patellar tracking and to help compensate for the usual lateral collateral laxity.

There are several methods of achieving good rotatory position. The method we prefer requires identification of the epicondyles. It has been found that by referencing the epicondylar line we obtain an automatic external rotation of a few degrees (average 4 degrees, range −1–7) in relationship to the posterior condylar line. The degree of external rotation varies according to the deformity and averages 3.5 degrees in the varus and 4.4 degrees in the valgus knee (20). This method has the advantage that the epicondyles represent the collateral ligament insertion and the axis of flexion. The epicondylar line is always to the tibial axis at all degrees of flexion.

The epicondyles are exposed at surgery by removing the synovium and dividing the lateral patellofemoral ligament. The lateral epicondyle is identified more easily because it is a more pointed structure. On the medial side identification is more difficult, because the epicondyle is larger and fan-shaped. The surgeon must identify its center (the bull's eye technique) or find the depression located between the separate insertion ridges for the superficial and deep medial collateral ligament. The epicondylar line is drawn on the resected distal femur using methylene blue (Fig. 22-3), and a slotted instrument is aligned along the line itself. A saw is used to produce a slot in the bone perpendicular to the epicondylar line in the center of the resected surface of the distal femur. This is 5 mm deep and does not damage the PCL. An anteroposterior cutting block of the appropriate size is engaged in the slot. The cutting block is moved in an anteroposterior direction using the anterior femoral cortex and the posterior condyles as reference. An anterior "boom" and a posterior "finger" connected to the block help in this purpose. The anterior boom should touch the anterior femoral cortex on its lateral and more prominent aspect. The posterior finger should indicate an average resection of 10 mm from the posterior condyles. Because a few degrees of external rotation are desired, resection of the posterior condyles is usually more than 10 mm medially and less than 10 mm laterally.

The proximal tibial cut is accomplished using an extramedullary guide. This guide references the malleoli, distally. The true center of the ankle is about 5 to 10 mm medial to the midpoint between the subcutaneous palpable medial and lateral malleoli. Proximally the alignment of the cut is perpendicular to the tibial axis in the coronal plane, with a 7-degree posterior slope. We try to remove 8 to 10 mm of bone from the normal tibial plateau. After the tibial cut, using laminar spreaders, we remove any remnants of the menisci and all the osteophytes that are present at the level of posterior femoral condyles and around the PCL. At this point the flexion and extension gaps have been established and are sized with spacers. At the same time, mediolateral stability and overall limb alignment are evaluated with the knee in the fully extended position. If a medial or a lateral ligament release is required, this is performed in a gradual fashion at this time. It can be completed then or adjusted after trial reduction if necessary.

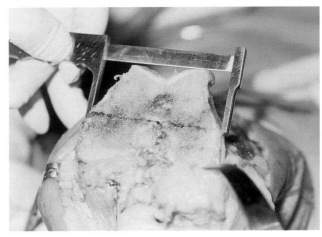

There are several methods for achieving good rotatory position. Our prefered method is to draw the epicondylar line on the flat surface of the distal femur. We have found that by referencing the epycondylar line we obtain an automatic external rotation.

■ FIGURE 22-3

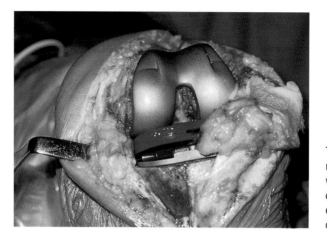

Tension in the posterior cruciate ligament is seldom correct; more frequently with the meniscal bearing knee it is excessive, causing limitation of flexion, excessive rollback, or an anterior liftoff of plastic insert.

The PCL is protected during the femoral and the tibial bone cuts. In particular during the proximal tibial cut an osteotome may be inserted in front of the posterior spine to protect the PCL tibial insertion. Alternatively the surgeon may choose to cut across the proximal tibia and therefore automatically obtain a partial release of the PCL at least to the level of the cut. After the insertion of the trial components, the knee is taken through a range of motion and the tension in the PCL assessed. Tension in the PCL is seldom correct. More frequently with the meniscal bearing knee it is excessive, causing limitation of flexion, excessive rollback, or an anterior liftoff of the plastic insert (Fig. 22-4). The liftoff is exaggerated if the patella is everted, and therefore it should be assessed with the patella reduced. In the case of excessive tension the PCL is released. This can be done off the femur, by selectively cutting the anterior fibers, or from the tibia, by releasing the insertion either with the knife or with a periosteal elevator. We prefer to release it from the tibial side, because it leaves the PCL attached to the posterior capsule so that it may later heal to the back of the tibia (Fig. 22-5). We feel that, in this way, at least the fundamental function of the PCL, stopping posterior tibial subluxation, is maintained.

The patellar osteotomy is performed using a saw or a reaming device that produces an even thickness, leaving sufficient bone to anchor the patellar prosthesis without increasing the original thickness. Caliper measurements of patellar thickness before and after resurfacing are very important. The patellar thickness with the trial should be equal to or slightly less than the original thickness of the patella. Three fixation holes are produced in the resected patellar surface, and the trial is inserted to observe patellar tracking with the component in place. The "no thumb" test is used: The patella should track with its medial

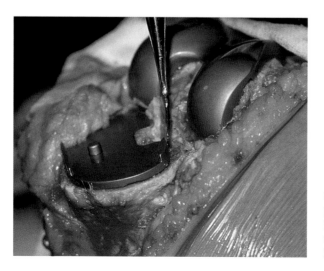

In case of excessive tension the posterior cruciate ligament is released. We prefer the release from the tibial side, because it leaves the ligament attached to the posterior capsule so that it later may heal to the back of the tibia.

border in contact with the femoral component throughout the range of motion without the pressure of the surgeon's thumb. We take the slack out of the quadriceps tendon coming from flexion to extension by applying longitudinal tension to the rectus with a Kocher clamp. If the patella tracks laterally, a lateral retinacular release is performed employing the oblique-cut technique or the multiple-puncture technique, saving the superolateral genicular vessels.

Before final fixation an overall check of limb alignment is made using external (proximal and distal) landmarks. Then, after careful bone cleaning by pulsatile lavage, the fixation of the final components is achieved with cement. The femur is cemented first. Excess cement must be removed completely, for fear that cement particles might become trapped under the mobile platform. After component fixation, knee stability, arc of motion, and patellar tracking are checked once again to ensure accuracy of the procedure.

The midline incision is closed by suturing the divided expansion side to side. Separation and retraction of the vastus medialis is not expected, and the knee can be mobilized early without fear of capsular separation. Finally, after skin closure, a light dressing is applied, and radiographs of the knee are obtained in the recovery room.

In total knee replacement surgery, achieving properly balanced flexion and extension gaps and smooth patellar tracking is mandatory for a good outcome with the prosthesis. In this respect a correct rotatory position of the femoral component is extremely important.

There are several methods of achieving good rotatory position of the femoral component. The traditional method involves referencing the posterior condylar line (21). Using this method is difficult in knees with posterior condylar erosion or dysplasia. In valgus deformities, erosion of the posterior aspect of the lateral condyle may lead to a relative internal rotation of the femoral component. Erosion of the posterior aspect of the medial condyle (in varus knees) may lead to an excessive external rotation of the femoral component.

The second method of adjusting the femoral component rotation (the parallel flexion gap method) involves creating the tibial cut first, tensing the collateral ligaments in flexion, and resecting the posterior condyles parallel to the tibial cut (22,23). Laminar spreaders or other specialized devices (tensors) may be used to tense the ligaments in flexion that obviously need to be properly balanced prior to adjust femoral rotation.

The third method is to measure the bone resections from distal and posterior cuts, equalizing them to achieve a suitable rotation (Gerald Engh, personal communication). With this method the proper rotation seldom is obtained, because of the different bone deficiencies at different levels of the condyles.

The fourth method requires drawing of the trochlear anteroposterior line (Whiteside's line), which is usually perpendicular to the epicondylar line. This method has been found to be particularly useful in the valgus knee (24). In our opinion the anteroposterior line shows too much variability compared with the posterior condylar line.

It is our opinion that referencing to the epicondylar line is the best method to achieve a reproducible and proper rotatory position of the femoral component. As previously reported, by referencing the epicondylar line we are able to obtain an automatic external rotation of a few degrees (average 4 degrees, range −1–7) in relationship to the posterior condylar line. The degree of external rotation varies according to the deformity and averages 3.5 degrees in the varus knee and 4.4 degrees in the valgus one (20).

This method has the advantage that the epicondyles represent the collateral ligament insertion and the axis of flexion. The epicondylar line is always perpendicular to the tibial axis at all degrees of flexion.

The anatomy of the epicondyles and their relationship with other distal femoral landmarks have been accurately described by Griffin et al. (25) using magnetic resonance imaging in 104 knees without boney pathology. He found that the distance from the distal joint line to the medial epicondylar sulcus averaged 27.4 ± 2.9 mm, with a statistically significant difference between genders (females: 26.3 mm; males: 29.2 mm); the distance between the posterior joint line and the medial sulcus averaged 29.0 ± 2.7 mm, again significantly

■ TECHNICAL ALTERNATIVES AND PITFALLS

different between females (27.8 mm) and males (30.8 mm). The distance between the distal joint line and the lateral epicondyle was 24.3 ± 2.6 mm on average (females: 23.4 mm; males: 25.6 mm), and between the posterior joint line and lateral epicondyle averaged 25.0 ± 2.6 mm (females: 23.9 mm; males: 26.7 mm). The angle between the surgical epicondylar axis (medial epicondylar sulcus–lateral epicondyle) and the tangent to the posterior condyles, defined as the posterior condylar angle, averaged 3.11 ± 1.75 degrees (26). This angle was measured by Griffin et al. (26) in another study in 107 osteoarthritic knees using a posterior reference and rotation guide. Varus knees measured 3.3 ± 1.9 degrees on average, valgus knees 5.4 ± 2.3 degrees, the difference a result of deficient lateral posterior condyles.

The epicondyles are exposed at surgery by removing the synovium carefully and dividing the lateral patellofemoral ligament. The lateral epicondyle is identified more easily because it is well pointed. On the medial side there are more difficulties, because the epicondyle is larger and fan-shaped and the surgeon has to identify its center (bull's eye technique) or find the depression (sulcus technique) located between the separate insertion ridges for the superficial and deep medial collateral ligament (19). Moreover, a small vessel often is present at the sulcus level . We found that this vessel does not correspond always to the sulcus.

■ REHABILITATION

In our clinic, rehabilitation begins on the first postoperative day with a continuous passive motion machine, allowing approximately 30 to 40 degrees of motion during the first day. The range of motion is advanced daily, with the objective of obtaining 90 degrees in 4 or 5 days.

Usually we allow the patient to stand on the second postoperative day, and if this is well accepted a few steps with a walker are encouraged. Progress is variable and age-dependent. Ambulation is done with a walker until the patient is steady enough to use a single cane. Full weight bearing without canes is suggested only after the patient has gained confidence.

Muscle exercises are prescribed immediately postoperatively for feet and ankles, and isometrics for quadriceps and gluteus muscles. Straight leg raising commences as soon as the patient is able to do it. Bicycle exercises are useful and begin soon if the patient has sufficient flexion (normally after the first 2 weeks).

The patient is discharged from the hospital normally after 7 to 10 days, if able to walk unaided, flex to 90 degrees, and climb stairs using a handrail. Physical therapy with emphasis on bicycling and range-of-motion and quadriceps exercises is continued at home for approximately 6 weeks.

■ OUTCOMES AND FUTURE DIRECTIONS

Two series of patients have had the meniscal bearing knee prosthesis implanted. The first series includes 23 patients operated on between October 1993 and October 1994. The second series includes 22 patients operated on during 1995. The average age of the 45 patients at surgery was 65.4 years (range 56–83). There were seven males and 38 females. The diagnosis was osteoarthritis in 42, rheumatoid arthritis in two, and osteonecrosis in one patient. The condition of the PCL at the end of surgery was as follows: In 22 patients (49%) the PCL was intact, in 18 (40%) it was released, and in five (11%) it was attenuated. A lateral retinacular release was performed in 14 patients (31%).

We were able to follow 44 patients for at least 1 year (Figs. 22-6 and 22-7). One patient died for unrelated reasons. The knee score according to the Knee Society rating system increased from an average of 40 points preoperatively to 89 points at follow-up. There were 28 patients (64%) with excellent results, 10 (23%) with good results, five (11%) with fair results, and one (2%) with poor results. The Knee Society functional score improved from an average of 55 points preoperatively to 86 points at follow-up. There were excellent results in 26 patients (59%), good in 23 (27%), fair in five (11%), and poor in one (2%). On a visual analogue scale from 1 to 10 for subjective satisfaction, 39 patients (89%) gave a score of 8 or more and no patients gave below 5. A visual analogue scale for pain revealed approxi-

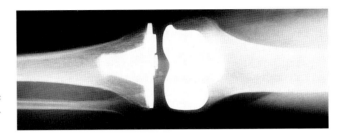

The anteroposterior radiographic view of an implanted meniscal bearing knee.

mately the same findings. The average postoperative flexion was 110 degrees, with a range of 90 to 130 degrees. Extension loss was present in three knees postoperatively. It measured 5 degrees in two knees and 8 degrees in one. Walking distance was unlimited in 29 patients (66%) and more than 10 city blocks in 10 (23%). Twenty-one patients (48%) could manage stairs normally, nine (20%) could walk downstairs holding the rail, and 13 (30%) could walk up- and downstairs using the rail.

Radiographic analysis of the angle between the mechanical axes of the femur and the tibia in long standing films showed that in 34 knees (77%) the angle was within 2 degrees from neutral, in six knees (14%) there was 3 to 5 degrees of varus, one knee (2%) was in 7 degrees of varus, two knees (4.5%) were in 3 to 5 degrees of valgus, and one knee (2%) was in 6 degrees of valgus. Tibial radiolucent lines were studied accoding to the Knee Society evaluation system. Radiolucent lines were present in zone 1 in 18 patients (41%), in zone 2 in 11 (25%), and in zone 4 in one patient (2%). The thickness of the radiolucency was 1 mm in all patients except one, in whom it was 2 mm. Patella symptoms were absent in 42 patients (95%). In two knees (4.5%) there was a moderate patellofemoral crepitation.

There were five fair and one poor results. The reasons for the five fair results were as follows: Three patients complained of knee pain, one had hip pain, and one had objective mediolateral instability. There was one poor result, which resulted from varus alignment of the limb (7 degrees) in an otherwise asymptomatic knee.

Two knees of Mark I (or first version of the prosthesis) series had some instability approaching extension. This did not cause symptoms in the patients but could be felt by the examiner. The phenomenon was attributable to anterior tibial subluxation, because the prosthesis did not allow for sufficient hyperextension. It should be emphasized that implantation of the tibial component with 7 degrees of posterior slope and the femoral component with 3 degrees of flexion already requires a prosthesis that allows 10 degrees hyperextension for the knee to come to full extension. More extension is required to obtain some recurvatum. This problem was corrected in a subsequent version of the (Mark II) prosthesis by moving the condylotrochlear groove of the femoral component anteriorly and proximally. The prosthesis now allows a total of 15 degrees of hyperextension. A further modification recently was introduced in the most recent version (Mark III) prosthesis. In this model the height of the intercondylar eminence of the plastic insert has been raised to prevent translocation of the components, which we observed to occur (in a posterolateral direction) in few cases at surgery, but not in our clinical follow-ups.

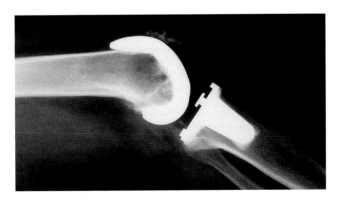

The L-L radiographic view of an implanted meniscal bearing knee.

References

1. Goodfellow JW, O'Connor J. Clinical results of the Oxford knee. *Clin Orthop* 1986; 205:21–42.
2. Buechel FF, Pappas MJ. Long-term survivorship analysis of the cruciate-sparing versus cruciate sacrificing knee prostheses using meniscal bearings. *Clin Orthop* 1990; 260:162–169.
3. La Fortune MA, Cavanagh PR, Sommer MS, et al. Three dimensional kinematics of the human knee during walking. *J Biomech* 1992; 25:347–357.
4. Nahass BE, Madson MM, Walker PS. Motion of the knee after total condylar resurfacing: An in vivo study. *J Biomech* 1991; 24:1107–1117.
5. Barnes CL, Sledge CB. Total knee arthroplasty with posterior cruciate ligament retention designs. In: Insall JN, Windsor RE, Scott NW, Kelly MA, Aglietti P, eds. *Surgery of the knee.* New York: Churchill Livingstone, 1993:815–827.
6. Thompson WO, Thaete FL, Fu FH, et al. Tibial meniscal dynamics using three-dymensional reconstruction of magnetic resonance images. *Am J Sports Med* 1991; 19:210–216.
7. Freeman MA, Railton GT. Should the posterior cruciate ligament be retained or resected in condylar nonmeniscal knee arthroplasty? *J Arthroplasty* 1988;(suppl 3):3–12.
8. Elias SG, Freeman MA, Gokcay EI. A correlative study of the geometry and anatomy of the distal femur. *Clin Orthop* 1990; 260:98–103.
9. Hollister AM, Jatana S, Singh AK, et al. The axes of rotation of the knee. *Clin Orthop* 1993; 290:259–268.
10. Walker PS. Design of total knee arthroplasty. In: Insall JN, Windsor RE, Scott NW, Kelly MA, Aglietti P, ed. *Surgery of the knee.* New York: Churchill Livingstone, 1993:723–738.
11. Lotke PA, Corces A, Williams JL, et al. Strain characteristics of the posterior cruciate ligament after total knee arthroplasty. *Am J Knee Surg* 1993; 6:104–107.
12. Cash RM, Gonzales MH, Garst J, et al. Propioception after arthroplasty: Role of the posterior cruciate ligament. *Clin Orthop* 1996; 331:172–178.
13. Franchi A, Zaccherotti G, Aglietti P. Neural system of the human posterior cruciate ligament in osteoarthritis. *J Arthroplasty* 1995; 10:679–682.
14. Wilson SA, McCann PD, Gotlin RS, et al. Comprehensive gait analysis in posterior-stabilized knee arthroplasty. *J Arthroplasty* 1996; 11:359–367.
15. Sthiel JB, Komistek RD, Dennis DA, et al. Fluoroscopic analysis of the kinematics after posterrior cruciate retaining knee arthroplasty. *J Bone Joint Surg Br* 1995; 77:884–889.
16. Dennis DA, Komistek RD, Hoff WA, et al. In vivo kinematics derived using an inverse perspective tecnique. *Clin Orthop* 1996; 331:107–117.
17. Aglietti P, Buzzi R, De Felice R, et al. The Insall-Burstein total knee replacement in osteoarthritis: A ten-year minimum follow-up. *J Arthroplasty* 1999; 14:560–565.
18. Colizza WA, Insall JN, Scuderi JR. The posterior stabilized total knee prosthesis: Assessment of polyethylene damage and osteolysis after a ten-year minimum follow-up. *J Bone Joint Surg Am* 1995; 77:1713–1720.
19. Berger RA, Rubash HE, Seel MJ, et al. Determining the rotational alignment of the femoral component in total knee arthroplasty using epicondylar axis. *Clin Orthop* 1993; 286:40–47.
20. Poilvache PL, Insall JN, Scuderi GR, et al. Rotational landmarks and sizing of the distal femur in total knee arthroplasty. *Clin Orthop* 1996; 331:35–46.
21. Hungerford DS, Kenna RV. Preliminary experience with a total knee prosthesis with porous coating used without cement. *Clin Orthop* 1988; 226:49.
22. Stiehl JB, Cherveny PM. Femoral rotational alignment using the tibial shaft axis in total knee arthroplasty. *Clin Orthop* 1996; 331:47–55.
23. Arima J, Whiteside LA, McCarty DS, et al. Femoral rotation alignment, based on the anteroposterior axis, in total knee arthroplasty in a valgus knee. *J Bone Joint Surg Am* 1995; 77:1331–1334.
25. Griffin FM, Math KM, Scuderi GR, et al. Anatomy of the epicondyles of the distal femur: MRI analysis of normal knees. In press.
26. Griffin FM, Insall JN, Scuderi GR. The posterior condylar angle in osteoarthritic knees. *J Arthroplasty* 1998; 13:812–815.

23

Soft Tissue Releases for the Valgus Knee

Ever since the importance of restoration of proper limb alignment first was appreciated, techniques have been developed to realign and also stabilize knee arthroplasties in the correct position: a neutral mechanical axis. In this position, a line connecting the center of the femoral head with the center of the knee is parallel to another line joining the center of the knee with the center of the ankle. The first coherent description of soft-tissue releases on the lateral side of the knee was aggressive. A Bennet retractor was placed in the lateral compartment of the flexed knee and pushed towards the foot. This elevated the lateral femoral condyle from the tibial articular surface, placing the lateral structures, prominently the lateral collateral ligament, under tension. These structures including the iliotibial band were transected. As the release progressed from the anterior aspect of the lateral structures more posteriorly, the retractor was rotated externally until the entire lateral complex had been released, including the popliteus. This was effective in correcting deformity, differed tremendously from the approach to the medial side in the varus knee, but occasionally resulted in posterior tibial instability, particularly in flexion (1). What followed was a sometimes confusing array of techniques that recommended different sequences of releases according to different surgeons. The surgical technique described here acknowledges that different structures are responsible for deformity in different knees. It makes sense then to evaluate which structures are tight, and to release them preferentially.

Choosing when and where to perform releases on the lateral side of a valgus knee depends heavily on understanding the pathology of the deformity and rationale of the surgical technique for correction of deformity. Valgus malalignment presents some of the greatest challenges to the arthroplasty surgeon. It is a distinct clinical problem and should never be considered to be the "mirror image" of the varus knee. Any deformity induces significant stresses on the collateral ligaments. Varus alignment threatens the lateral structures, which are of less importance to the final arthroplasty but protect the all-important medial collateral ligament, which can be released at the time of arthroplasty. The valgus knee, however, may stretch and even damage or destroy the medial ligament, to the point at which the arthroplasty cannot be stabilized easily with conventional techniques.

The pathology of the knee with a valgus deformity includes an aberration of limb alignment and an imbalance of the length and tension of the soft-tissue envelope around the joint (2). The usual osseous morphology that accompanies valgus deformity is hypoplasia of the lateral femoral condyle. Surgeons are accustomed to recognizing this aspect of the valgus knee from evaluation of anteroposterior radiographs. The smaller lateral femoral condyle creates a valgus orientation of the distal femur and accordingly of the limb (Fig. 23-1).

The lateral femoral condyle, however, is generally smaller, in almost every dimension. The posterior extent of this condyle is smaller or shorter as well, with significant implications for the rotational positioning of a femoral component. Simply describing these knees as valgus may be inadequate. We must think of them in three dimensions, as knees with hypoplastic lateral femoral condyles.

The smaller nature of the condyles is of course exacerbated by arthritic changes. Cartilage has been worn off to a greater extent on the lateral side, rendering the apparent deficit greater.

■ HISTORY OF THE TECHNIQUE

■ INDICATIONS AND CONTRAINDICATIONS

231

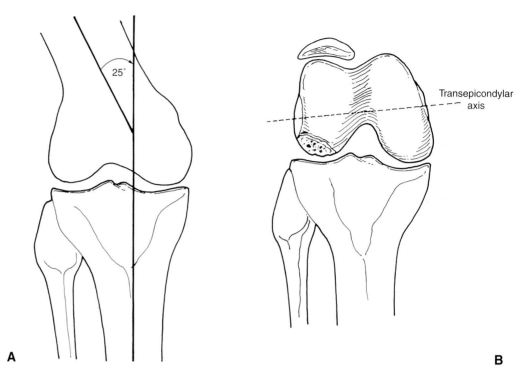

■ FIGURE 23-1   **A**   **B**

A: Pathology of the varus knee. Surgeons are accustomed to the hypoplastic lateral femoral condyle as the site of the valgus deformity. This is readily appreciated on anteroposterior radiographs. **B:** The posterior aspect of the lateral femoral condyle is similarly hypoplastic. This may result in inadvertent internal rotation position of the femoral component if the unsuspecting surgeon orients this component parallel to the posterior condyle bone. The transepicondylar axis is a more reliable orientation.

Creating the distal femoral cut at the appropriate angle is relatively easy. If the distal bone is so lacking that a defect persists after the distal femoral cut has been made, then a modular augmentation, available with most prosthetic systems, is required. The deficient posterior condylar bone may deceive the surgeon into positioning the femoral component in internal rotation, if the cutting block is aligned with the posterior condyles, as many instruments have been designed to do. Identification of the epicondyles on the distal femur is essential to avoid this complication. The femoral component should be aligned parallel to the epicondylar axis, which joins the two condyles. This line corresponds to the anatomic joint line in flexion, as dictated by the location of the collateral ligaments. The femoral component that is rotated internally with respect to this axis produces a dead arthroplasty, susceptible to the range of patellar complications that follow from maltracking, as well as pain and poor motion.

Considering the knee in the two dimensions that correspond to the anteroposterior radiograph, however, we are concerned immediately with the collateral ligaments. The structures on the medial side are relatively longer or more lax than those on the lateral side. Not all valgus knees are similar—in some, the normal tension in each side is the same until the deformity is corrected with an arthroplasty. In others, there may be a contracture of the lateral structures with histologically normal medial structures. In yet others, which are the most difficult to deal with, soft-tissue structures on the medial side have suffered plastic deformation. Because of the incessant tension that results from valgus deformity, the collagen yields and becomes stretched. In the first two instances, releases to elongate the lateral side easily create similar tension on both sides of the joint; it may not be possible in the third instance to elongate the lateral side to the extent that it is as long or as lax as the failed medial collateral ligament.

Releases therefore are indicated in the valgus knee if the lateral structures are tighter than the medial collateral ligament, so that it is impossible to have the knee well aligned and stable without elongating the lateral ligaments with a release. Contraindications to ligament releases are relative. Overly aggressive releases, as were practiced previously, may leave the knee unstable, especially in the flexion. In other circumstances, although release is indicated, it may be inadequate if, for example, the medial structures have suffered plastic deformation. No amount of lengthening on the lateral side can place the medial structures under tension. A constrained implant or reconstruction of the medial ligament is required to restore functional stability to the joint.

This concept of failure of the medial structures may be visualized as the "disabling pathology" of the valgus knee. Although the vast majority of valgus knees can be realigned and stabilized with conventional releases, there are a few in which damage to the medial structures represents disabling pathology. This situation usually is remedied with a more constrained, though nonlinked, implant, a particularly easy decision in the elderly or physically inactive (low-demand) patient. Linked devices or hinges are indicated very rarely and should be avoided if an option exists.

The younger or more active patient is problematic. In the unusual situation in which the medial ligament is damaged, conventional releases are inadequate, and constraint is undesirable, innovation may be necessary. Ligament-advancement techniques have been described for use in knee arthroplasty surgery, and some clinical results have been reported.

Devising the appropriate surgical technique for correction of deformity begins with the surgical approach. It is agreed generally that the "pathology" of the valgus knee resides on the lateral side—often lateral compartment arthritic disease or relative tightness or even contracture of the lateral stabilizers of the knee. This has been the motivation to develop and use a lateral parapatellar surgical approach to the valgus knee (3). This has the advantage of bringing the surgeon immediately into contact with the lateral structures that may require release, and it is further promoted as a facile means of providing a lateral patellar retinacular release simply by leaving parts of the arthrotomy open.

■ SURGICAL TECHNIQUES

The approach yields inferior exposure of the joint, however, and jeopardizes the extensor mechanism, because part of the patellar tendon must be elevated from the tubercle for eversion. The closure is less secure and depends on interposition of part of the patellar fat pad to avoid drainage. The compelling reason to avoid this approach in any knee, however, is that the disabling pathology of the medial structures is remote from the incision. The lateral structures can be released easily with a standard medial approach. The medial structures cannot be reconstructed so easily from the lateral side. Should revision arthroplasty be required, the lateral skin incision proves problematic, often necessitating a tubercle osteotomy.

Although there are committed proponents of the lateral arthrotomy for the valgus knee, the standard medial approach favored by most surgeons invariably works well. This may be a standard medial parapatellar, Insall straight anterior, subvastus, midvastus, or trivector arthrotomy. Whichever approach is favored, the medial collateral ligament must be protected through the procedure. Unlike the varus knee, in which exposure can be enhanced early on by completing part or all of the medial releases, exposure of the valgus knee must be accomplished by removing the capsule at most from the medial tibia. Forceful knee flexion and external rotation, so useful in dislocating the tibia forward in a varus knee, may compromise an already stretched medial collateral ligament and should be avoided.

Which structures should be released if conventional techniques are planned (4)? The first techniques that were applied to the correction of the valgus knee during arthroplasty surgery have been abandoned in deed if not concept. The releases were aggressive, complete, and performed immediately after the knee had been exposed. The lesson to be learned from this technique, however, is that these knees generally remained very stable in extension, demonstrating the tremendous importance of valgus alignment and the medial structures. Simply stated, if an arthroplasty is aligned in valgus, the medial collateral ligament functions as a tension band with each step the patient takes.

Lateral releases for the valgus knee have become more selective and less aggressive There still is not general agreement in the arthroplasty literature as to which of the lateral structures is responsible for a valgus deformity. Different surgeons have described different sequences of releases. It is true that some structures impart different deforming forces to the valgus knee: The iliotibial band contributes to valgus alignment in extension but not flexion, in which it may be responsible for external rotation deformity. This is seen most commonly in rheumatoid arthritis. Clearly, in the valgus knee with an external rotation deformity of the tibia, the iliotibial band must be released. The lateral collateral ligament creates tightness on the lateral side of the valgus knee in all positions of flexion. Releasing this structure removes not only a potent deforming force but a major stabilizing force as well. Accordingly, the risk of posterior tibial instability, especially in nonconforming arthroplasties, but also in posterior stabilized implants, is greatest once this structure has been transected. For this reason, multiple puncture techniques have supplanted the transection that was once practiced for the release of ligaments.

Could the lack of agreement as to which structures should be released in which order stem from the fact that not every valgus knee suffers the same pathology? If a different constellation of ligament pathology may occur in each knee with valgus deformity, then perhaps it is not so much a difference in philosophy that is important as a difference in the personality of these knees.

How then can we determine which structures would benefit from release in which patient? This hinges on palpation or observation of each of them in the functional position of extension. There generally has been an understandable reluctance on the part of surgeons to perform releases with the knee extended, given that this creates tension on the neurovascular structures in the back of the joint. Nonetheless, by extending the valgus knee after preliminary bone cuts have been completed we can assess the tension in each structure and selectively release those that are tight. Multiple puncture techniques mitigate against destabilization of the joint.

The need for releases can be evaluated after bone cuts have been made. The basic bone cuts that provide static alignment for the joint can be completed without undue concern over stability. *Static alignment* refers to the angulation of the cuts so that a neutral mechanical axis is restored. This means that, without considering stability or soft-tissue balance for the moment, if a spacer block is inserted between the cut distal femur and the proximal tibia, then a line (usually indicated by the electrocautery cord) placed over the center of the ankle and knee passes over the center of the hip joint, usually approximated as several inches medial to the anterior superior iliac crest.

Valgus knees are characterized by hypoplasia of the lateral femoral condyle, which is easy to appreciate in extension on an anteroposterior radiograph. The condyle is also smaller, posteriorly, which is difficult to visualize, except with computed tomographic scanning. The implications for rotational positioning of the femoral component are profound, however. If the posterior articular surface of the lateral femoral condyle is small, then the conventional instruments that reference this surface leave the component internally rotated relative to the epicondylar axis, which generally is regarded as a more accurate reference line for rotational positioning.

We accept that with classic alignment techniques in knee arthroplasty the orientation of the proximal tibial cut should lay at right angles to the long axis of the tibia. We know that the distal femoral cut should lay at right angles to a line drawn from the center of the hip to the center of the knee. The amount of bone removed from the distal femur, in accord with the concept of "measured resection," equals the thickness of the proposed implants, referenced from the more "normal" medial distal femur. This alignment must exist in the arthroplasty, irrespective of the magnitude or orientation of the preoperative deformity.

A spacer block is used to evaluate the knee after the proximal tibial, distal, and posterior femoral cuts have been made. One should try to use the next thinnest block if possible. If the knee is prepared using the thinnest block, the plan obviously is to use the thinnest tibial polyethylene. Although this may not be ideal in terms of polyethylene wear, there is a more immediate concern: If the thinnest insert is planned for, the surgeon has no choice of an even thinner insert if the final result is tight. Although the thinnest block and the thinnest insert may function well with the spacer blocks and then the trial components, if the cement on the final components takes up some space a flexion contracture or poor motion is the inescapable result. Time taken to resect a small additional amount of proximal tibia does not affect the balance of the knee from flexion to extension but provides an appealing option if the final arthroplasty is too tight.

The static alignment with a spacer block is confirmed in the extended joint using an electrocautery cord or alignment rod. One should ensure that the femoral component has been rotated parallel to the epicondylar axis. The relative medial to lateral stability of the joints is evaluated: Is the lateral side tighter than the medial, as one would expect in a significant valgus deformity? If the knee is balanced we might assume that the ligament tension is ideal and that the preoperative valgus deformity is a result exclusively of bone and cartilage deficiency. It may also result from failure to correct the valgus deformity. One should be critical of the static deformity.

More typically, the lateral side is tighter, implying the need for a release of some or all of the lateral structures. Consider the medial side for a moment. Is there still some structural integrity to them? If the deformity has exceeded 20 degrees and the medial structures feel attenuated, although a lateral release is still essential it may not be enough. Anticipation of what ultimately may become necessary is advantageous.

One should compare the situation in extension with that in flexion by inserting the spacer block into the flexed knee, now between the posterior cut femoral surface and the cut proximal tibia. If the knee was well aligned and stable in extension, and if this is replicated in flexion, no more need be done. The surgeon can proceed to finishing cuts and implantation of the prosthesis.

More than likely the knee in flexion resembles how it was in extension: tighter on the lateral side than the medial. This implies generally a need for a release, but also that the lateral collateral ligament and perhaps the popliteus are the offending structures. Remember that the iliotibial band externally rotates the tibia in flexion but anatomically cannot make the flexion gap tighter on the lateral side.

What if the knee, though requiring a lateral release in extension, is nicely balanced from medial to lateral in flexion? It may be that the iliotibial band is the offending structure, because it tightens the lateral side in extension but not flexion. The surgeon should not settle for this assessment, however, until he or she checked the rotational position of the femoral component. An internally rotated femoral component, so damaging to the arthroplasty result, selectively tightens the medial side of the flexion gap without affecting the extension gap appreciably. Overlooking this scenario is a grave error.

Three criteria should be satisfied at this point: The knee should extend fully, have good valgus alignment (neutral mechanical axis), and, after the soft tissue has been managed, have good varus–valgus stability in extension. Another method of evaluating the medial and lateral sides of the flexion and extension gaps is with laminar spreaders. This is best done after the spacer block has been removed (Fig. 23-2).

There are several approaches to releasing tight structures on the lateral side of the valgus knee. It makes sense to release those that are palpably tight. This is appreciated most easily through the insertion of laminar spreaders, with both handles angled away from the surgeon, with the knee in full extension. Tension on the lateral structures can be appreciated, and they easily are released with a multiple-perforation technique using a pointed scalpel (no. 11 blade).

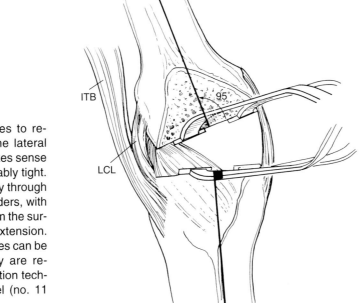

■ FIGURE 23-2

■ TECHNICAL
ALTERNATIVES AND
PITFALLS

The technical alternatives are constrained implants, in which the prosthesis provides mechanical stability, in patients in whom ligament balance cannot be achieved by the collateral ligaments despite releases. Linked constrained or hinged implants should be avoided. Early work with ligament reconstructions and advancements has been described as a means to avoid constraint. These techniques are required infrequently. Failure to recognize the incompetence of the medial structures may result in the continued performance of aggressive releases on the lateral side and then the use of progressively thicker polyethylene inserts in an attempt to stabilize the joint. This cannot be achieved if the medial collateral ligament is incompetent. The knee in that case develops a flexion contracture, because the posterior structures remain tight as thicker polyethylene is inserted.

The most common pitfall in dealing with the valgus knee is rotational malalignment of the femoral component. This commonly is internal rotation, which creates patella-tracking problems and difficulties with arthroplasty stability and motion (5,6). The epicondylar axis or anteroposterior axis (7) is a superior guide to rotational positioning. The internally rotated femoral component may be responsible for a wide range of patellar complications. If these occur, it is usually necessary to perform a complete revision knee arthroplasty (8). If surgeons use lateral approaches the valgus knee, the usual landmarks for positioning are somewhat more difficult to orient, and care must be taken. In addition, the exposure may be more difficult, and the patellar tendon attachment is in jeopardy.

Medial stability may be lacking; such a lack may go undetected. This can occur if the surgeon evaluates medial stability with the knee locked in full extension. The sensation of good medial stability in this setting results from tight posterior structures. The same assessment performed with the knee slightly flexed produces more information about the integrity of the medial side.

Overly aggressive release of the lateral structures, without close attention to the balancing of flexion and extension gaps, may result in posterior tibial instability, even dislocation (9). Failure to recognize problems above and below the knee may cause the surgeon to choose a more valgus alignment in the arthroplasty than is necessary. For example, an older-style total hip arthroplasty ipsilateral to the knee replacement, which has a marked valgus neck–shaft angle, has displaced the femoral shaft medially. Accordingly, the knee arthroplasty in this limb requires only a few degrees of valgus to achieve neutral mechanical alignment. Any more may create an excessive valgus moment at the knee, which either disrupts the collateral ligaments or dislocates the constrained implant.

Pes planus secondary to rupture of the posterior tibialis tendon is a frequent complication of valgus knee alignment. This requires at a minimum an orthotic to balance the foot. Otherwise a destructive medial moment is induced at the knee, resulting in failure. The definitive treatment for this deformity is a hindfoot (calcaneal) osteotomy.

■ REHABILITATION

The valgus knee should be aligned with a neutral mechanical axis and be stable with intact collateral ligaments. This arthroplasty should be capable of standard rehabilitation with protected weight bearing for comfort only, encouraging the patient to progress rapidly to full weight bearing. The emphasis as always during rehabilitation is on increasing flexion and ensuring that full extension is achieved. This is more important than trying to increase walking distance, which induces swelling and makes it more difficult to regain motion.

In those cases in which the medial collateral ligament has been stretched, constrained arthroplasties may have been used. These are mechanically stable immediately, and patients should be encouraged to progress rapidly with rehabilitation. If a ligament reconstruction has been performed, it may be necessary to brace the knee temporarily until the surgeon feels that adequate healing has occurred. In the techniques that we have developed for ligament advancement, the intraoperative fixation has proven sufficiently strong to proceed aggressively with rehabilitation, according to our standard protocol.

The classic complication in correction of the valgus knee always has been peroneal nerve palsy (10). This problem is not unique to the valgus knee, however. It results from lengthening of the knee on the lateral side with collateral ligament releases and occurs most frequently in conjunction with correction of concomitant flexion contractures. Patients with valgus knees must be warned of this potential complication. It is not useful to explore the nerve at the time of surgery, despite such recommendations in the earlier literature. Such a knee may be placed in a continuous passive motion machine immediately after surgery, with the knee extending about 30 degrees short of full extension. Gradually, with the patient awake, the extension may be increased. If a peroneal nerve palsy is diagnosed, the bandages and dressing should be loosening or changed if dried blood has hardened them. The knee should be placed in continuous passive motion in extension and followed closely. If a palsy persists after 6 weeks, surgical exploration and decompression has proven effective (11).

Careful attention to basic principles yields excellent results, even in the severely deformed knee. Restoration of neutral mechanical axis and creation of adequate soft-tissue stability are mandatory. Good functional results may be achieved with constrained implants, but the long-term durability may be in question.

■ OUTCOMES AND FUTURE DIRECTIONS

Miyasaka et al. (12), reviewing cases of Ranawat, observed that in 60 valgus knees in 46 patients followed for 10 years in whom the iliotibial band and capsule were released first, followed by detachment of the lateral collateral ligament and popliteus tendon from the femur, the results were generally good. Some degree of instability occurred, however, in 24%, which led to the development of less aggressive techniques for ligament releases.

Krackow and colleagues (13) evaluated 99 knees in 81 patients with valgus deformity in 1991. They categorized the valgus knees according to pathology of deformity, enhancing our understanding of the pathology. Type I was defined as valgus deformity secondary to bone loss in the lateral compartment and soft-tissue contracture with medial soft tissues intact; type II as obvious attenuation of the medial capsular ligament complex; and type III as severe valgus deformity with valgus malpositioning of the proximal tibial joint line after overcorrected proximal tibial osteotomy. Results with ligament-tightening techniques were reported for some of theses knees and were generally good for all three types. These results were slightly inferior, however, to those in a control group without deformity.

Stern et al. (14), reporting on surgery performed by Insall, conclude that alignment and stability can be corrected with standard release in most patients, with posterior stabilized implants. They concluded that "total knee arthroplasty is a reliable and durable procedure in the treatment of valgus knee arthritis. However, valgus-deformed knees represent a greater challenge than their varus counterparts to the implant surgeon in terms of the intraoperative balancing required" (14).

References

1. Insall J. *Surgery of the knee*. Edinburgh: Churchill Livingston, 1984.
2. Vince KG. Leg length discrepancy after revision total knee sarthroplasty. *Techniques in Orthopedics* 1988; 3:35.
3. Keblish PA. The lateral approach to the valgus knee: Surgical technique and analysis of 53 cases with over two-year follow-up evaluation. *Clin Orthop* 1991; 271:52–62.
4. Buechel FF. A sequential three-step lateral release for correcting fixed valgus knee deformities during total knee arthroplasty. *Clin Orthop* 1990; 260:170–175.
5. Nagamine R, White SE, McCarthy DS, et al. Effect of rotational malposition of the femoral component on knee stability kinematics after total knee arthroplasty. *J Arthroplasty* 1995; 10:265–270.
6. Arima J, Whiteside LA, McCarthy DS, et al. Femoral rotational alignment, based on the anteroposterior axis, in total knee arthroplasty in a valgus knee: A technical note. *J Bone Joint Surg Am* 1995; 77:1331–1334.
7. Whiteside LA, Arima J. The anteroposterior axis for femoral rotational alignment in valgus total knee arthroplasty. *Clin Orthop* 1995; 321:168–172.
8. Briard JL, Hungerford DS. Patellofemoral instability in total knee arthroplasty. *J Arthroplasty* 1989; 4(suppl):87–97
9. Sharkey PF, Hozack WJ, Booth RE Jr, et al. Posterior dislocation of total knee arthroplasty. *Clin Orthop* 1992; 278:128–133.

10. Idusuyi OB, Morrey BF. Peroneal nerve palsy after total knee arthroplasty. Assessment of pre-disposing and prognostic factors. *J Bone Joint Surg Am* 1996; 78:177–184.

11. Mont MA, Dellon AL, Chen F, et al. The operative treatment of peroneal nerve palsy. *J Bone Joint Surg Am* 1996; 78:863–869.

12. Miyasaka KC, Ranawat CS, Mullaji A. 10- to 20-year followup of total knee arthroplasty for valgus deformities. *Clin Orthop* 1997; 345:29–37.

13. Krackow KA, Jones MM, Teeny SM, et al. Primary total knee arthroplasty in patients with fixed valgus deformity. *Clin Orthop* 1991; 273:9–18.

14. Stern SH, Moeckel BH, Insall JN. Total knee arthroplasty in valgus knees. *Clin Orthop* 1991; 273:5–8.

KELLY G. VINCE

24

Soft Tissue Releases for the Varus Knee

Varus deformity is the malalignment that surgeons encounter most frequently in knee arthroplasty surgery, and loosening was regarded as the most common problem in knee arthroplasty surgery for many years. These observations are related: There was persistent varus alignment after arthroplasty, which in turn loaded the medial tibial bone to the point at which it yielded and the component subsided.

It long has been recognized that knee arthroplasties that are left in varus face a higher-than-average rate of component loosening and rapid demise from polyethylene wear (1). This point originally was established by Lotke and Ecker (2) and reinforced by Vince et al. (3). Insall is credited with devising the surgical techniques that enabled surgeons to stabilize knees in neutral alignment through ligament releases (4).

Some patients suffer increasingly severe varus deformity as a result of arthritis. Many of these patients, however, started life with a tendency towards mechanically varus knees. In correcting their deformity, we are at times going beyond the alignment that was at one time natural for them in order to achieve a neutral mechanical axis for the entire lower extremity. The neutral axis means that we have aligned the leg so that the hip, knee, and ankle are colinear.

Medial ligament releases are indicated in a knee arthroplasty in which the patient has varus alignment. The mechanical pathology of the arthritic varus knee (whether the patient has had a varus knee for his or her entire life or not) is that articular cartilage damage initiates problems in the medial compartment. As further erosion of cartilage occurs, bone also is ground away, until the knee collapses into the medial compartment. At times, this allows for the contracture of the medial collateral ligaments and eventual stretching of the structures on the lateral side.

The medial structures must not be transected during the release but rather should be detached progressively from the proximal medial tibia, keeping them in continuity as a sleeve. Releases on the medial side may have to lengthen the medial structures beyond their original lengths for two reasons:

1. Varus alignment may have been the normal status for a given patient, and his or her medial collateral ligament may have always been abnormally shorter.
2. The medial structures may require lengthening so that they are as long as the stretched lateral structures.

The preoperative planning for correction of varus deformity is instrumental in achieving satisfactory valgus alignment and knee stability. Long radiographic cassettes that show the hips, knees, and ankles on the same film are extremely helpful in detecting anatomic deformities in either the femur or tibia outside of the knee joint. Anatomic bowing of both the femur and tibia, in most cases, can be corrected with the appropriate releases in the joint. The correct static alignment of the components can be planned only from full-length radiographs. Classical alignment of knee arthroplasties dictates that the proximal tibia be resected at 90 degrees of the long axis of the tibia. Similarly, the distal femoral cut should be

■ HISTORY OF THE TECHNIQUE

■ INDICATIONS AND CONTRAINDICATIONS

at a right angle to a line that is drawn from the center of the hip to the center of the knee. For the patient with excessive femoral bowing, this mandates a distal femoral resection exceeding the normal 6 to 7 degrees of valgus.

The anatomy of the medial structures dictates the nature of the technique for their release. The medial collateral ligament has superficial and deep layers (5). These structures that we refer to as medial collateral ligament actually represent consolidations of the capsular tissues. The deepest layer, the deep medial collateral ligament, is released in the vast majority of knees as part of the surgical exposure. There is some disagreement among experienced surgeons as to whether these releases should be done in a progressive fashion, with more extensive release for the more extensively deformed knee, or whether each knee simply should have a complete release. The technique described here favors progressive releases for increasingly severe varus deformity. There is also disagreement as to whether the medial release can create medial instability to valgus stresses even if the technique has been performed properly. Although rare, overrelease can occur.

Medial releases are contraindicated in patients with valgus deformities. They are never planned in this setting but may be performed inadvertently during the surgical exposure, if excess amounts of medial capsule are elevated from the tibia or the saw blade transects the medial collateral ligament during the tibial cut.

■ SURGICAL TECHNIQUES

The surgical exposure for a varus knee depends largely on surgeon preference. A medial approach, whether it is parapatellar, transpatellar, subvastus, or midvastus, suffices. The very important aspect of surgical technique, however, is strict attention to detail. The fact that these medial structures may have been contracted and that the medial side is being lengthened explains why some of these knees become very difficult to close securely at the completion of the arthroplasty. The contracted medial tissues often retract posteriorly and make it difficult to achieve a secure closure. Irrespective of the arthrotomy preferred, the skin incision should lay 1 cm medial to the base of the tibial tubercle. In this location, the surgeon protects the patellar tendon, is certain not to elevate fibers of the patellar tendon with the arthrotomy, and enjoys thicker periosteum for the later closure. The capsular tissues medial to the arthrotomy must be elevated from bone with periosteum as an intact sleeve. The initial arthrotomy, made with a scalpel, should proceed directly down to bone. This incision in the periosteum must be respected so that an intact sleeve of tissue can be furnished. Further elevation of the medial tissue is best accomplished with a periosteal elevator and perhaps a small mallet. Attempting to elevate the medial structures with a scalpel alone risks the making a series of parallel incisions through the periosteum, converting this intact sleeve of tissue into a series of ribbons. Failure to elevate risks drainage in the immediate postoperative period. Once the patella has been everted, the tibia should be rotated externally as the knee is flexed. This brings the released anteromedial portion of the tibia forward. Release of soft tissue on the most proximal aspects of the tibia is standard for the vast majority of knees. Releasing the capsular tissue and perhaps some of the deep medial collateral ligament does not always result in significant correction of the varus deformity. Greater lengthening of the medial structures occurs as the surgeon proceeds distally with the elevation.

The Key elevator may be used to elevate a triangular piece of anteromedial capsule. Orienting the elevator distally makes it easier to separate the periosteal fibers from bone where they convert. Osteophytes may be removed from the medial tibia as this part of the bone is brought forward by increasing knee flexion and external tibial rotation. Eventually, as flexion is forced, some pressure may be placed by the assistant on the anteromedial femur. This brings the posteromedial corner of the tibia forward, facilitating the release with a scalpel of the insertion of the semimembranosus tendon. Small amounts of thick bursal fluid may be released from the bursa overlying the semimembranosus in the posteromedial corner. This degree of release is adequate as a preliminary realignment and as a means of facilitating the exposure. Once the basic bone cuts have been made, spacer blocks can be inserted into the knee joint to evaluate the need for more extensive release and lengthening of structures on the medial side. With the basic exposure of the varus knee complete, the instrument systems particular to the chosen prosthesis are employed to make bone cuts. As described previously, a right-angled cut on the proximal tibia and a cut on the distal femur lying at right angles to the mechanical axis of the bone (usually 5 to 7degrees of valgus relative to the intramedullary axis of the femur) are satisfactory to align the knee in extension. The femoral component size has been selected and the posterior condyles resected to create a flexion gap. The rotational positioning of the femoral component is extremely important regardless of the design selected. As a rough guide, the most prosthetic components should be rotated externally relative to the articular surface of the posterior femoral condyles. This is not as reliable an indicator of the desired position, however, as the epicondylar axis extending from the medial to femoral epicondyle. This axis, based on the length of the collateral ligaments, is a far more accurate guide to correct rotational positioning of the femoral component.

Assessment of stability in motion commences with reduction of the knee in flexion with a spacer block inserted. This can be accomplished once the distal, anterior, and posterior femoral cuts have been made in conjunction with the proximal tibial resection. With the knee flexed at 90 degrees, a tight medial side is to be expected. A large discrepancy, however, between tension on the medial and lateral sides indicates a need to reevaluate the femoral component's rotational position. Internal rotation of this component causes a multitude of problems with the arthroplasty, especially with patellar tracking. One can visualize that an internally rotated femur preserves bone on the posteromedial condyle and creates a knee that is tight selectively on the medial side in flexion.

The knee can be extended safely with the spacer block in place by performing the equivalent of an anterior drawer maneuver and bringing the knee into extension. If medial tension is similar in both flexion and extension, then further release of medial structures can be expected to restore alignment, stability, and motion to the arthroplasty. Medial tension in flexion, which is not present in extension, is an indicator of an internally rotated femoral component.

Most commonly, the knee with the significant varus deformity is tighter on the medial side in extension. There is no technique for selectively releasing the medial structures that would have a differential effect on the knee in flexion and extension. Simply stated, whatever release is performed on the medial side has an equivalent effect in both flexion and extension. Accordingly, one of the two positions must be regarded as more important than the other. Because of weight bearing and ambulation, it is desirable to adjust the ligament tension so that the knee is stable and correctly aligned in extension in preference over flexion. Although small amounts of increased medial laxity in flexion can be tolerated, the knee must not be left tight on the medial side in flexion or the patient will be unable to bend the joint.

Further releases of medial tissues may be accomplished in stages if the knee continues to be tighter on the medial than the lateral side in extension. A more complete release of the deep proximal tissue at the cut bone surface of the tibia would be appropriate. The joint capsule and deep medial collateral ligament are released posteriorly until muscle fibers are revealed. Osteophytes must be excised from under the medial collateral ligament on the femur as well as the tibia.

In principle, all tight structures on the medial side of the midline are potential varus deforming forces. This is the basis for proceeding with releases around the posteromedial and towards the posterior aspect of the tibia. Within 1 cm of the resected tibial bone, all of the posteromedial capsule can be released from the posterior tibia. It is common to see flexion contractures in conjunction with varus deformity, and release of this tissue helps correct both. A complete release reveals muscle of the posterior tibial compartment. Any more distal release does not help correct deformity and is dangerous, because of the proximity of the anterior tibial artery. It is wise to reassess the knee before embarking on a more aggressive release of the medial structures, specifically the superficial medial collateral ligament and sometimes even the tendons of the pes anserinus. Some knees, especially those with extensive tibia vara, internal tibial torsion, or femoral bowing require a very aggressive release. In particular, the internally rotated "bandy legged" tibia almost needs to be untwisted or derotated by the releases to restore alignment and stability. In contrast, however, if the static alignment of the bone cuts is in excessive valgus, the surgeon is driven to overrelease the knee in order to balance this new deformity. Reconfirmation of the static alignment of the bone cuts is important at this point. Complete release of the superficial medial collateral ligament with an osteotome extended distally underneath this structure may be necessary but can be expected to produce an arthroplasty without the solid endpoint to valgus stress testing that is characteristic of most reconstructions (Fig. 24-1).

The knee will remain stable, but valgus stress testing will reveal a softer, more spongy endpoint. This extensive release of the superficial collateral ligament covers a large surface of anatomic attachment to the tibia. In all probability, this ligament reattaches later in a new position and perhaps without the original strength of attachment. If even further release is required, the pes anserinus tendons may be detached from the tibia. This is accomplished best with sharp dissection or the aggressive use of an osteotome.

Even the most severely deformed arthroplasty should now be balanced on the medial and lateral sides in flexion and extension. The knee must be balanced preferentially in extension, with reliable stability to varus and valgus stresses. It should not be excessively tight on either side. It may be necessary to tolerate some small increased laxity on the medial side in flexion, especially if the femoral component has been rotated parallel to the epicondylar axis. Surgeons who are unaccustomed to the aggressive release of medial structures may find the appearance of the knee disconcerting. The magnitude of the release creates doubt as to whether the arthroplasty can ever be rendered stable again. The results in terms of correction of deformity and restoration of stability with good valgus alignment are, however, dramatic. Overrelease of the medial side is distinctly unusual, and medial in-

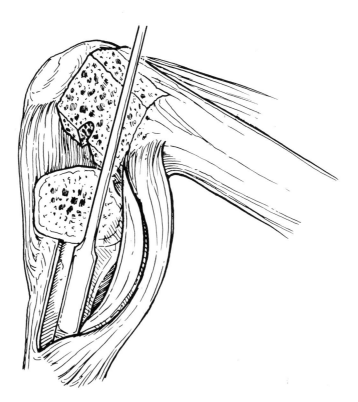

■ FIGURE 24-1

Exposure and preliminary elevation of the medial capsule. With the knee flexed maximally, and the leg externally rotated, the posteromedial corner of the tibia comes out from behind the femur. Near the proximal tibia, using cautery, the medial structures can be released from the tibia, extending posteriorly and including the semimembranosus. For more extensive releases, an osteotome is inserted under the medial structures and advanced gently with a mallet to release the superficial medial collateral ligament.

stability is likely to result from excessive valgus alignment only in conjunction with inadvertent transection of the medial structures rather than their detachment from the tibia.

Once trial components have been inserted, many of the releases can be refined. With trial components in place and the knee extended, three criteria must be satisfied:

1. Absolutely full extension.
2. Satisfactory valgus alignment.
3. Dependable varus–valgus stability

If the knee does not extend fully, the components must be removed and the arthroplasty reassessed, either with further posterior releases or in some cases resection of a few millimeters of additional distal femoral bone.

Once the actual components have been introduced into the knee, these criteria again should be applied. Closure of the distal arthrotomy in an arthroplasty in which an extensive medial release has been performed can prove difficult. The tissue, tight prior to the arthroplasty, is even more difficult to close because the bones have been separated on the medial side. Closure is facilitated by placing and not tying sutures until the last one has been positioned in the distal aspect of the wound. In this way, the medial capsular tissue and both superficial and deep medial collateral ligaments are easier to grasp than if they are tied. The capsule in this area is less tight if the knee is flexed to 90 degrees.

The medial collateral ligament, though often in need of release to correct varus deformity, generally is protected by the varus alignment of the knee. The lateral structures in these knees, however, are subjected to severe tensile forces, which can lead to plastic failure. In many cases, the collateral ligaments are intact but very lax, because of either loss of medial tibial bone in the arthritic knee or collapse of the medial tibial plateau underneath a component in the failed arthroplasty. Restoration of substance to the bone either with graft or modular implants goes a long way toward restoring stability in the joint. In very rare cases, there can be so much varus deformity that the lateral structures fail significantly because of stretching. Some of these may require constrained though nonlinked implants. Initial work has been reported on techniques for ligament advancement or tightening on the convex side of angular deformity in conjunction with extensive releases of the contracted side.

There are no practical alternatives to release of the medial collateral ligament in a varus knee. Although some may argue that, in theory at least, stretching of the lateral collateral ligament is the true pathology, advancing or tightening lateral structures is rarely practical. Reconstruction may be considered following a good release of the tight medial structures. In some situations, a surgeon may choose a constrained implant to provide stability if a large deformity is present, as an alternative to conventional releases. This can be described only as misguided.

There are a few pitfalls that may endanger the knee arthroplasty if a medial release is performed. One is inadequate release, which may occur because the surgeon is concerned about destabilizing the knee; although overrelease can occur, it is unusual and occurs far less frequently than underrelease. Medial instability, if it occurs, more often results from transection of the ligament near the joint line. The technique is clear: The medial structure should be stripped from the tibia, intact, as a sleeve. Underrelease also may occur if the bone cuts do not correct the static alignment adequately in the joint.

Some patients with varus knees have malalignment, which extends into the diaphysis of the tibia or is accompanied by varus bowing of the femur. Others may have suffered a malunion of a diaphyseal fracture above or below the knee. Regardless of the shape of the bones above and below the knee, a line from the center of the femoral head to the center of the knee must be parallel to a line extending from the center of the knee to the center of the ankle. Failure to accomplish this realignment means that a limited medial release provides stability to the malaligned knee. These are two errors that create a bone that feels stable but which is malaligned, an unacceptable situation. Corrective osteotomies may be indicated in some of these patients (6). Aggressive soft-tissue techniques have been described that release the ligaments on the medial side and advance those on the lateral.

■ TECHNICAL
ALTERNATIVES AND
PITFALLS

Many surgeons who have not seen aggressive medial releases are concerned about the amount of release that often is performed posteriorly. All structures on the medial side of the midline contribute to the varus deforming force and should be released.

■ REHABILITATION

Varus deformity is so common that it should be considered almost the norm for knee arthroplasty. The releases must be performed in such a way that the arthroplasty is stable and balanced from the moment the patient leaves the operating room. The knee should be capable of bearing weight as soon as comfort permits. There is no role for bracing of the arthroplasty after release. If a brace is required, then by definition stability has not been achieved, and there is no reason to expect that it will be achieved later. The arthroplasty that is unstable after surgery requires revision surgery.

Flexion and extension remain the top priorities after all knee arthroplasties, including those in which there has been correction of deformity. Patients who try to gauge their progress by how far they can walk create swelling that impedes motion in the short term, possibly leading to a permanently stiff knee.

■ OUTCOMES AND FUTURE DIRECTIONS

The results from correction of varus deformity have been gratifying in clinical practice (7). In fact, these techniques have been responsible for the success of knee arthroplasty surgery generally.

Future directions are difficult to predict. Unusual circumstances, including intraarticular correction of extraarticular deformity with a combination of medial releases and lateral ligament advances, have been reported by Vince (8). These applications, however, are very limited. Technical variations on the classic technique have been described, usually involving removal of the ligament from the medial femoral condyle. The release techniques may be calibrated by electronic devices that can measure tension across the joint, affording the surgeon a means of assessing the adequacy of releases during surgery (9).

References

1. Windsor RS, Moran MC, Insall JN. Mechanisms of failure of the femoral and tibial components in total knee arthroplasty. *Clin Orthop* 1989; 248:15–19.
2. Lotke PA, Ecker ML. Influence of positioning of prosthesis in total knee replacment. *J Bone Joint Surg Am* 1977; 59:77–79.
3. Vince KG, Insall JN, Kelly MA. The total condylar prosthesis: 10- to 12-year results of a cemented knee replacement. *J Bone Joint Surg Br* 1989; 71:793–797.
4. Insall J. *Surgery of the knee.* Edinburgh: Churchill Livingston, 1984.
5. Warren LM. The supporting structures and layers on hte medial side of the knee: An anatomical analysis. *J Bone Joint Surg Am* 1979; 61:56–62.
6. Wolff AM, Hungerford DS, Pepe CL. The effect of extraarticular varus and valgus deformity on total knee arthroplasty. *Clin Orthop* 1991; 271:35–51.
7. Teeny SM, Krackow KA, Hungerford DS, et al. Primary total knee arthroplasty in patients with severe varus deformity: A comparative study. *Clin Orthop* 1991; 273:19–31.
8. Vince KG. Collateral ligament reconstructions in difficult primary and revision total knee arthroplasty. Presented at the Annual Meeting of the Knee Society, January 1997, San Francisco, CA.
9. Takahashi T, Wada Y, Yamamoto H. Soft-tissue balancing with pressure distribution during total knee arthroplasty. *J Bone Joint Surg Br* 1997; 79:235–239.

SEVAN GREGORY
ORTAASLAN
KELLY G. VINCE

25

Reconstruction of Tibial Defects

In primary and revision total knee arthroplasty, the surgeon faces technical challenges if presented with bone defects. Distinct differences exist in both of these types of surgery based on quality of the host bone, as well as bone available for reconstruction. Certain principles must be respected, however, in all situations. In essence, it is preferable to reconstruct a defect in the tibia rather than sacrifice healthy bone in order to restore the angle of the tibial bone.

In total knee arthroplasty, one of the earliest approaches to resolving the problem of tibial defects was to perform a cut below the level of the defect. This method compromised healthy bone, and consequently, because the strength of the trabecular bone weakened as the distance increased from the joint, conventional instruments and components proved unsatisfactory for the resurfacing of the tibia. With the invention of newer techniques, surgeons concentrated on reconstructing or bypassing the defect rather than building on a flat but lower tibial surface. For instance, with the use of polymethylmethacrylate (PMMA) or screw-reinforced PMMA, small defects were filled easily with cement, and thereafter the tibial surface underwent conventional treatment (1).

In larger defects, it was found that bone grafting (either autograft or allograft) improved the biomechanics of the construct, based on its potential for union and enhanced bone stock. Several of these bone-grafting techniques have been used, including particulate or structural autograft and morseled or large structural allograft; these are described subsequently in this chapter. In addition, modular implants and custom components expanded the armamentarium of devices for the reconstruction of these defects. These included a variety of wedges and blocks that worked adequately in the situation of a primary total knee arthroplasty. For the larger deficiencies in revision surgery, however, these components were found to be insufficient, and thus they required the support of various bone-grafting techniques. The defects that appear with primary and revision arthroplasty are distinctly different, as are the sources of graft material. With the combination of these different surgical options, the majority of tibial defects have been treated successfully, with excellent results.

■ HISTORY OF THE TECHNIQUE

The management of tibial defects differs depending on the size and location of the deficiency with respect to the tibial surface. Several classifications exist to aid the surgeon with reconstruction guidelines. The Anderson Orthopaedic Research Institute created a bone-defect classification for revision total knee surgery, based on preoperative radiographs and intraoperative assessment (2,3), outlining three types of defects (Table 25-1). The Anderson classification has been applied to both the femoral and tibial sides, and a treatment protocol was suggested for each type (Table 25-2). Another classification of tibial bone deficiencies (Table 25-3) (4), described for both primary and revision knees, contains many similarities to the Anderson classification; however, it is simpler in both description and outline of treatment.

Among the choices already discussed, the use of PMMA, alone or with screw enhancement, is technically the simplest (5). PMMA easily conforms to the irregular shapes of bony

■ INDICATIONS AND CONTRAINDICATIONS

246   Techniques in Knee Surgery

TABLE 25-1. ANDERSON ORTHOPAEDIC RESEARCH INSTITUTE CLASSIFICATION OF BONE DEFECTS

Type	Defect
1	Metaphyseal bone is intact, with minor bone defects that do not compromise the component's stability
2	Metaphyseal bone is damaged, with cancellous bone deficiency, involving:
A	One plateau
B	Both plateaus
3	Large metaphyseal deficiency, compromising a major segment of one or both plateaus

TABLE 25-2. ANDERSON ORTHOPAEDIC RESEARCH INSTITUTE MANAGEMENT OF BONE DEFECTS

Type	Treatment
1	Standard nonstemmed implants
2	Augmentation or bone graft to restore joint line and stability
3	Reconstruction with major bone grafts, custom components, or hinges

TABLE 25-3. RECONSTRUCTING BONE DEFECTS

Defect	Technique
Contained	Cement, particulate autograft or allograft chips
Noncontained	Modular augmentation implant
Massive	Structural allograft
Metaphyseal–diaphyseal expansion	Impaction grafting

From ref. 4.

deficiencies, creating a flat surface for the foundation of the component. Because of its limited biomechanical properties, however, PMMA is best suited for shallow defects 5 mm or less in depth and involve less than one third of the tibial plateau (6). In larger defects, PMMA has poor durability, even with the reinforcement of corticocancellous screws, and eventually fails. Hence, for any tibial deficiency that is greater than 5 mm in depth, bone grafting should be considered (3).

If it is available, autogenic bone graft is preferred over allograft because of its ideal biologic qualities (7,8). In primary knee arthroplasty, the routine bone cuts provide excellent autograft for reconstruction. This bone graft can be used in either particulate or corticocancellous forms. Evidently, this supply is present infrequently in revision cases because of bone deficiency, although conversion of a standard cruciate ligament–retaining prosthesis to a constrained condylar type of implant often yields bone from the intercondylar notch.

In primary knee arthroplasty, bone grafting is indicated for tibial defects 5 mm or greater in depth that involve up to two thirds of the tibial plateau (9). Whereas particulate autograft can be used in contained lesions, the noncontained defects necessitate the use of corticocancellous segments from the routine bone cuts. Insall and Sculco originated techniques that use bone from the intercondylar notch and distal femoral cut, respectively

(10,11), with favorable results. Laskin described an approach of autogenic bone graft for tibial defect reconstruction, using bone from the posterior femoral resection (12). He reported relatively poor results, however. Thirty percent of his study group demonstrated either fragmentation of the graft or lack of incorporation, which may have resulted from the contact between cortical (graft) and subchondral (articular) surfaces in this technique.

The Insall and Sculco autografting techniques generally work well in primary knee arthroplasties (10,11), provided that sufficient bone exists from the cuts. If the defect is too large, allograft may be used with these same techniques. No clinical results are available, however, using these techniques with allograft. Modular wedges and blocks can be used instead of bone graft in some situations, depending on the match between the defect and the available augments in regards to size and shape (13).

Revision surgery, in contrast to primary knee arthroplasty, often involves larger tibial deficiencies. Thus, the surgeon almost always is obligated to use allogenic bone graft for reconstructive purposes. The same Insall or Sculco techniques may be employed with allograft, although the host bed is usually quite deficient in a patient undergoing revision surgery. For larger defects, however, massive structural allografts may be necessary, especially in younger individuals, because they improve tibial bone stock. These types of allograft are indicated for lesions ranging from 50% of metaphyseal bone loss to complete proximal tibial replacement.

There exists concern with the use of massive structural allografts, however, stemming from acetabular reconstruction studies that show high failure rates because of collapse (14–16). To date, in the 10-year history of proximal tibial defect reconstruction using massive allograft, there are no published data depicting failures as were reported for structural acetabular allografts in hip arthroplasty surgery (17–21).

Certain issues must be addressed in the use of large allograft bone in revision knee surgery. Although it is ideal to replenish bone stock in young patients, modular components may be of greater benefit in older or immunodeficient patients. There exists a relative contraindication for the use of allograft, because of the small but present risk of infectious transmission. In accordance, allograft and, of course, revision surgery itself, are contraindicated in patients with active knee sepsis. In the reimplantation phase of two-stage reconstructions for infection, however, the advantages of structural allografts may outweigh their disadvantages. As an alternative, some surgeons favor hinged prostheses instead of allografts. I do not hold this opinion, however. Failure of stemmed revision components or hinges poses a unique problem. In addition to extensive bone loss at the cut surface, there may be intramedullary expansion resulting from the loose stem. Impaction grafting of the tibia, a technique adopted from hip reconstruction, shows promise as a solution (22).

Modular components can be of great benefit to both the surgeon and patient in revision knee surgery. They easily augment smaller (10-mm) defects or facilitate the application of bone graft in larger ones. Customized components can be used, because they can replace the entire deficiency. Because of the cost and difficulty in devising their shape and size, however, these prostheses remain a less favorable option for tibial reconstruction.

Cement and Particulate Bone Graft   Polymethylmethacrylate and particulate bone graft can be used similarly to reconstruct small tibial defects (Fig. 25-1). Contained defects of up to 5 mm and 10 mm can be rebuilt with PMMA and particulate graft, respectively (Fig. 25-2). In each case, the surfaces of the tibial defects must be prepared to optimally accept the new filler (cement or bone graft). Usually, the surface of these defects is densely sclerotic, which provides excellent support but a poor interface for components and the fillers. Techniques including multiple small drill holes or shallow criss-crossing saw cuts can improve both the cement–bone and graft–bone interdigitation. Screw augmentation has been used to reinforce this construct, with the added advantage of limiting how low the component can sink into the defect.

■ SURGICAL TECHNIQUES

Autograft for Primary Total Knee Arthroplasty   Several bone-grafting techniques exist using autograft sources. Scuderi et al. (11) uses a self-locking principle to secure autograft,

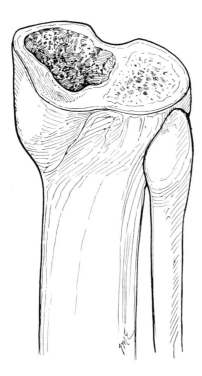

■ FIGURE 25-1

Peripheral, contained tibial defects of up to 5 and 10mm can be rebuilt with polymethylmethacrylate and particulate bone graft, respectively.

shaped from bone removed from the intercondylar notch in posterior cruciate ligament–substituting knees without any permanent metal fixation. In central defects of the tibial condyles, the curved contour of the femoral condyle is often responsible for eroding into the tibia. This defect must be reshaped into a rectangular or trapezoidal construct, thus excising all sclerotic bone until healthy cancellous bone is exposed (Fig. 25-3). Using methylene blue, the bone block taken from the intercondylar notch bone is marked in the same dimensions as the recipient site. After reshaping the graft with a saw or burr, the bone block then is tapped gently into place. In principle, a snug fit should be obtained in order to prevent cement from entering the interface. In addition, a small preliminary batch of ce-

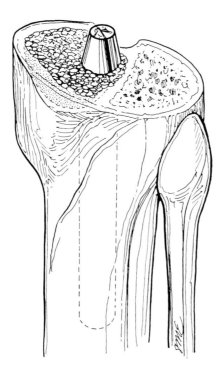

■ FIGURE 25-2

A contained tibial defect smaller than 10 mm (most often seen in revision arthroplasty) is filled and packed with particulate bone graft, after an intramedullary rod or guide is introduced to keep graft from falling into the canal.

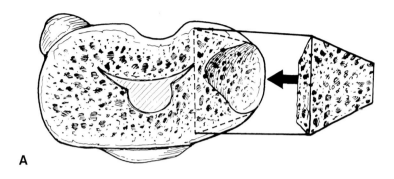

A

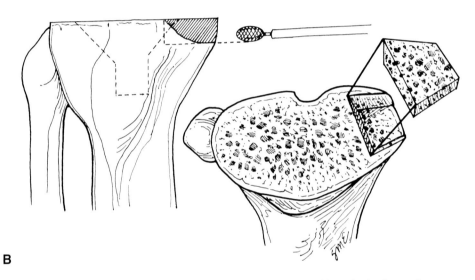

B   ■ FIGURE 25-3

Insall "dovetail" technique. **A:** The defect is reshaped, using a high-speed burr, in the form of a trapezoid, with its largest base towards the center of the tibia. **B:** Autograft bone (from the intercondylar notch) is shaped to fit into this trapezoidal defect and is tapped home in a self-locking fashion.

ment may be prepared to "grout" the interface and prevent intrusion of large amounts of polymethylmethacrylate bone cement (PMMA).

For noncontained, peripheral lesions, Insall suggests that a trapezoidal or dovetail construct be created, with its widest base directed centrally on the tibia (11). Then the bone block is seated and held in place temporarily with two smooth horizontally placed Kirschner wires. These wires should not be removed until the tibial component is cemented and all excess bone has been removed. This step prevents undesired movement of the graft. Again, the shape of the graft, with its widest base aimed over the center of the tibia, helps secure it in place. In this fashion, only compressive forces are exerted on the graft.

Windsor et al. (10) describe a technique using bone shaped from the distal femur. They suggest preparing the tibia by cutting the minimum 5 mm of bone from the proximal tibia, and then using a reciprocating saw to excise the sclerotic surface over the tibial defect until healthy cancellous bone is exposed. The defect thus is converted to a flat, but sloping, surface (Fig. 25-4). Then, the cancellous surface of the distal femoral bone cut is placed over the defect and secured using threaded Steinman pins or wires from a cannulated screw set. Excess bone is removed, leaving a level tibial surface. After a trial component is tested for

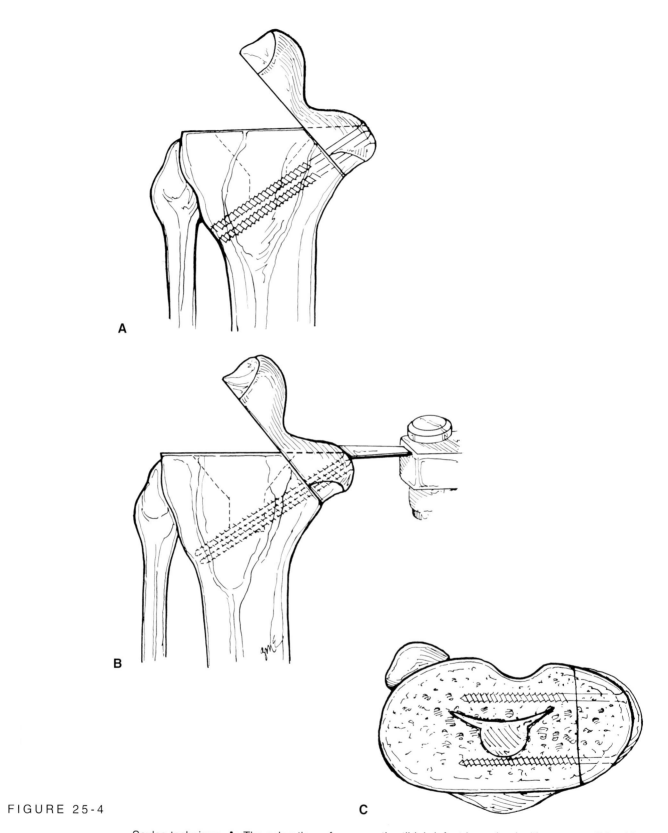

Sculco technique. **A:** The sclerotic surface over the tibial defect is excised with a saw until healthy cancellous bone is exposed. **B:** The cancellous surface of the distal femoral bone cut is placed over the defect and secured with cancellous screws, ensuring that they do not interfere with the tibial component's stem or keel. **C:** The excess bone is removed with an oscillating saw, leaving a level tibial surface.

fit, the Steinman pins are cut flush with the graft, or cancellous screws are used to compress the surfaces together firmly before the component is cemented (Fig. 25-4B,C). It is suggested that two batches of PMMA be used during cementing. Once the first batch becomes doughy (after about 3 or 4 minutes), it is spread on top of the graft–tibia interface to act as a sealant between this interface and the tibial surface. Shortly before the first batch of cement cures, a second batch is used in the standard fashion to cement the component on the tibial surface. This cementing technique, in conjunction with screw fixation, helps keep the graft interface clear of cement, thus aiding graft incorporation.

The technique described by Laskin (12) uses bone removed from the posterior femoral condyles during standard femoral resections (Fig. 25-5A). In spite of the high failure rate noted by the author, it still may be useful in some patients with stronger bone. This procedure involves an initial cut of the tibial surface, 4 to 6 mm as measured from the normal side. Bone from the posterior femoral resection then is prepared as graft by denuding it of cartilage and scarring its subchondral surface. Securing the entire bone block with cancellous screws or Kirschner wires may help prevent fragmentation (Fig. 25-5B). The fixation then is countersunk. By trimming the graft at the level of the remaining tibial surface, a foundation is left for cementing the tibial component. Laskin suggests using doughy cement to minimize intrusion into the graft interface.

The Laskin technique is well suited to the type of defects created by rheumatoid arthritis. Unfortunately, the bone quality in these patients often leads to poor results. The Sculco

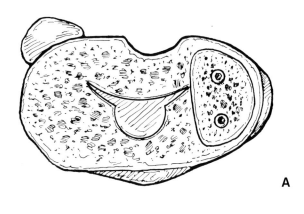

A

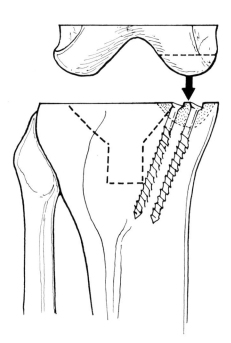

Laskin technique. **A:** After preparing bone from the posterior femoral surface as graft by denuding it of cartilage and scarring its subchondral surface, the entire bone block is secured with cancellous screws. **B:** The fixation then is countersunk, and the graft is trimmed to the level of the remaining tibial surface.

B ■ FIGURE 25-5

technique has the advantage of opposing two cancellous surfaces for superior healing and can be used for large defects. Screws or pin fixation are required. The Insall technique does not require fixation but can be used only for small defects. The cancellous autograft used generally incorporates well.

Modular and Special Implants   Custom prostheses can be costly and difficult to design and ultimately may not fit the patient. Modular prostheses with augmentation, however, such as wedges or blocks, can be obtained readily at a marginally higher cost than standard implants. They work well for defects sized 10 to 20 mm. Preoperative radiographs dictate the type of augmentation necessary, as templates for each size and type of augment exist for use with standard knee films. Occasionally, bone-grafting techniques in conjunction with augmented prostheses improve the final result, especially if irregularly shaped deformities exist. Overall, the use of augmentation has simplified the management of the majority of tibial defects, and good results are obtained consistently (13).

Allograft   Massive allograft reconstructions appear complex, but with preoperative planning and application of surgical principles during the procedure, excellent results can be obtained (17). Ideally, a distal femoral or proximal tibial allograft serves well for the reconstruction of tibial deficiencies. Duplication of the correct side helps with a tibial graft. Size is important, and a radiograph of the graft should be compared with that of the host proximal tibia. These films actually can be used as templates, to assess the shape of the allograft needed preoperatively as well as the final size and type of implant (18).

After exposure of the knee and debridement of the proximal tibia, the final evaluation begins regarding allograft requirements. Certain principles must be respected in shaping the allograft. The overall height of the host proximal tibia should be restored, and either an intact plateau or the fibular head acts as a guide. The shape of the allograft should provide maximal contact between itself and the host bone (17). By preserving an anteromedial cortical strip, the graft–host interface increases, and rotational control is improved greatly. Overall, the allograft should be sculpted to the host bone surface, so that the fit confers rotational stability (21).

Intramedullary fixation, in the form of stems, is highly recommended for additional support of the graft–host bone interface (21). Offset stems are very helpful in this circumstance, because the allograft has a tendency to displace the component with respect to the intramedullary canal. With the use of offset stems, this malalignment of the component is avoided and intramedullary stability is maximized. Additional fixation in the form of plates and screws should be avoided, because they prevent subsidence and may even distract the allograft host interface (21). Cerclage wires are preferred (Fig. 25-6), because they provide stability without the impedance of screws in the intramedullary region and do not act as stress risers.

Once the allograft is sculpted, the allograft and host bone require preparation for the tibial implant. Bone clamps can be used to hold the graft in place as an oscillating saw cuts the tibial surface at the final correct level. Tibial component sizing and preparation should proceed in the usual manner. During implantation, the cement technique using two batches of PMMA (as described previously) can be used to avoid getting PMMA in the allograft–host interface. The stemmed implant then should be inserted, while the prepared cerclage wires are tightened. It is critical to note the final alignment of both the tibial component and allograft with respect to the host bone, because the altered tibial anatomy can prove misleading. We favor cementation of the tibial component as the mode of fixation, because the use of porous surfaces adjacent to avascular allograft offers little chance of osseous integration (18).

Soft-tissue management remains important during knee arthroplasties that require massive allograft techniques. The soft-tissue sleeve should be maintained for the stability of the reconstruction, so that posterior cruciate ligament–substituting (posterior stabilized) and not constrained articulating surfaces can be used. The former are preferred, because the latter transfer additional stress to the bone–implant interface, which may resulting in a higher

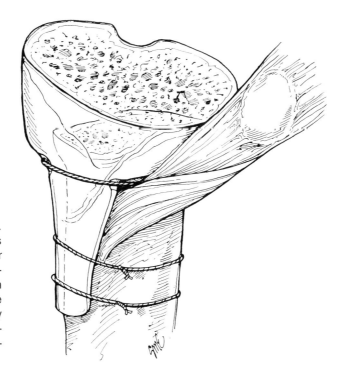

Massive structural reconstruction. After sculpture of the allograft, it is held in place with bone clamps or cerclage wires (as shown), maintaining the correct alignment with the host tibial bone, while the stemmed tibial component is finally inserted. The cerclage wires are secured at the end, providing additional stability.

■ FIGURE 25-6

failure rate. In essence, with proper soft-tissue balance, correct alignment, and solid stability of the allograft and component, excellent results can be achieved with massive allograft reconstruction of significant tibial deficiencies.

Impaction Grafting   In cases of failed knee arthroplasties in which only a shell of metaphyseal–diaphyseal bone remains, a technique adopted from hip revision surgery can be applied in order to reconstruct this defect (22). As described by Ullmark and Hovelius (23), this procedure begins with complete removal of the prosthesis, cement, debris, and fibrous membrane. The sclerotic inner surface of this metaphyseal–diaphyseal shell then should be roughened and irrigated. With a canal plug in place, a centralizing device is screwed into it, maintaining position for the duration of the graft impaction procedure. Using femoral heads for allograft, Ullmark and Hovelius (23) suggest using a special bone mill, which osteotomizes the heads into small chips of different sizes, adding stability to the impaction. After partially defatting the morseled graft, by washing in 40°C saline solution, it is packed firmly onto the plug with distal impactors. This maneuver continues until graft chips reach a few centimeters above the planned level of the tip of the stem. Serial cannulated impactors are used to fill and gently press graft in the remainder of the shell. With the final impactor well seated distally over the centralizer, additional graft is impacted proximally to a level just below the edges of the tibial condyle. The centralizer device then is removed. A small suction catheter removes all fluid from the canal, which then is extracted immediately before cementing in retrograde fashion, using a cement gun with a conical tip. Pressurization is maintained for a few seconds, followed by the insertion of the tibial component while the cement's viscosity is still low.

Because most lesions are on the medial tibial plateau, defects can be overcome using a smaller tibial component and shifting it laterally on the plateau (23). In this fashion, grafting, PMMA, and modularity may not be required, and thus standard instrumentation and implantation techniques are used for the knee arthroplasty. Significant undersizing of the tibial component, however, should not be permitted.

PMMA and modular components may be used as alternatives to bone grafting. They generally are used for smaller contained defects or larger defects, respectively. Iliac crest

■ TECHNICAL ALTERNATIVES AND PITFALLS

autograft can be used in place of local autograft, if there is inadequate bone from the knee (10,11). The iliac crest can be used with the techniques described previously for grafting tibial defects.

Certain problems occur commonly during knee reconstruction. Excising excess bone, by cutting too low on the tibia, is an error that can be avoided with proper preoperative planning. If reconstruction of a defect is anticipated from radiographic templates, one should be suspicious of the intraoperative cut of the proximal tibia if the defect no longer "appears" to require such intervention. This observation may suggest varus alignment of the tibial surface, which if unrecognized results in malalignment and premature failure of the knee.

There often exists confusion regarding the indications for augmented intramedullary fixation with reconstruction of defects, or the use of constrained polyethylene inserts. Stems are useful for bone-defect reconstruction to unload the tibial surface supporting the implant. Adequate fixation of bone grafts is critical, and intramedullary fixation provides this by unloading the surface sufficiently (24,25) but allowing some subsidence. With proper soft-tissue management, the knee usually can be balanced, providing stability without constraint. Constrained inserts are recommended if this ligamentous balance is inadequate. Intramedullary fixation may be used with nonconstrained implants to protect bone reconstitution of a graft.

■ REHABILITATION

The goal of all rehabilitation programs is to minimize adverse sequelae and maximize functional results. Complications, which include wound problems, sepsis, deep venous thrombosis, hematoma, bleeding, and poor pain control, need disciplined preventative attention in both primary and revision cases (26). All patients benefit from properly placed incisions, with careful tissue handling and meticulous closure technique. Prophylactic antibiotics should be used routinely, as should mechanical and pharmacologic prophylaxis for thromboembolic disease (27). These requirements are particularly true for the patient with bone defects, because there probably exist previous incisions and the surgery may be extensive, and thus the risk of wound problems and infection can be greater.

Bone-graft reconstructions have been regarded as vulnerable, with conservative postoperative physical therapy, specifically protected weight bearing and limited motion, preferable. Windsor et al. (10) suggest partial weight bearing with crutches for 4 to 8 weeks in patients with "large defects" that have been grafted. Patients undergoing cementless revisions with massive tibial allografts also have been placed categorically in toe-touch therapy for 3 months, with full weight bearing allowed only 6 months after the operation (28). Other surgeons feel that all patients should be mobilized as soon as possible, and high-flexion continuous passive motion and weight bearing as tolerated should be implemented as long as "no contraindications" (25) exist. Indeed, intramedullary fixation should protect the reconstruction, and it is unusual for bone graft to be any stronger several months after surgery. There is no clear consensus on the guidelines for rehabilitating patients with bone-graft reconstruction of tibial defects.

On this controversial subject of postoperative management, we have adopted conventional rehabilitation for all revision total knee arthroplasties with tibial defect reconstruction, use of PMMA and bone graft, and modular augmentation, without contraindication to weight bearing as tolerated, with full range-of-motion exercises. With both autografts and allografts (including massive structural technique), bone resorption may occur over time, because of an inflammatory response, and remodeling may take months to years (7). This suggests that the bone-graft reconstruction is mechanically at its peak in the immediate postoperative period. Thus, it is our impression that with solid graft and implant fixation, weight bearing should be implemented as tolerated. In our experience, this approach has not yielded failures.

■ OUTCOMES AND
FUTURE DIRECTIONS

Although today's technology seems to provide the solutions to tibial defects, the future may reveal shortcomings. Modularity has simplified reconstructions, but long-term results have yet to be appreciated fully. Although no major complications have surfaced thus far, fretting that results in metal-particle generation has been suggested as a theoretic mode of failure.

Implants and instruments continue to be improved, resulting in a wider range of choices. The biology of bone grafting is being studied and understood better with time. Bone substitutes, such as growth factors and bone morphogeneic protein, also are being developed. With time, they may supplant allograft and autograft, thus providing new ways to manage the problem of bone loss in knee arthroplasty surgery.

References

1. Ritter MA. Screw and cement fixation of large defects in total knee arthroplasty. *J Arthroplasty* 1986; 1:157–163.
2. Engh GA, Parks NL. The management of bone defects in revision total knee arthroplasty. *Instr Course Lect* 1997; 46:227–236.
3. Rorebeck CH, Smith PN. Results of revision total knee arthroplasty in the face of significant bone deficiency. *Orthop Clin North Am* 1998; 29:361–371.
4. Vince KG. Revision knee arthroplasty. In: Chapman MW, ed. *Operative orthopaedics*, 2nd edition. Philadelphia: JB Lippincott Co, 1993:1981–2010.
5. Windsor RE, Bono JV. Management of bone loss in total knee arthroplasty. In Callaghan JJ, et al., eds. *Orthopaedic knowledge update: Hip and knee reconstruction.* AAOS, 1995:277–282.
6. Chen F, Krakow KA. Management of tibial defects in total knee arthroplasty: A biomechanical study. *Clin Orthop* 1994; 305:249–257.
7. Goldberg VM, Stevenson S. Natural history of autografts and allografts. *Clin Orthop* 1987; 225:7–16.
8. Lotke PA, Wong R, Ecker M. The management of large tibial defects in primary total knee replacement. *Ortho Transactions* 1985; 9:425.
9. Garbuz DS, Masri BA, Czitrom AA. Biology of allografting. *Orthop Clin North Am* 1998; 29:199–204.
10. Winsdor RE, Insall JN, Sculco TP. Bone grafting of tibial defects in primary and revision total knee arthroplasty. *Clin Orthop* 1986; 205:132–137.
11. Scuderi GR, Insall JN, Haas SB, et al. Inlay autogeneic bone grafting of tibial defects in primary total knee arthroplasty. *Clin Orthop* 1989; 248:93–97.
12. Laskin RS. Total knee arthroplasty in the presence of large bony defects of the tibia and marked knee instability. *Clin Orthop* 1989; 248:66–70.
13. Brand MG, Daley RJ, Ewald FC, et al. Tibial tray augmentation with modular metal wedges for tibial bone stock deficiency. *Clin Orthop* 1989; 248:71–79.
14. Jasty M, Harris WH. Salvage total hip reconstruction in patients with major acetabular deficiency using structural femoral head allografts. *J Bone Joint Surg Br* 1990; 72:63–67.
15. Mulroy RD Jr, Harris WH. Failure of acetabular autogenous grafts in total hip arthroplasty: Increasing incidence. A follow-up note. *J Bone Joint Surg Am* 1990; 72:1536–1540.
16. Kwong LM, Jasty M, Harris WH. High failure rate of bulk femoral head allografts in total hip acetabular reconstructions at 10 years. *J Arthroplasty* 1993; 8:341–346
17. Dennis DA. Structural allografting in revision total knee arthroplasty. *Orthopaedics* 1994; 17:849–851.
18. Mow CS, Wiedel JD. Structural allografting in revision total knee arthroplasty. *J Arthroplasty* 1996; 11:235–241.
19. Tsahakis PJ, Beaver WB, Brick GW. Technique and results of allograft reconstruction in revision total knee arthroplasty. *Clin Orthop* 1994; 303:86–94
20. Harris AI, Poddar S, Gitelis S, et al. Arthroplasty with a composite of an allograft and a prosthesis for knees with severe deficiency of bone. *J Bone Joint Surg Am* 1995; 77:373–386.
21. Engh GA, Herzwurm PJ, Parks NL. Treatment of major defects of bone with bulk allografts and stemmed components during total knee arthroplasty. *J Bone Joint Surg Am* 1997; 79:1030–1039.
22. Gie GA, Linder L, Ling RS, et al. Contained morselized allograft in revision total hip arthroplasty. Surgical technique. *Orthop Clin North Am* 1993; 24:717–725.
23. Ullmark G, Hovelius L. Impacted morsellized allograft and cement for revision total knee arthroplasty: A preliminary report of 3 cases. *Acta Orthop Scand* 1996; 67:10–12.
24. Bourne RB, Finlay JB. The influence of tibial component intramedullary stems and implant-cortex contact on the strain distribution of the proximal tibial following total knee arthroplasty. An in vitro study. *Clin Orthop* 1986; 208:95.

25. Bourne RB, Crawford HA. Principles of revision total knee arthroplasty. *Orthop Clin North Am* 1998; 29:331–337.

26. Vince KG. Fractures, neurovascular complications, and wound healing problems after total knee arthroplasty. In Callaghan JJ, et al., eds. *Orthopaedic knowledge update: Hip and knee reconstruction.* AAOS, 1995:291–296.

27. Paiement GD, Green H. Thromboembolic disease in hip and knee replacement patients. In Callaghan JJ, et al., eds. *Orthopaedic knowledge update: Hip and knee reconstruction.* AAOS, 1995:1–8.

28. Whiteside LA. Cementless reconstruction of massive tibial bone loss in revision total knee arthroplasty. *Clin Orthop* 1989; 248:80–86.

ANDREW G. URQUHART
CLIFFORD W. COLWELL

26

Correction of Fixed Flexion Contracture in Total Knee Replacement

Fixed flexion contracture represents a formidable challenge to the orthopedic surgeon. The degree of deformity may range from mild (less than 10 degrees), as often is seen in the osteoarthritic knee, to severe (more than 90 degrees) in a wheelchair-bound patient with inflammatory arthritis. The cause can be one of several, from a preference of a rheumatoid patient for a flexed position of the knee to assist in pain control, to hamstring tightness limiting motion in an osteoarthritic patient. Secondary soft-tissue and bony changes exaggerate the deformity (1). A significant contracture usually exceeds 20 degrees and typically involves deformity of both bone and soft tissue. A fixed flexion contracture persists despite anesthesia, whereas a functional contracture corrects with anesthesia.

■ HISTORY OF THE TECHNIQUE

All flexion contractures should be addressed and corrected prior to wound closure. Despite contentions to the contrary, one cannot assume that persistent deformity under anesthesia at the time of closure will be corrected with postoperative rehabilitation (2). Mild to moderate contractures (less than 25 degrees), which often result from degenerative arthritis, often can be corrected with routine surgical techniques of total knee replacement (3–6). With more severe contractures, significant anatomic deviation occurs as follows: The collateral ligaments pass posterior to the midline of the femur and tibia in the sagittal plane, where they shorten. In addition, the posterior capsule and posterior cruciate ligament (PCL) shorten and can lay over posterior osteophytes of the femur and tibia, respectively, effectively exaggerating the contracture. With more severe deformities, there is are bony defects of both the posterior tibia and posterior femoral condyles (Fig. 26-1).

■ INDICATIONS AND CONTRAINDICATIONS

Anesthesia for fixed flexion contracture does not differ from that for a routine total knee arthroplasty but should be adequate to allow for a prolonged duration of operation if needed. The skin incision for fixed flexion contraction surgery generally is unchanged from that used for routine total knee replacements: a straight midline incision extending from the medial tibial tubercle proximally 10 cm superior to the patella performed with the knee flexed. During deeper exposure a "subvastus" approach may be utilized but is far more difficult for the tight knee. A midline median parapatellar rectus-splitting incision or a "midvastus" vastus-medialis-obliquus-splitting incision is preferred, with the latter offering adequate exposure for most deformities. With relative elongation of the quadriceps mechanism, the patella usually is everted easily. If not, incision of the patella femoral ligaments and a lateral patellar retinacular release that spares the superior lateral geniculate artery if possible should be performed early to assist exposure. Medial dissection does not vary from that for routine knee arthroplasty. The medial collateral ligament should be elevated subperiosteally in a continuous sleeve, with care taken to preserve its integrity (Fig. 26-2). The more distal fibers can be elevated easily from the metaphysis with a periosteal elevator. Sharp dissection may be required of Sharpey's fibers at the more adherent,

■ SURGICAL TECHNIQUES

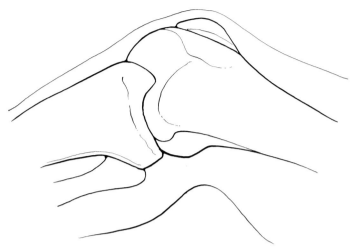

With severe flexion contractures, there is a defect not only of the posterior tibia but also of the posterior femoral condyles.

■   FIGURE 26-1

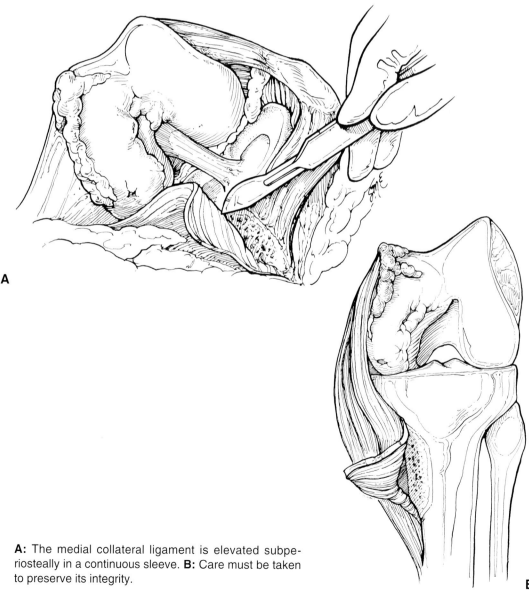

A

A: The medial collateral ligament is elevated subperiosteally in a continuous sleeve. B: Care must be taken to preserve its integrity.

■   FIGURE 26-2

B

deeper, proximal medial collateral ligament. The dissection must be carried posteriorly around the proximal medial corner of the tibia to the insertion of the semimembranous. These releases may be performed as part of the initial surgical exposure or after some bone cuts have been made. It is frequently only after trial reductions have been performed that the full extent of releases can be determined. Osteophytes should be removed from both the medial femur and tibia, effectively lengthening the medial collateral ligament. The infrapatellar fat pad, meniscal–tibial ligaments, and anterior cruciate ligament are sacrificed prior to addressing osseous deformity. Bone cuts of the femur and tibia typically can be made without releasing the lateral structures or the PCL. A standard distal femoral resection is usually adequate; larger distal resections may be required in more severe flexion deformities. The preferred limit to the distal resection of the femur is at the level of the PCL origin on the femur (Fig. 26-3), because more generous resections effectively raise the joint line and can affect patellar biomechanics as well as the flexion–extension balancing of the lateral and medial collateral ligaments adversely. Anterior, posterior, and chamfer cuts can be referenced off the anterior cortex to prevent "notching" and maintain appropriate flexion gap. External rotation positioning of the femoral component to match the epicondylar axis improves patellar tracking.

After performing the distal, anterior, posterior, and chamfer cuts on the femur, the tibia can be subluxated anteriorly to allow thorough removal of the menisci and remaining anterior cruciate ligament. A standard tibial cut then can be made to match the implant specifications. Routinely this is a 4- to 10-mm cut with a 5-degree posterior slope (Fig. 26-4).

Completion of the posterior femoral and proximal tibial cuts allows excellent visualization of the posterior knee. With intramedullary instrumentation on the femoral side, a "femoral lifter" can be used with the knee flexed at 90 degrees to assist with the posterior exposure (Fig. 26-5). All posterior osteophytes must be removed. A curved osteotome is used to aide differentiation between posterior condyle and osteophyte. A curved "right-angle" curette should be employed to protect the neurovascular structures of the posterior

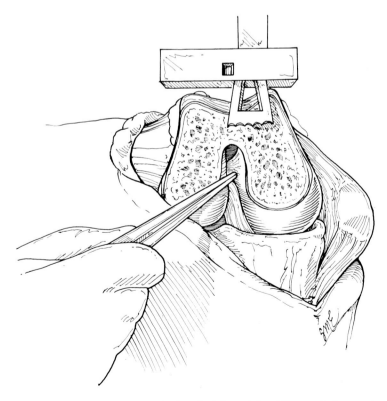

■ FIGURE 26-3

The preferred limit to the distal resection of the femur is the level of the origin of the posterior cruciate ligament on the femur.

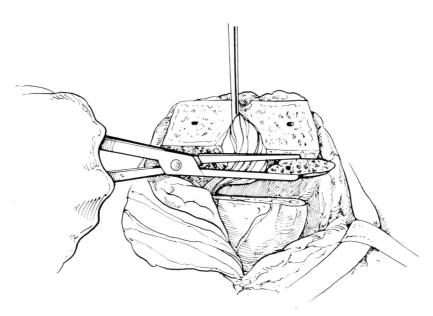

A standard tibial cut (routinely 4–10 mm, with a 5-degree posterior slope) is performed to match implant specifications.

knee (Fig. 26-6). After disruption of the osteophyte attachments, the curette can be used to sweep the osteophytes from the posterior knee. If a flexion contracture persists despite complete posterior osteophyte removal, a periosteal elevator can be used to elevate the capsule from the posterior distal femur. The femoral attachments of the gastrosoleus complex may require elevation in the same fashion.

With trial components in place, medial and lateral flexion and extension gaps can be assessed. The tension of the PCL should be assessed primarily in flexion (Fig. 26-7) to rule out contracture and the PCL should be recessed or excised if necessary. In PCL-substituting designs, the PCL is removed completely. In cruciate ligament–retaining arthroplasties, the

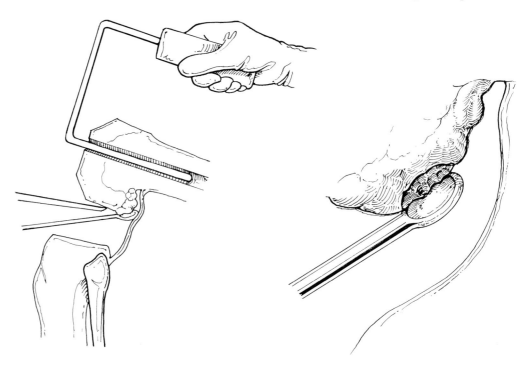

■   FIGURE 26-5

A "femoral lifter" is used to assist with the posterior exposure.

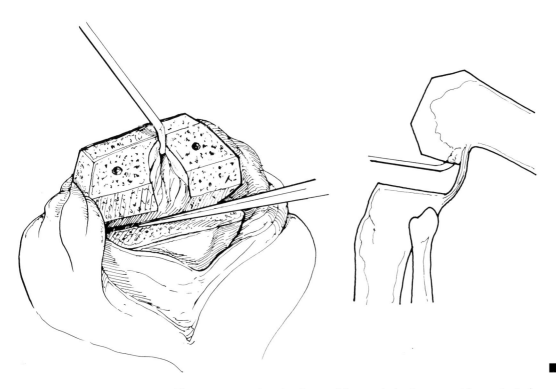

The neurovascular structures of the posterior knee must be protected.

PCL probably is contracted and requires release, lengthening, or recession. The PCL can be recessed from either the femoral or tibial side if needed (Fig. 26-8). Sacrifice of the PCL can be reserved for the most severe deformities, in which it often is required, necessitating a PCL-substituting or deep-dish cruciate ligament–sparing design. In the attempt to gain full extension, if the knee remains tight laterally, lateral femoral osteophytes should be removed. If lateral tension is not relieved, the lateral collateral ligament and popliteus can be

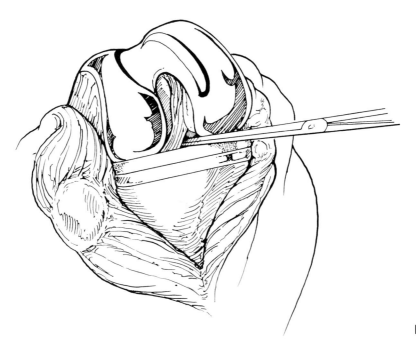

■   FIGURE 26-7

Assessing the tension of the posterior cruciate ligament in flexion.

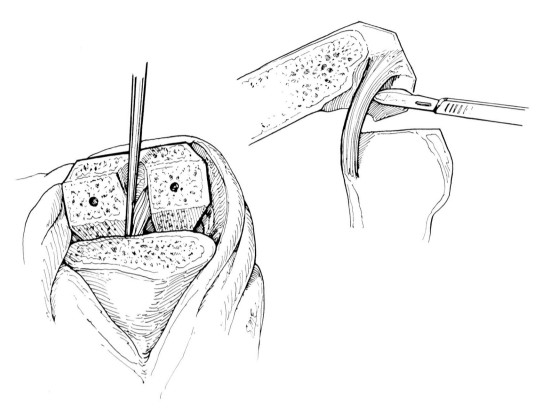

■ FIGURE 26-8

The posterior cruciate ligament is recessed if necessary.

elevated subperiosteally from the lateral femoral condyle (Fig. 26-9), in a method analo-
gous to the elevation of the medial collateral ligament from the tibia for tight medial compartments. With a tight lateral compartment, a lateral patellar retinacular release is often
necessary and should be extended to Gerdy's tubercle. Isolation and protection of the superior lateral geniculate artery is encouraged.

   Trial components are used to assess the knee stability in flexion and extension and to ensure full correction of the flexion deformity. A PCL-substituting design should be used if
the PCL is deficient and the knee is unstable in flexion.

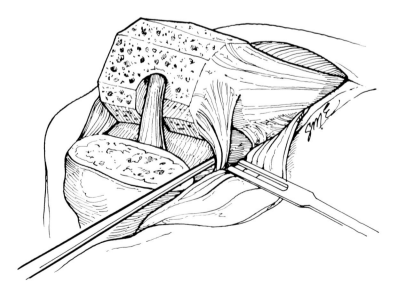

■ FIGURE 26-9

The lateral collateral ligament and popliteus are elevated from the lateral femoral condyle.

Although the routine total knee replacement procedure is closed in flexion, the surgeon may prefer to close the knee with a preoperative flexion contracture in extension. The closure can be either before or after tourniquet release, depending on the surgeon's preference. A drain is used at the discretion of the surgeon.

With inflammatory arthritides, flexion contractures often are associated with valgus deformity, with an increased risk of stretching the peroneal nerve. Although the iliotibial band often requires release in these knees, prophylactic exposure and release of the peroneal nerve may interfere with its blood supply and induce a palsy. Routine exposure of the peroneal nerve therefore is not recommended.

■ TECHNICAL ALTERNATIVES AND PITFALLS

Rehabilitation is unchanged from that for a routine total knee arthroplasty, except for emphasis placed on knee extension. The knee is placed initially in an extension immobilizer, with no pillows behind the joint. Attention is directed to maintaining a fully extended position for at least part of the day, until extensor lag is overcome. Active and passive motion begins on postoperative day 1. Long-term studies have shown no benefit of routine continuous passive motion treatment, and such treatment may be harmful in the patient with a preoperative fixed flexion deformity.

■ REHABILITATION

Patients with contractures have a higher manipulation rate. If the patient is to be manipulated, this should be done early, within the first 3 or 4 weeks following surgery. Manipulation typically improves flexion defects more predictably than flexion contractures, however, and is therefore uncommon.

■ OUTCOMES AND FUTURE DIRECTIONS

References

1. Daniel DM, Akeson WH, O'Connor JJ, eds. *Knee ligaments: Structure, function, injury and repair.* New York: Raven Press, 1990.
2. McPherson EJ, Cushner FD, Schiff CF, et al. Natural history of uncorrected flexion contractures following total knee arthroplasty. *J Arthroplasty* 1994; 9:499–502.
3. Firestone TP, Krackow KA, Davis JD, et al. The management of fixed flexion contractures during total knee arthroplasty. *Clin Orthop* 1992; 284:221–227.
4. Insall JN. Knee arthroplasty. In: Insall JN, ed. *Surgery of the knee.* New York: Churchill Livingstone, 1984:587–695.
5. Krackow KA: *The technique of total knee arthroplasty.* St. Louis: CV Mosby, 1990:249–372.
6. Rand JA, ed. *Total knee arthroplasty.* New York: Raven Press, 1993:115–153.

27

Supracondylar Fractures Following Total Knee Replacement

■ HISTORY OF THE
TECHNIQUE

A supracondylar fracture following a total knee replacement not only is an unforeseen complication but also frequently is associated with devastating problems of limited range of motion and pain. The various modalities for treatment consist of conservative approaches with high nonunion rates and surgical approaches associated with limited range of motion, infections, and nonunion. The ultimate result for the total knee replacement becomes compromised. Factors that predispose to fracture as a result of sometimes minor trauma include: osteopenia, notching, revision surgery, and stress reactions. The only factors that seem to be common to all are trauma and osteopenia. The surgeons in our institution looked at 670 posterior cruciate condylar total knee replacements and found that 28% had major notching of the anterior femur (1). There were four fractures with no notching and two fractures with a notch. Also, if notching were a factor in fracture, then the fractures probably would have occurred within the first 6 weeks, but the majority of fractures in our group of patients occurred an average of 5 years after the total knee replacement.

Merkel et al. (2) demonstrated a 100% complication rate in patients treated by operative means and recommended closed methods of treatment. Cain et al. (3), however, looking at both open and closed methods of treatment, found a 25% rate of union with the open method and a 17% rate with the closed method. It was because of the diversity of opinion as to which method was most favorable that we elected to begin using Rush rods.

■ SURGICAL
TECHNIQUE

Since 1980, I have used percutaneous *in situ* intramedullary Rush rods for the fixation of all supracondylar fractures following total knee replacements. I am pleased with this means of fixation, and as time has passed, the techniques that I have learned have allowed me to perform procedures with few complications, excellent union, and return to function not unlike the previous results with total knee replacement.

All fractures, whether displaced or comminuted, can be treated by this method. The patient is anesthetized and positioned on a fracture table with a bolster under the distal thigh. Multiple evaluations of the fracture alignment with image intensification are made, until the the fracture is in the appropriate anatomic valgus alignment associated with a normal functioning knee (Fig. 27-1). This is confirmed on the anteroposterior and lateral radiographic views, after which the knee is prepped and draped aseptically. Two 1.5-inch incisions are made on the medial and lateral side of the knee from just above the joint line distally. Visualized under the image intensifier, a Rush awl is passed into the epicondyle just proximal to the prosthesis (Fig. 27-2). A Rush pin then is passed up along the groove of the awl into the hole and directed toward the proximal fragment, with the bevel flat against the opposite endosteal cortex (Fig. 27-3). The same procedure is performed on the other side of the knee, and then the rods are passed up so that they cross once but not twice. This usually means that the rods need to be just past the midportion of the femur. The rods then are relieved of stress just before implantation (Fig. 27-4). The level of the stress relief should be the distance from the epicondyle to the metaphyseal–diaphyseal junction, the distance

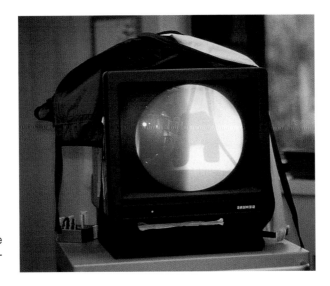

Image intensification of the fracture following closed reduction and the initial placement of a Rush awl.

■ FIGURE 27-1

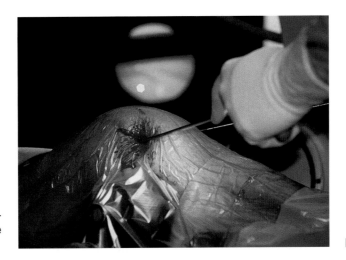

A Rush awl being fixed into the epicondyle and visualized on the image intensifier.

■ FIGURE 27-2

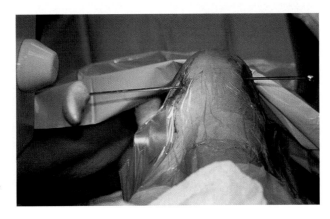

A Rush awl is in one side of the knee and a Rush pin in the other.

■ FIGURE 27-3

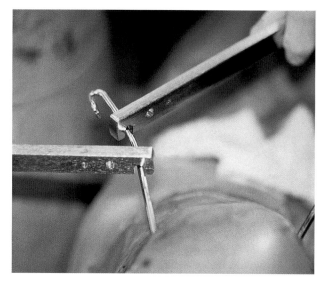

■ FIGURE 27-4   Stress relief of the Rush pin.

from the distal hook to the level of the bevel or relief (Fig. 27-5). This has to be estimated. If on is trying to correct alignment, then less relief must be put on one side or the other. The rods used have supracondylar flat surfaces rather than the hooks. Next the wounds are closed, the patient is taken out of the traction, and range of motion is checked under the image intensifier for stability.

■ REHABILITATION

Postoperatively, patients are maintained in compression dressings, and ambulation with the foot flat on the ground, easy range-of-motion exercises, and use of a knee immobilizer, if necessary for pain relief, are begun. Because of the comminution that frequently is associated with these fractures, one has a tendency to be more worried about the fixation with these rods; however, comminution may be the best indication for this technique.

■ OUTCOMES AND
FUTURE DIRECTION

Since we began utilizing Rush rods, we have treated 35 fractures, and all have healed (Fig. 27-6). Two fractures were left in too much valgus. This was noticed postoperatively and should have been corrected instantly, because the rods hold the patient in the position in which he or she is left.

In the 35 fractures we have treated, the prefracture total knee alignment was 5 degrees of anatomic valgus, and the postfracture alignment was the same. The range of motion pre-

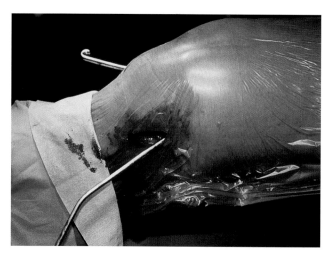

■ FIGURE 27-5

Both pins have been relieved of stress before application.

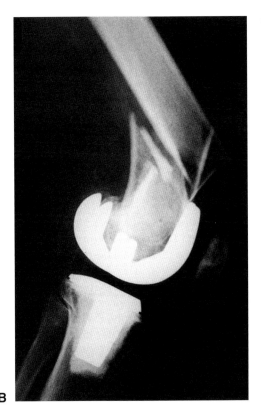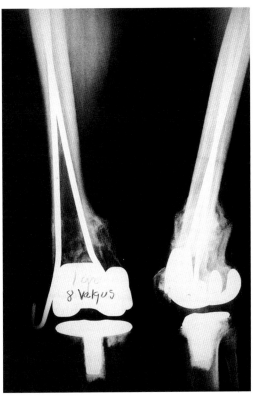

A, B   ■ FIGURE 27-6

A: A 67-year-old white man with a supracondylar fracture with 100% displacement, following a fall from some steps. **B:** One year postoperative. The fracture is healed, the anatomic alignment is about 8 degrees of valgus, and the lateral rod is beginning to migrate distally where it became prominent under the skin prior to removal.

fracture was 0 to 102 degrees; postfracture it was 0 to 101 degrees. There have been no instances of nonunion, and only two knees have been left in more than 10 degrees of valgus (4).

The utilization of Rush rods for supracondylar fractures is a simple means of fixing a complicated problem with the least amount of morbidity and allows the surgeon to regain the success of the total knee replacement prior to the fracture.

References

1. Ritter MA, Faris PM, Keating EM. Anterior femoral notching with ipsilateral supracondylar femur fracture in total knee arthroplasty. *J Arthroplasty* 1988; 3:185–187.
2. Merkel KD, Johnson EW Jr. Supracondylar fracture of the femur after total knee arthroplasty. *J Bone Joint Surg Am* 1986; 68:29.
3. Cain PR, Rubash HE, Wissinger HA, et al. Periprosthetic femoral fractures following total knee arthroplasty. *Clin Orthop* 1986; 208:205.
4. Ritter MA, Keating EM, Faris PM, et al. Rush rod fixation of supracondylar fractures above total knee arthroplasties. *J Arthroplasty* 1995; 10:213–216.

DOUGLAS A. DENNIS
ANNE B. SZYMANSKI

28

Removal of Metal-backed Patellar Button

■ HISTORY OF THE
TECHNIQUE

Patellar complications have been shown to be a predominant cause of failure of total knee arthroplasty (TKA) (1–13). Brick and Scott (4) noted that patellar complications can account for up to 50% of TKA revisions. With the advent of metal-backed patellar designs, patellar complications have risen substantially, particularly as a result of polyethylene wear and dissociation from the underlying metal plate (2,3,13). Mathematic contact-stress analysis subsequently has predicted premature failure of these devices, because contact stresses exceed the yield strength of ultra–high molecular weight polyethylene (14). Revision of well-fixed polyethylene patellar components in condylar TKA has been infrequent. If necessary, the bone–cement interface and peg–plate junction simply are divided with thin osteotomes or thin saw blades, providing access to the pegs. The incidence of cementless metal-backed patellar component failure has been substantially higher, particularly as a result of polyethylene wear and dissociation (1–5,8,9,12,13,15). With this mode of failure, fixation of the metal backing to the bone, particularly the fixation pegs, often remains rigid. Turner et al. (16) have demonstrated variable bone ingrowth (12–85%) into the supporting metal plates, but predictable bone ingrowth into the fixation pegs in canine studies. Additional histologic evaluation has confirmed that similar predictable osseous ingrowth into the anchoring pegs occurs in humans (15). In patients with rigid bone ingrowth into the fixation pegs, component removal can be difficult, because of impeded access to the fixation interface surrounding the pegs. After the metal plate–fixation interface is divided, trying to pry out fixation pegs by applying angular forces to thin osteotomes risks patellar fracture. Because of this problem, a new and safer technique of removal of the well-fixed metal-backed patellar button was developed.

■ INDICATIONS AND
CONTRAINDICATIONS

The indications for the described surgical technique include removal of any failed metal-backed patellar button that demonstrates rigid fixation through bone ingrowth into the fixation pegs. The procedure also has been utilized in removal of well-fixed, cemented, metal-backed patellar components, for which removal with traditional methods proved difficult. This technique is not required for removal of metal-backed patellar components in which fixation is not rigid.

■ SURGICAL
TECHNIQUES

The goals of this surgical technique for removal of rigidly fixed components are to preserve remaining patellar bone, provide easy access to the bone-ingrown anchoring pegs, and lessen the risk of patellar fracture during patellar button extraction. These are accomplished by division of the metal plate–fixation peg junction of the metal-backed patellar component, thereby allowing direct access to the well-fixed anchoring pegs.

The knee may be exposed with any of the surgical approaches customary for TKA. The patella is everted, and peripatellar soft tissues are debrided to gain clear visualization of the bone–prosthesis (metal plate) interface. Fixation of the polyethylene to the underlying metal plate in most metal-backed patellar component designs is not rigid. This may allow removal of the polyethylene from the metal plate by sectioning with an oscillating saw or simply by grasping and removing the polyethylene with a rongeur. This provides excellent

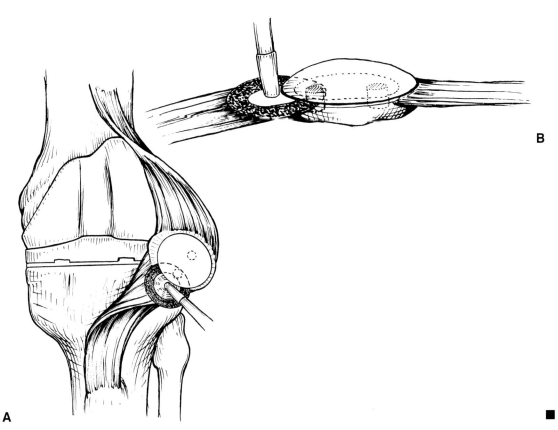

A

B

■ FIGURE 28-1

Diagrams demonstrating use of the pneumatic tool with a diamond-edged circular saw disrupting the peg–plate junction of a metal-backed patellar component.

visualization of the bone–metal plate interface. The patella then is held with two bone tenaculi for firm control during the use of power instruments. The peripatellar soft tissues are covered with surgical sponges to collect metallic debris resulting from division of the peg–plate junction. The periphery of this interface is minimally disrupted with flexible osteotomes to develop a plane for a diamond-edged circular saw blade (Midas Rex, Fort Worth, TX) that is used to cut through the anchoring pegs at the peg–plate junction (Figs. 28-1 and 28-2). The circular saw blade slowly is passed circumferentially around the periphery of the patellar component, disrupting both the bone–plate interface and peg–plate

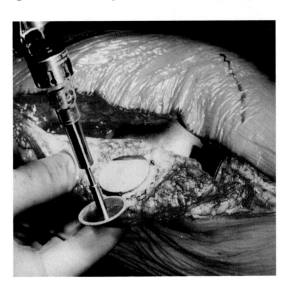

Intraoperative photograph of division of the peg–plate junction.

■ FIGURE 28-2

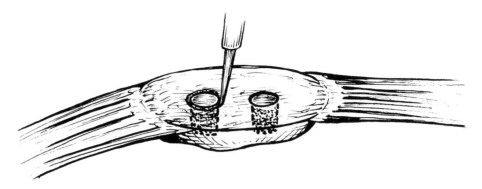

■ FIGURE 28-3

Diagram demonstrating use of the pneumatic tool with a pencil-tip drill utilized to circumferentially disrupt the bone-anchoring peg interface. (From Dennis DA. Removal of well-fixed cementless metal-backed patellar components. *J Arthroplasty* 1992;7:217, with permission.)

junction. The metal-plate portion of the patellar component is removed, providing easy access to the well-fixed anchoring pegs. Utilizing a pencil-tip, side-cutting, high-speed drill, the bone–peg interface is disrupted in a circumferential fashion, and the pegs are extracted (Figs. 28-3 and 28-4). Continuous irrigation is used to prevent thermal necrosis during use of the high-speed saw and drill. Following completion of patellar component removal, the debris-collecting sponges are removed and the patella and wound are thoroughly irrigated with pulsatile lavage fluid. The patella then is prepared for repeat resurfacing utilizing a patellar component of the surgeon's choice.

■ TECHNICAL
ALTERNATIVES AND
PITFALLS

The described technique of peg–plate disruption using a diamond-edged circular saw provides a safe and expeditious method of cementless patellar component removal. Patellar bone stock, often deficient in revision TKA, is preserved, and fracture is avoided. A potential disadvantage of this technique is the creation of microscopic metallic debris. The majority is collected on the peripatellar sponges or removed via pulsatile lavage. No adverse effects attributed to debris formation, such as chronic postoperative effusion or periprosthetic osteolysis, have been observed in the author's 10-year experience with this technique.

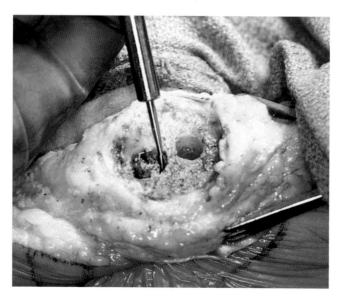

■ FIGURE 28-4

Intraoperative photograph of the pencil-tip drill being used to disrupt the ingrown pegs.

An alternative to division of the metal plate–fixation peg junction is removal with thin osteotomes. The use of conventional extraction techniques with thin osteotomes risks fracture, because of the inability to gain access to anchoring pegs well fixed with osseous ingrowth. This is especially apparent if osteotomes are twisted against the bone and metal plate in an attempt to lever out the pegs. Additionally, passage of osteotomes through the bone–plate interface may prove challenging, because of interference by the pegs, particularly in triangularly oriented three-peg designs.

Standard rehabilitation protocols appropriate to revision TKA are utilized. No deviation from standard rehabilitation methods is required.

■ REHABILITATION

The described surgical technique for removal of well-fixed, cementless, metal-backed patellar components has been utilized in 52 patients, involving seven different metal-backed designs (both titanium and cobalt–chromium alloys). The average time from patellar component insertion to subsequent extraction was 49 months (range 18–109 months). Thirty-eight patients were found to have chronic patellofemoral pain and effusion associated with lateral patellar subluxation. In the majority of these cases, a review of Merchant patellar radiographs suggested the presence of polyethylene wear (Fig. 28-5). In the remaining 14 patients, the patellar component was functioning well at the time but was removed during revision TKA for failure of either the femoral or tibial component. Preoperative radiographic assessment suggested rigid fixation of all patellar components. At the time of revision TKA, all patellar components were found to be fixed rigidly and were removed without fracture. In all cases, sufficient bone stock remained for successful replantation of a new, all-polyethylene, three-pegged resurfacing patellar component. Anchoring pegs from the initial five patients were submitted to pathology for assessment of bone ingrowth. Histologic analysis of these fixation pegs demonstrated extensive osseous ingrowth (Fig. 28-6), which confirmed the rigid fixation observed at operation (15).

■ OUTCOMES AND FUTURE DIRECTIONS

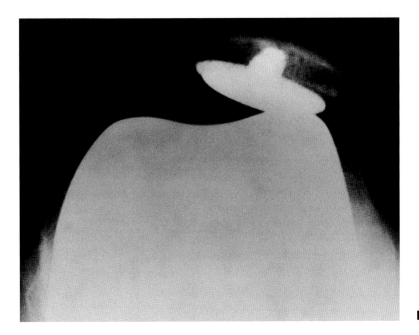

■ FIGURE 28-5

Merchant radiograph of a failed cementless patellar component with lateral subluxation, which had functioned well for 3 years until polyethylene wear occurred, exposing metal. (From Dennis DA. Removal of well-fixed cementless metal-backed patellar components. *J Arthroplasty* 1992;7:217, with permission.)

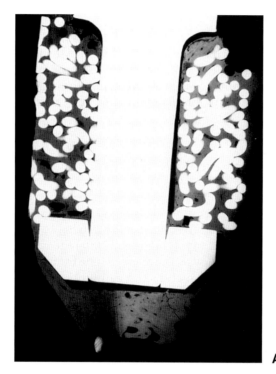

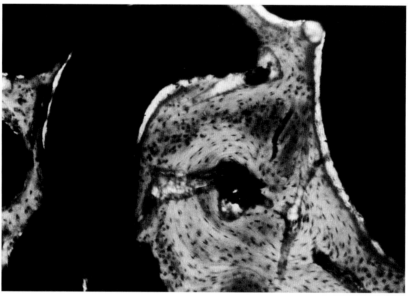

■ FIGURE 28-6

A: Typical microradiograph of a patellar component anchoring peg demonstrating ingrowth of bone into the porous fiber–metal surface. **B:** Typical histologic hematoxylin and eosin–stained section of a patellar component anchoring peg demonstrating substantial ingrowth of bone into the porous fiber–metal surface (magnified ×400). (From Dennis DA. Removal of well-fixed cementless metal-backed patellar components. *J Arthroplasty* 1992;7:217, with permission.)

References

1. Baech J, Kofoed H. Failure of metal-backed patellar arthroplasty: Forty-seven total knees followed for at least 1 year. *Acta Orthop Scand* 1991; 62:166.
2. Bayley JC, Scott RD. Further observations on metal-backed patellar component failure. *Clin Orthop* 1988; 236:82.
3. Bayley JC, Scott RD, Ewald FC, et alB. Failure of the metal-backed patellar component after total knee replacement. *J Bone Joint Surg Am* 1988; 70:668.

4. Brick GW, Scott RD. The patellofemoral component of total knee arthroplasty. *Clin Orthop* 1988; 231:163.
5. Doolittle KH, Turner RH. Patellofemoral problems following total knee arthroplasty. *Orthop Rev* 1988; 17:696.
6. Goldberg VM, Figgie HE III, Inglis AE, et al. Patellar fracture type and prognosis in condylar total knee arthroplasty. *Clin Orthop* 1988; 236:115.
7. LeBlanc JM. Patellar complications in total knee arthroplasty. *Orthop Rev* 1989; 18:296.
8. Lombardi AV Jr, Engh GA, Volz RG, et al. Fracture/dissociation of the polyethylene in metal-backed patellar components in total knee arthroplasty. *J Bone Joint Surg Am* 1988; 70:675.
9. Petrie RS, Hanssen AD, Osmon DR, et al. Metal-backed patellar component failure in total knee arthroplasty: A possible risk for late infection. *Am J Orthop* 1998; 27:172–176.
10. Rand JA, Gustilo RB. Technique of patellar resurfacing in total knee arthroplasty. *Tech Orthop* 1988; 3:57.
11. Rand JA. Patellar resurfacing in total knee arthroplasty. *Clin Orthop* 1990; 260:110.
12. Rosenberg AG, Andriacchi TP, Barden R, et al. Patellar component failure in cementless total knee arthroplasty. *Clin Orthop* 1988; 236:106.
13. Stulberg SD, Stulberg BN, Hamati V, et al. Failure mechanisms of metal-backed patellar components. *Clin Orthop* 1988; 236:88.
14. Buechel FF, Pappas MJ, Makris G. Evaluation of contact stress in metal-backed patellar replacements: A predictor of survivorship. *Clin Orthop* 1991; 273:190.
15. Dennis DA. Removal of well-fixed cementless metal-backed patellar components. *J Arthroplasty* 1992; 7:217.
16. Turner TM, Urban RM, Sumner DR, et al. Tibial component fixation in canine total knee arthroplasty. *Trans Soc Biomater* 1986; 9:173.

29

Extensor Mechanism Reconstruction with a Semitendinosus Graft

■ HISTORY OF THE
TECHNIQUE

Rupture of the patellar tendon during or after total knee arthroplasty occurs infrequently but is a potentially catastrophic complication. Neither direct suture repair nor staple fixation of the ruptured or avulsed tendon is a reliable method of repair. With appropriate surgical reconstruction of the tendon, however, a profound disability of the knee can be avoided. The concept of "supplementing the torn patellar tendon with a kindred structure" first was advocated in 1957 by Kelikian et al. (1) for delayed repairs of the tendon. Cadambi and Engh (2) advocated and reported successful results of patellar tendon repair with a semitendinosus graft as the kindred structure in total knee arthroplasty.

■ INDICATIONS AND
CONTRAINDICATIONS

Early patellar tendon rupture can occur as an intraoperative complication during total knee arthroplasty or while the patient is regaining knee flexion in postoperative therapy. A knee with limited preoperative flexion is particularly prone to tendon rupture with an overzealous release of the tendon from the tibial tubercle during surgical exposure. Simple suture repair or staple fixation alone does not provide the stability necessary to the reattached tendon for early motion, particularly in patients with limited preoperative knee flexion (3). If the patellar tendon is avulsed intraoperatively, a semitendinosus graft augmentation and reattachment of the patellar tendon are indicated.

Rupture of the patellar tendon from the patella can occur months to years after total knee arthroplasty. Most patients with this type of complication are elderly, and often they suffer from underlying connective-tissue diseases such as rheumatoid arthritis. The patellar tendon is more prone to rupture following multiple operations or revision total knee arthroplasty that may devascularize and thin the patella.

Late patellar tendon rupture often involves the avulsion of a small fragment of bone from the inferior pole of the patella. The rupture usually occurs as an acute episode and often is associated with a fall, in which the knee gives way because of disruption of the extensor mechanism. The rupture may be the primary cause of the fall, which results from a sudden contracture of the quadriceps mechanism, or may be secondary to the fall, a result of acute knee flexion. The patient usually presents with an emergent condition and is unable to support weight on the extremity. On rare occasions, the clinical symptoms are insidious. The patient may complain of buckling of the knee, an inability to climb stairs or walk up an incline, or difficulty getting up from a chair. The diagnosis of patellar tendon rupture is confirmed by loss of complete knee extension, a palpable tendon defect, and an abnormal clinical and radiographic position of the patella (patella alta). These physical findings confirm the need for surgical repair.

The semitendinosus is the strongest and most robust of the pes anserine tendons. Its yield strength has been measured in cadaveric specimens to be approximately one half that of the patellar tendon (4). The "two sides" of a semitendinosus graft theoretically create a structure with the strength of the patellar tendon. Because it is an autogenous structure, a semitendinosus graft should be considered the material of choice to repair most patellar tendon disruptions. Two options should be reserved for patients who have lost so much of the patella and patellar tendon that the proximal attachment of a tendon graft would be compromised: replacement with an allograft extensor mechanism, and reconstruction with a synthetic graft material.

A ruptured patellar tendon should be repaired as soon as possible. Minor knee abrasions from a fall are not contraindications to surgery, but deep abrasions over the front of the knee should be healed fully before surgery is performed. Repair of the extensor mechanism is contraindicated in cases of deep sepsis, severe ankylosis, or soft-tissue loss that would jeopardize a surgical repair. A knee fusion is indicated in these situations.

The surgical reconstruction of a ruptured patellar tendon with a semitendinosus graft is carried out under epidural, spinal, or general anesthesia. Preoperative patellar traction to stretch the quadriceps tendon is not necessary. A tourniquet is applied to the proximal thigh, and the knee is draped for an anticipated counterincision 6 to 8 cm proximal to the popliteal space. The semitendinosus tendon should be released at its musculotendinous junction if maximum graft length is necessary.

■ SURGICAL TECHNIQUES

The knee is exsanguinated with an elastic wrap and the tourniquet inflated with the knee at 90 degrees of flexion to tension the extensor mechanism as much as possible. The anterior midline incision from the previous total knee arthroplasty is extended distally along the medial border of the tibial tubercle. This incision ends at the lower border of the tibial metaphyseal flare.

The defect in the patellar tendon is identified and the scar tissue excised. Adhesions in the suprapatellar region should be freed from the quadriceps tendon and extensor mechanism to maximally mobilize the patella toward the tibial tubercle. The knee is placed in a varus posture and in 90-degree flexion (a "figure-four" position) to identify the pes anserine group of tendons. The gracilis and semitendinosus are distinct and easily palpated through their investing fascia at the inferior border of the tibial metaphyseal flare. The semitendinosus tendon is the more distal of the two tendons. The tendons shift or roll with palpation by sliding an index finger across them tendons near their insertion. An incision is made directly in line with the semitendinosus tendon, beginning at its insertion to the tibia and extending proximally a distance of 6 cm. Metzenbaum scissors are used to free the semitendinosus tendon from its distal insertion in a proximal direction. The semitendinosus insertion near the inferomedial border of the tibial tubercle is maintained. It is common to encounter slips of tendon that must be released from the inferior margin to free the tendon.

The semitendinosus tendon can be harvested with a tendon stripper or dissected from its muscle in the posterior thigh. In most patients, approximately 20 cm of tendon graft can be harvested with a stripper, compared with the 25 cm of graft harvested using a second incision. A separate incision is required if maximum graft length is needed for delayed repairs involving patella alta, or if tendon grafts must be anchored through the quadriceps tendon above the patella.

The location of the semitendinosus tendon at its musculotendinous junction proximal to the popliteal space is identified by palpating the tendon. First, the knee is positioned in 90 degrees of flexion. A hemostat is passed beneath the tendon near its insertion, and tension is applied to the tendon while it is palpated behind the knee. Next, a 4- to 6-cm posterior incision is made transversely through the skin and subcutaneous tissue superficial to the tendon, four finger widths proximal to the popliteal space. The tendon sheath is opened with the knee in flexion, and the relaxed tendon and adjoining musculotendinous junction are delivered from the incision. Muscle fibers are dissected from the tendon in order to harvest as much graft as possible. The tendon then is released completely proximally and delivered into the distal, primary incision. A locking loop ligament suture of nonabsorbable no. 2 or heavier material is placed in the free end of the tendon.

The optimal anchor for a tendon graft is the inferior one third of the patella if adequate bone is present. A 0.5-cm transverse drill hole is made at the junction of the lower one third of the patella. One must be careful to avoid disrupting the fixation interface of the patellar component if it is to be retained. The semitendinosus tendon then is brought proximally

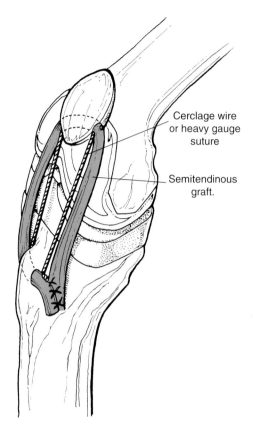

Cerclage wire
or heavy gauge
suture

Semitendinous
graft.

■ FIGURE 29-1

The semitendinosus graft is routed through a 0.5-cm drill hole in the inferior pole of the patella. A second drill hole in the tibial tubercle is optional. The free end of the graft is sutured to the periosteum and the intact insertions of the pes anserine tendon. A cerclage wire or suture is optional.

along the medial border of the patellar tendon remnant, and the tendon passed through the drill hole in the patella with a tendon passer. The graft is routed distally from the patella, and the free end of the is graft anchored to the periosteum and the patellar tendon remnant along the medial border of the tibial tubercle. Another option is to pass the graft through a second 0.5-cm transverse drill hole in the tibial tubercle (Fig. 29-1).

The graft is advanced through the drill holes with the knee in 60 degrees flexion. Tension then is applied to the free end of the graft, and the graft is anchored to the periosteum and bone. First the lead suture is tied, then additional slowly absorbable (Vicryl) or nonabsorbable sutures are passed through the graft, the patellar tendon remnant, and the adjacent periosteum. The semitendinosus tendon can be sutured back to its insertion and to the gracilis insertion. A nonabsorbable (no. 5) heavy suture or cerclage wire is passed through the drill hole in the patella and through a second drill hole in the tibial tubercle to reinforce and protect the patellar tendon reconstruction. The repair should be tested by passively flexing the knee to 90 degrees before wound closure. It is important to pay particular attention to the location of the patella relative to the femoral component and the tibial tubercle. The patella should rest on the anterior femoral flange and follow the patellofemoral groove as the knee is flexed.

■ TECHNICAL
ALTERNATIVES AND
PITFALLS

As previously mentioned, patellar tendon avulsions can occur during the surgical exposure of the knee. If this occurs and the defect can be closed without undue tension at 60 degrees of knee flexion, a locking loop ligament suture is placed in the patellar tendon for reapproximation of the tendon to bone (5). A nonabsorbable or slowly absorbable suture (no. 3 or heavier) is preferable. Two oblique drill holes should be made through the tibial tubercle with a 3.2-mm drill bit, and the sutures passed through the holes with either a Keith needle or a Beath pin. A hemostat should be applied to the suture ends, but the suture should not be tied until a semitendinosus graft has been harvested and routed to reinforce this direct tendon repair. If the tendon avulsion cannot be anchored without limiting knee flexion, the tendon can be reapproximated to the adjacent semitendinosus graft.

Technical errors can result in a detached or badly frayed graft, or in a graft of insufficient length. If a tendon stripper is used, the graft length may be compromised. If the tendon stripper does not capture fully and slide easily along the semitendinosus tendon, this technique should be abandoned and a separate posterior incision made that preserves the maximum graft length. The graft can be lengthened by releasing some of the fibers of the semitendinosus insertion to the tibia. A broad periosteal sleeve is preserved by releasing some of the tendon graft fibers on its deep surface and dissecting the base of the graft forward toward the tibial tubercle.

Because the graft may be detached inadvertently from its insertion to the tibia, incisions should not be made in the periosteum anterior to the insertion of the pes tendons into the tibia. Sharpey's fibers and the semitendinosus insertion in this location must be preserved to provide an anchor for the free end of the tendon graft. If the graft becomes detached, then a transverse drill hole in the tibial tubercle is required. The free graft is passed through drill holes in both the patella and tibial tubercle, and then the tendon graft is overlapped and sutured to itself (side-to-side) (Fig. 29-2). A cerclage no. 5 suture is routed with the tendon graft to protect the repair.

Extensor mechanism disruption also occurs with displaced transverse fractures through the body of the patella. In this case, the tendon graft must be routed to a transverse drill hole in the proximal fracture fragment or through the quadriceps tendon just above the patella. A posterior incision should be used to harvest as much tendon from its musculotendinous junction as possible and to achieve the maximum graft length. The semitendinosus insertion is raised on a periosteal sleeve toward the tibial tubercle to obtain additional graft length. The graft still may be of insufficient length to complete a full loop back to its insertion on the tibia. The repair then may be augmented by including a second graft using the gracilis tendon or by using a strip of the iliotibial band. If the iliotibial band is used, its insertion to Gerdy's tubercle must be maintained. This additional strip of tendon or iliotibial band is routed in the opposite direction and sutured to the side of the semitendinosus graft (side-to-side).

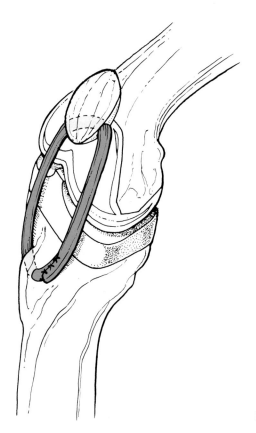

If the attachment of the semitendinosus tendon to the tibia is avulsed, the graft can be sutured to itself. A second drill hole for anchoring the graft to the tibia is essential for patellar tendon grafting with a detached graft.

■ FIGURE 29-2

Tendon grafts looped over the top of the patella cause the lower end of the patella to tilt or lift up. There are several methods of controlling patellar tilt:

1. The patella can be held against the femur by turning a central strip of the quadriceps tendon distally and incorporating it in the repair.
2. The "two sides" of the graft can be brought together and sutured to the lower end of the patella.
3. Synthetic biocompatible materials can be used to reinforce the surgical repair.
4. Dacron vascular grafts (6), filamentous carbon fiber as a stint, and the Leeds–Keio artificial ligament (7) have been used successfully for patellar ligament ruptures.

■ REHABILITATION

After surgery, the knee is immobilized in a 16- to 19-inch knee splint, a cylinder cast, or a hinged knee brace locked in full extension for 6 weeks. Quadriceps control is almost always present the first day after surgery. The patient should perform leg lifts without weights and be encouraged to begin full weight bearing with crutches.

Knee flexion and leg lifts with weights should not be permitted until after the 6-week follow-up examination. The integrity of the repair is confirmed by removing the cast or knee splint and asking the patient to perform a straight leg lift. A lateral radiograph of the knee should be obtained to determine the position of the patella relative to the knee. The patient may begin gradual antigravity knee flexion to 60 degrees in physical therapy. A brace should be used to maintain full knee extension with weight bearing for an additional 6-week interval.

Three months after surgical repair of the tendon, the leg should be fitted for a hinged rehabilitation knee brace, with a dial-lock set to allow 0 to 60 degrees knee flexion. The patient is encouraged to walk without a cane. At this point, the patient can progress in physical therapy to exercises with weights and to graduated range-of-motion exercises.

■ OUTCOMES AND FUTURE DIRECTIONS

In 1992, we reported seven cases of patellar tendon rupture or avulsion treated with an autogenous semitendinosus graft (2). All of the patients regained quadriceps strength and satisfactory overall function. Although all seven patients were older than 65 years of age, four had rheumatoid arthritis, and one had insulin-dependent diabetes mellitus, there were no postoperative complications. Three patients achieved greater than 90 degrees of knee flexion. Additional knee surgery has not been necessary in any of the cases (2). In an earlier review by the Mayo Clinic, 18 patellar tendon ruptures following total knee arthroplasty were treated by a variety of methods. This review included one case of a semitendinosus graft that failed (3).

The Anderson Clinic experience (1985–1996) includes 17 cases of extensor mechanism rupture. Four ruptures were of the quadriceps mechanism and 13 were patellar tendon ruptures. The patellar tendon ruptures included 11 repaired with a semitendinosus graft and two repaired with an extensor mechanism allograft that included the patella.

The location of rupture in the 11 knees repaired with semitendinosus grafting was as follows: five through the tibial tubercle, four through the patella, and two midsubstance ruptures. The average age of these patients at the time of the rupture was 76 years (range 68–85).

The average follow-up interval is 47 months (range 5–99). None of the patients have required any additional surgery on the knee. Six patients have no extension lag, three have less than a 10-degree extension lag, and two have greater than a 10-degree extension lag. Although the tendon repair restored continuity and stability to the extensor mechanism, the overall knee flexion in these patients is significantly less than that of patients who have undergone total knee replacement. Only four patients achieved greater than 90 degrees knee flexion, three patients achieved 70 to 89 degrees of knee flexion, and four patients achieved only 50 to 74 degrees of knee flexion. It is important to note, however, that many of these patients had very limited preoperative ranges of motion.

Most of these semitendinosus reconstructions did not include a cerclage wire or suture to protect the graft. We now advocate placing a synthetic tape or heavy gauge suture to reduce tension on the repair. No other changes have been added to our surgical technique for managing patellar tendon ruptures.

References

1. Kelikian H, Riashi E, Gleason J. Restoration of quadriceps function in neglected tear of the patellar tendon. *Surg Gynecol Obstet* 1957; 104:200–204.
2. Cadambi A, Engh GA. Use of a semitendinosus tendon autogenous graft for rupture of the patellar ligament after total knee arthroplasty: A report of seven cases. *J Bone Joint Surg Am* 1992; 74:974–979.
3. Rand JA, Morrey BF, Bryan RS. Patellar tendon rupture after total knee arthroplasty. *Clin Orthop* 1989; 244:233–238.
4. Noyes FR, Butler DL, Grood ES, et al. Biomechanical analysis of human ligament grafts used in knee-ligament repairs and reconstructions. *J Bone Joint Surg Am* 1984; 66:344–352.
5. Krackow KA, Thomas SC, Jones LC. A new stitch for ligament tendon fixation. *J Bone Joint Surg Am* 1986; 68:764–766.
6. Levin, PD. Reconstruction of the patellar tendon using a Dacron graft. *Clin Orthop* 1976; 118:70–72.
7. Fujikawa K, Ohtani T, Matsumoto H, et al. Reconstruction of the extensor apparatus of the knee with the Leeds-Keio ligament. *J Bone Joint Surg Br* 1994; 76:200–203.

30

Choices in Coverage for Wound Problems Following Total Knee Replacement

■ HISTORY OF THE TECHNIQUE

The advent of muscle flaps and free flap tissue transfers in the mid-1970s improved our ability to salvage a functioning knee joint following soft-tissue complications of total knee replacement. The most useful reconstructive techniques are the medial and lateral gastrocnemius muscle transposition flaps (1) and free-flap muscle transfers (rectus abdominis [2,3], latissimus dorsi [4], or gracilis [5]). On rare occasions soft-tissue expanders may be helpful, particularly for prophylactic coverage in anticipation of total knee replacement after numerous prior knee surgeries.

Drainage from the knee arthroplasty wound may indicate a superficial necrosis, hematoma, mechanical wound problem, or sepsis. Complications may occur despite the most cautious surgery. Although rapid and accurate diagnosis of any wound problem is imperative, determining in particular whether the joint is infected is paramount. Deep infection invariably requires removal of the prosthesis.

■ INDICATIONS AND CONTRAINDICATIONS

The extent and location of soft-tissue deficiency must be determined. A tiny draining sinus may conceal a significant deeper soft-tissue deficit (Figs. 30-1 and 30-2) The size of the defect often can be determined only during surgical debridement. The most common location for problems following total knee replacement is the inferior portion of the wound, usually around the tibial tubercle, where the bone is subcutaneous and there is a paucity of soft tissue. The medial gastrocnemius muscle transposition flap covers this area easily in most patients.

The lateral gastrocnemius muscle flap may reach as far as the patella, but its lateral head is smaller and its axis of rotation is more limited than the medial gastrocnemius. The common peroneal nerve is in jeopardy during the dissection of the lateral gastric flap and when the flap is transposed over the nerve. Because of the risk to the nerve, the lateral gastrocnemius is reserved for lateral defects in which the flap may be transposed without tension on the common peroneal nerve.

Preoperative evaluation of the soft tissue around the knee is of the utmost importance in patients with multiple incisions, especially in anticipation of revision arthroplasty. Multiple scars that adhere to underlying bone, tendon, or muscle presage disaster (Fig. 30-1). Prophylactic soft-tissue coverage may be indicated. The actual deep soft-tissue deficit may be sizable, beyond the capacity of local muscle transposition flaps. Similarly, extensive loss of soft tissue that exposes the components of a total knee replacement requires coverage with a larger flap. The exposed prosthesis usually is infected, by definition, and requires removal. Free flaps may be the only way to salvage a disastrous situation.

In considering a free flap for a salvage procedure, I prefer to use the rectus abdominis, latissimus dorsi, or ipsilateral gracilis muscle. The gracilis is dissected easily, creates no functional deficit from its absence, and being on the ipsilateral extremity does not cause difficulties with the healthy opposite leg should a complication arise in the donor site. The main disadvantage of the gracilis muscle is that its pedicle vessels are relatively small. The

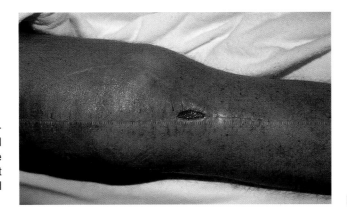

An apparently small defect represents a draining sinus following total knee replacement. Note that the draining sinus is located at the point of intersecting scars over the tibial tubercle.

inferior portion of the rectus muscle, supplied by the deep inferior epigastric vessels, is an excellent choice for coverage around the knee. The muscle size is adequate to cover a fairly considerable defect, and the dissection is relatively simple. Either the contralateral or the ipsilateral rectus muscle may be used, depending on the choice of recipient vessels, for the free-flap anastomosis. The latissimus dorsi muscle is the flap of choice for an extensive defect. This muscle can cover the anterior knee from medial to lateral axis on a patient with a circumferential soft-tissue deficit.

Soft-tissue expanders are useful not for an acutely draining wound but rather in the prevention of problems. Soft-tissue expanders rely on stretching of skin and subcutaneous tissue for coverage, rather than the introduction of healthy muscle to the area. A muscle flap bringing new blood supply is more desirable, in particular if sepsis is a problem (6).

Free-tissue transfers provide excellent coverage but depend heavily on the patient's vasculature and general health. A free flap requires a prolonged and delicate operative procedure, with the patient in good medical condition. Although local flap procedures are less arduous, good medical condition and a healthy circulation are still important.

Coverage of necrotic tissue, dead bone, or infected components cannot be successful; therefore, appropriate preparation of the wound is a prerequisite. The procedures outlined previously have been used to salvage noninfected arthroplasties with wound problems but are not recommended in the presence of established sepsis. If drainage persists after flap coverage, the components generally are contaminated and must be removed. This does not preclude future reimplantation, and the improved coverage following a flap procedure may be advantageous.

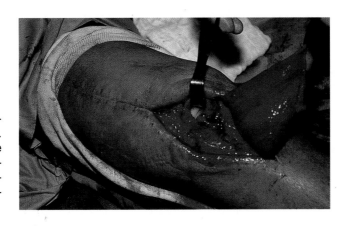

The actual capsular defect associated with the draining sinus in Fig. 30-1, following debridement of the wound. Note the arthroplasty components and the medial gastrocnemius muscle flap to be used for coverage.

Medial Gastrocnemius Muscle Transposition Flap

Anatomy   The medial gastrocnemius muscle originates from the medial condyle of the femur and inserts through the Achilles tendon into the calcaneus (Fig. 30-3). It is supplied by branches of the tibial nerve. The vascular pedicle arises from the popliteal artery and enters the muscle proximally with the nerve. This muscle head may be donated for coverage with impunity in the presence of a functioning soleus, particularly if the lateral head of the gastrocnemius muscle is intact.

The muscle may be used as a simple transposition flap, as a musculofascial or musculocutaneous unit, or in any of these capacities as an island flap—that is, with all attachments to the muscle divided excepting its vascular pedicle. The medial gastrocnemius muscle is not practical as a free flap, compared with other muscles.

Technique   The procedure is performed with the patient supine. The knee and hip are flexed, in a frog's-leg position, to facilitate dissection. Prior to elevation of the flap, the recipient defect should be prepared by debridement and elevation of surrounding skin and subcutaneous tissue flaps, to allow insetting of the muscle under the skin surrounding the defect. The usual recipient site is the proximal tibia and inferior patella. One should judge the length of flap to be used, usually the entire head of the medial gastrocnemius muscle distal to the pedicle. The arc of rotation may be estimated by folding a surgical sponge to roughly the size of the medial head of the gastrocnemius flap. The sponge is held fixed with

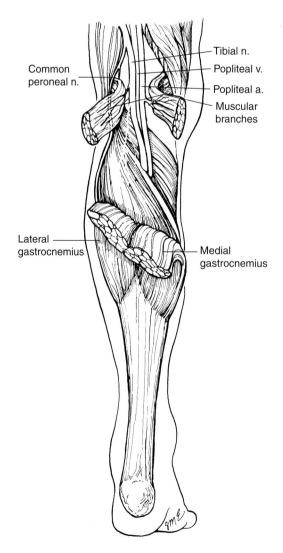

Common
peroneal n.

Lateral
gastrocnemius

Tibial n.

Popliteal v.

Popliteal a.

Muscular
branches

Medial
gastrocnemius

■ FIGURE 30-3   Anatomy of the popliteal fossa and posterior leg.

a finger at its point of rotation, the vascular pedicle to the muscle. This is roughly at the level of the posterior knee joint skin crease overlying the midhead of the medial gastrocnemius muscle. The sponge may be rotated into the defect to estimate if the muscle alone is sufficient for closure or if a fascial or cutaneous extension is required. In most cases simple muscle transposition is sufficient. If a musculocutaneous flap is used, a skin graft usually is needed to close the donor site.

An incision is made about 1 cm posterior to and parallel with the medial edge of the tibia, along the length of the medial head of the gastrocnemius muscle. Curving the incision slightly to the posterior at the inferior end aids in the dissection of the flap with the fascia divided; blunt digital dissection separates the gastrocnemius muscle from the overlying fascia and underlying soleus muscle. Once the belly of the muscle has been isolated to the median raphe between the medial and lateral heads of the gastrocnemius muscle, the two heads may be cut apart. Although it is often difficult to distinguish between the medial and lateral heads of the gastrocnemius muscle distally, the space between the heads of the muscle clearly is delineated proximally. The plantaris tendon is seen overlying the soleus muscle. The lesser saphenous vein and the sural nerve are in direct relation to the raphe between the medial and lateral heads of the muscle, and care must be taken to preserve these structures as the raphe is incised. The heads are separated most efficiently with electrocautery, proceeding from superficial to deep, with the finger beneath the raphe to protect the underlying structures.

A more proximal dissection may be desired, preserving the appropriate extension of the muscle, if an island flap or musculocutaneous or musculofascial extension is anticipated. Once the median raphe has been divided, the attachment of the medial head of the gastrocnemius muscle is separated from the Achilles tendon. The muscle flap then may be transposed into the defect at the knee via a subcutaneous tunnel (Figs. 30-4).

The tunnel may be opened to facilitate transfer of the flap. Cutting across the skin bridge and elevating skin and subcutaneous tissues at a fascial level proximally and distally allows transposition of the muscle flap into the defect without encumbrance (Fig. 30-5). The greater saphenous vein and branches lie within this skin bridge and should be preserved.

The muscle flap is sutured beneath the skin flaps that have been elevated around the defect with fine absorbable sutures. The knee should be extended and flexed to ensure that excessive tension has not been placed on the flap. A suction drain, placed in the bed of the donor site, is brought out through a stab wound inferior to the donor incision. The donor wound is closed. A split-thickness skin graft over the muscle flap may be held in place with fine absorbable sutures or staples.

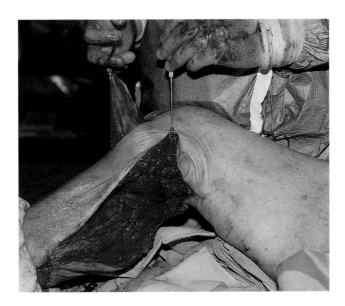

The medial gastrocnemius muscle flap passed beneath a skin bridge.

■ FIGURE 30-4

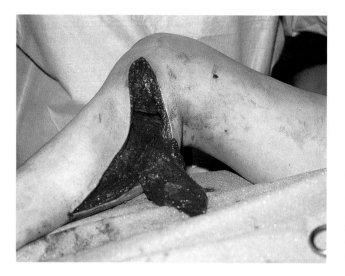

■ FIGURE 30-5

A divided skin bridge for placement of a medial gastrocnemius muscle flap onto a defect of the medial knee. Note the greater saphenous vein and the saphenous nerve in the wound in which the skin bridge was located.

A nonadherent bolus dressing consisting of petrolatum gauze covered by web absorbent cotton gently is pressed into the wound overlying the skin graft. Either a "tie-over" dressing or a cautiously applied circumferential wrap may be placed over the skin graft and flap. Excessive pressure must be avoided. This is merely a device to prevent shearing while the graft heals. Compression may compromise the blood supply to the flap as swelling occurs. Avoid constriction where the muscle flap dives beneath skin flaps or under a skin bridge to reach a recipient bed.

The knee should be splinted in extension, with precautions taken to pad and position the heel and ankle joint. Pressure on the flap must be avoided during splint application. An injudiciously applied splint can destroy a perfectly dissected and inset flap.

The wound is redressed in 5 days and the drain removed. The knee may be put through a range of motion gently at 2 weeks. The skin graft should be lubricated several times each day with a petrolatum gauze dressing or unguent to prevent drying. At 4 to 6 weeks full motion is permitted. The flap should be observed during motion to be sure that it is not stressed unduly. Once the skin has toughened, usually at 4 to 6 weeks, application of lubricant to the skin graft may be discontinued (Fig. 30-6). Weight bearing may be started after 2 weeks depending on the status of the knee joint.

Pitfalls of Dissection   Good planning, including choosing the proper flap for a given defect and being sure that it fits easily into the defect without tension, is mandatory. It is essential that tension on the flap be assessed through the full range of joint motion. If the skin

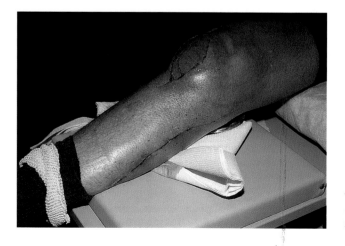

■ FIGURE 30-6

Healed gastrocnemius muscle flap with skin graft and healed donor site (patient from Figs. 30-1, 30-2, and 30-4).

bridge appears to place pressure on the flap, it should be divided. During the division of medial and lateral heads of the gastrocnemius muscle along the raphe, the lesser saphenous vein and the sural nerve should be protected. If the dissection extends proximally into the popliteal fossa, then the popliteal vessels and tibial nerve are at risk. Proximal dissection also may jeopardize the pedicle to the flap.

Lateral Gastrocnemius Muscles Transposition Flap

Anatomy   The lateral gastrocnemius muscle originates from the lateral condyle of the femur and inserts through the Achilles tendon to the calcaneus. The muscle is innervated proximally through branches of the tibial nerve. Blood supply enters the muscle proximally via a vascular pedicle from the popliteal vessels. The common peroneal nerve is adjacent to the proximal lateral muscle belly as it courses around the fibular head. The lateral head of the gastrocnemius muscle may be sacrificed as a donor flap with impunity, especially in the presence of a functioning medial head and soleus muscle.

Procedure   The patient is positioned supine with the hip and knee flexed. The defect (usually in the lateral knee area) is debrided and skin flaps elevated around the defect. An incision is made about 1 cm posterior to and parallel with the fibula along the length of the lateral gastrocnemius muscle. The location of the common peroneal nerve should be foremost in the surgeon's mind. Damage to this nerve is responsible for the majority of problems in transferring the lateral gastrocnemius flap.

The axis of rotation of the muscle is planned as described for the medial gastrocnemius flap. The lateral gastrocnemius muscle is separated from the underlying soleus and overlying fascia (Fig. 30-7). With awareness of the lesser saphenous vein and the sural vein, the raphe between the two muscle heads is divided and the attachment to the Achilles tendon is cut. The flap is transposed as was the medial gastrocnemius flap. The bridge of skin between the flap dissection and the defect may be elevated or divided.

During transposition, great care must be taken not to compress the common peroneal nerve around the neck of the fibula. If a more proximal dissection of the muscle is required so that the muscle must be dissected from the common peroneal nerve, extreme caution is indicated. A flap requiring this level of dissection is not recommended.

After the flap has been transposed, all the precautions recommended for medial gastrocnemius flap should be observed, especially testing through a range of knee motion. Skin-graft dressing, splinting, and rehabilitation are the same as for the medial gastrocnemius muscle transposition flap.

Pitfalls of Dissection   The greatest single danger with the lateral gastrocnemius muscle flap is injury to the common peroneal nerve. The lateral gastrocnemius muscle flap is

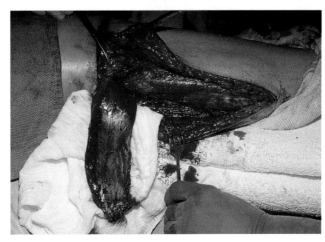

Elevated lateral gastrocnemius muscle flap. Note the common peroneal nerve (indicated by the hemostat tip), soleus muscle (#1) and median raphe (#2).

■ FIGURE 30-7

smaller, with less of an arc of rotation, than the medial flap. It should be limited to lateral defects of the knee that it can reach easily. Stretching the flap beyond what can be covered easily by its arc of rotation sets the stage for peroneal nerve palsy.

Injury to the sural nerve and lesser saphenous vein in dividing the muscle head and problems with skin bridges also occur. Cutaneous and fascial extensions of the lateral gastrocnemius muscle flap may be used if an extension of the flap is contemplated.

■ FREE FLAPS

If a defect is larger than can be covered by transposing local muscle flaps, one should consider a free muscle transfer. Although a free transfer of skin and subcutaneous tissue may be used, there are secondary benefits associated with the use of muscle, especially in the treatment of infectious problems (6), because muscle imports new vascularity. Although the ipsilateral gracilis and latissimus dorsi muscle flaps frequently are used, the inferior portion of the rectus abdominis muscle is used most often. Aside from the ease of patient positioning for knee coverage, the flap is versatile in terms of the length of its pedicle, the size of the vessels, and the size and shape into which the muscle itself can be fashioned.

Anatomy

Rectus Abdominis Muscle   Description of the dissection of latissimus dorsi or gracilis flaps may be found elsewhere (4,5). The rectus abdominis muscle may be found within the leaves of the anterior and posterior rectus sheath. The deep inferior epigastric vessels arise from the external iliac artery and vein. They enter the rectus sheath along the posterior surface of the rectus abdominis muscle and join the muscle belly inferiorly. The inferior epigastric artery and its venae comitantes are of relatively large diameters and the pedicle can be several centimeters in length, facilitating its transfer to the recipient site. The entire length of the rectus muscle may be taken if needed, but usually the portion inferior to the umbilicus suffices.

After the muscle is taken, it must be remembered that there is no posterior rectus sheath layer inferior to the arcuate (semicircular) line. The anterior rectus sheath fascia, however, may be closed directly; a solid closure in this area prevents hernia.

Recipient Site   Several of the vessels around the knee may be used to supply the free flap, but the anterior tibial vessels are preferred. The dissection is simple, the location of the ves-

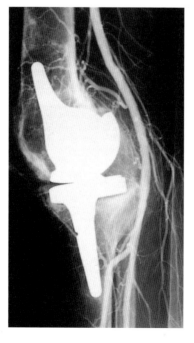

Lateral-view arteriogram of the right knee. Note anterior tibial artery).

■ FIGURE 30-8

sels is constant, and the patient does not have to be repositioned after harvesting if the rectus abdominis muscle is used as the donor flap.

Exposure of the anterior tibial vessels is relatively simple (7). The anterior tibial artery and veins lie deeply within the anterior compartment between the tibialis anterior muscle belly and the muscle belly of the extensor digitorum longus. The cleavage plane between these two muscles is difficult to discern proximally. At the midtibia level, however, the muscle bellies become distinct. By identifying the cleavage plane and dissecting proximally, the anterior tibial vessels are identified easily (Fig. 30-8). The anterior tibial nerve travels in close association with the vessels, and this structure must be protected.

Technique   It must be ensured that the recipient vessels are healthy and appropriate for anastomosis prior to taking the flap. An arteriogram of the involved extremity and the donor flap often if required. This should be done 2 weeks prior to the anticipated surgery, if possible, to avoid intimal irritation from the angiography dye.

The anterior tibial vessels are exposed with an incision as described by Henry (7), extending from the middle of the "gothic arch" formed by the junction of the tibia and fibula superiorly, directed inferiorly overlying the middle of the anterior compartment, to about the midtibia level. The fascia is divided and the plane between the bellies of the tibialis anterior and extensor digitorum longus muscles identified. These muscles are separated bluntly to the level of the anterior tibial vascular bundle (Fig. 30-9).

The artery and the venae comitantes are separated for several centimeters in the upper third of the dissection to allow for the anastomoses. The operating microscope is positioned and the vessels are prepared. The artery is anastomosed end-to-side, and the vein may be anastomosed either end-to-side or end-to-end. It is usually sufficient to anastomose one of the venae comitantes, although both may be connected if desired.

Once the vessels have been exposed, the recipient bed is prepared. The actual defect is exposed and measured. Skin flaps are elevated around the periphery of the defect to accept the donor muscle. Skin bridges present between the recipient vessel and the recipient bed should be divided. With the defect prepared and hemostasis obtained, attention is turned to the donor flap.

A paramedian incision is made over the middle of the inferior portion of the rectus abdominis muscle. The muscle ipsilateral to the defect has vessels properly oriented for the anterior tibial recipient vessels. The length of the incision is determined by the length of muscle needed for the defect. The anterior rectus sheath fascia is incised, and the lateral border of the rectus muscle is bluntly dissected away from the rectus sheath fascia. The deep inferior epigastric vessels are identified inferiorly. They are exposed from the point at which they enter the muscle to the point at which they enter the rectus sheath fascia. Once the vessels are identified and protected, the entire circumferential dissection of the

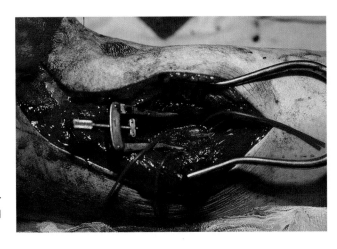

Anterior tibial vessels exposed for anastomosis. Note artery (#1) and vein (#2).

■ FIGURE 30-9

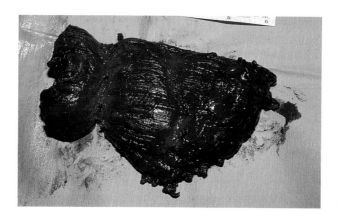

■ FIGURE 30-10

Inferior right rectus abdominis muscle free flap. Note the donor vessels.

rectus abdominis muscle may be completed. If only a narrow flap is required, the medial and lateral portions of the rectus muscle may be spared, taking only the central muscle where the vessels travel. If this is completed over the length of needed muscle, the inferior muscular attachment is divided just inferior to the entrance point of the vessels into the muscle. The superior muscle attachment is easily divided with electrocautery.

The muscle then is detached completely from surrounding structures except for its vascular pedicle. The pedicle is retained as long as possible, and the artery and the venae comitantes are divided between fine ligatures of permanent suture material. Once the vessels are ligated the flap is ischemic, and anastomosis must be performed rapidly (Fig. 30-10).

The flap is transported to its position on the leg and temporarily held with sutures. The donor vessels are oriented properly and draped into the wound, where the recipient anterior tibial artery and vein are reexposed. The microscope, previously adjusted, is returned to the operative field. The donor site may be closed temporarily with towel clips. After completing the anastomoses, the vascular clamps that have been placed on the recipient vessels are removed and flow through the anastomoses can be observed. The flap artery shoulder be anastomosed end-to-side to the anterior tibial artery to maximize flow to the leg. The venous anastomoses may be completed end-to-side or end-to-end, depending on the patient's anatomy (Fig. 30-11).

After flow through the arterial and venous anastomoses has been confirmed, the retractors exposing the vessels are removed and the position of the flap may be adjusted to fit the defect with the least tension on the vascular pedicle. The flap is sutured into place in the same way that the medial gastrocnemius muscle flap was set into its bed. The same procedure may be used for skin grafting. The wound exposing the anterior tibial vessels is

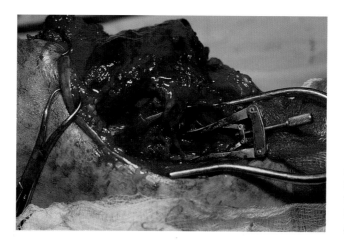

Anastomoses of rectus abdominis muscle free flap following removal of vascular flap and removal of vascular clamps. Note end-to-side arterial anastomosis.

■ FIGURE 30-11

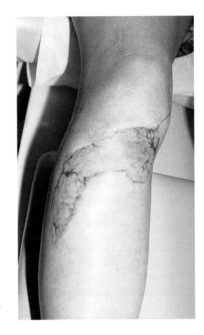

Healed rectus abdominis muscle free flap in patient from Figs. 30-9 through 30-11.

■ FIGURE 30-12

closed. In addition to avoiding pressure on the flap, the surgeon also must be certain that there is neither undue pressure nor tension on the newly anastomosed pedicle. There must be no torsion of the vessels (Fig. 30-12).

The donor site is closed by suturing all layers of the anterior rectus sheath fascia with a nonabsorbable fascial closure material. Skin-closure technique and the use of a drain depend on the preference of the surgeon.

There should be a minimum of 5 days' immobilization before movement of the knee and before redressing the wounds, unless conditions warrant earlier inspection. A 2 cm diameter opening in the dressing may be desirable for monitoring circulation to the free flap with a Doppler probe.

Rehabilitation is the same as described for the medial gastrocnemius muscle transposition flap, following the mandatory 5-day period of immobilization while the anastomoses reendothelialize.

■ REHABILITATION

Planning is the most important factor in success. If the right flap is chosen for a patient who has been prepared properly for surgery, the procedure should be successful. An incisional hernia may be avoided at the donor site by including all layers of the anterior rectus sheath in the fascial closure. Sacrifice of one rectus abdominis muscle should not cause significant functional deficit. At the recipient site, one needs to be cautious with the anterior tibial nerve and its muscular branches to prevent weakness of the anterior compartment muscles.

■ PITFALLS OF THE PROCEDURE

There is controversy as to the possibility of salvaging cases in which a prosthesis has been exposed. Some arthroplasties have been salvaged after exposure of the components, however. Success depends on the nature of the infecting organism (if infection is involved) and whether or not there is an osteomyelitis. Components in wounds with gram-positive infections may be salvaged. In the presence of gram-negative infection, mixed organism infection, or direct bone involvement, the components should be removed. The safer course, recommended by many experts, would be to remove all components and admit the patient to a two-stage protocol for the treatment of infected knee arthroplasty. Flap reconstruction

■ OUTCOMES AND FUTURE DIRECTIONS

is best performed once the resection arthroplasty has healed and before reimplantation of a prosthesis.

In all cases in my personal experience, if a flap or coverage from expanded tissue was used prophylactically, no wound complications developed in the prosthetic reimplantation. Of course, in any prophylactic procedure it is impossible to know whether there would have been a problem had the prophylaxis not been performed. It would seem that there is a place for prophylactic flap coverage prior to knee arthroplasty if the skin is compromised by multiple scars or problems with sepsis.

■ CONCLUSION

Several options are available for reestablishing soft-tissue coverage around the knee. An educated choice can salvage an arthroplasty or allow knee replacement to proceed with a greatly diminished risk of wound complications.

References

1. McGraw JB, Fishman JM, Sharzer LA. The versatile gastrocnemius muscle flap. *Plast Reconstr Surg* 1978; 62:15–23.
2. Moon HK, Taylor GI. The vascular anatomy of the rectus abdominis musculocutaneous flap based on the deep superior epigastric system. *Plast Reconstr Surg* 1988; 82:815–829.
3. Klein NE, Cox CV, Fu FH, Harner CD, Vince K, eds. *Knee surgery.* Baltimore: Williams & Wilkins, 1993:1539–1552.
4. Taylor GI, Daniel RK. The anatomy of several free flap donor sites. *Plast Reconstr Surg* 1975; 56:243–253.
5. Mathes SJ, Nahai F, Vasconez LO. Myocutaneous free flap transfer. *Plast Reconstr Surg* 1978; 62:162–166.
6. Calderon W, Chang N, Mathes SJ. Comparison of the effects of bacterial innoculation in musculocutanous and fasciocutaneous flaps. *Plast Reconstr Surg* 1986; 77:785–792.
7. Henry AK. *Extensile exposure*, 2nd edition. Edinburgh: Churchill Livingstone, 1973:272–276.

31

Technique of Three-step Revision Total Knee Arthroplasty

With the advent of primary knee arthroplasties several decades ago, the concept of revision surgery was not considered to be feasible. Knee replacement surgery was regarded as a last-ditch effort to salvage the profoundly arthritic knee in virtually nonambulatory patients. Eventually surgeons felt that it might be possible to revise a failed knee arthroplasty. Unfortunately, the techniques that were employed amounted to little more than repeat primary knee replacements. This was misguided, and the results were profoundly inferior.

A second phase in the understanding of revision knee arthroplasty came with the recognition that special techniques and implants would be required to revise the failed arthroplasty. Unfortunately, excessive constraint and fully cemented intramedullary stems were employed frequently. Nonetheless, these were improvements along the road to a modern understanding of revision total knee arthroplasty.

The next important step in revision knee arthroplasty came with the recognition that there are a variety of causes for failure of knee replacements. Every cause of failure must be diagnosed, and the technique and implants for the revision need to be chosen in accord with the cause of failure. For example, the knee that has failed because of tibial component loosening is different than the knee that has yielded because of instability. Jacobs et al. identified four important causes of failure in an early series of knee revisions. Prominent among their categories is the fact that the knee with undiagnosed pain is unlikely to benefit from a revision (1). If the surgeon is unable to establish a diagnosis that identifies the mechanical roots of failure and to propose a specific revision technique, further surgery should not be undertaken. In 1995, Vince and Long (2) proposed an additional four categories of failure. Since then, failure as a result of fracture has been added as a ninth cause.

Different techniques for revision knee arthroplasty have been described. Some focus on the importance of restoration of the joint line (3), others on the problems inherent in reestablishing stability. Inherent in revision knee arthroplasty surgery is the confusion that confronts the surgeon once a knee that has undergone a failed replacement is opened. Swirling in front of the surgeon are problems related to bone defects, instability, motion, fixation, and restoration of kinematics to the arthroplasty. It is often unclear where to start. The point of the three-step technique is to establish a path on which the surgeon can ascend from one level of reconstruction to the next. This three-step technique can be applied to any failed knee, regardless of why the primary arthroplasty failed.

The first step involves reconstruction of a tibial platform, which functions as a foundation for the knee arthroplasty. The knee then is stabilized in flexion while a femoral component and an articular polyethylene insert are selected. As a third step, the femoral component is seated on the femur, either more distally with augments or more proximally by resection of a distal femoral bone, to create an extension gap that is equal to the flexion gap (Fig. 31-1) (4).

■ HISTORY OF THE TECHNIQUE

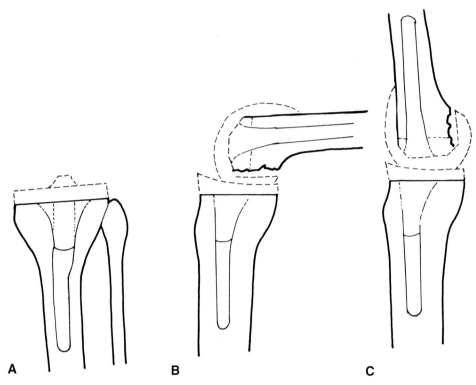

■ FIGURE 31-1   **A**   **B**   **C**

The three steps in revision of total knee arthroplasty. **A:** The tibia is reconstructed to establish a foundation for the rest of the knee. The tibial polyethylene insert is not selected at this point. **B:** The knee is stabilized in flexion by determining the correct rotational position of the femoral component, choosing the component size to stabilize the knee in flexion and then coupling the femoral component size with the appropriate thickness of polyethylene to establish the correct joint-line height. **C:** The knee then is stabilized in extension by seating the femoral component either more proximally or distally to create an extension gap equal to the flexion gap seen in **B**.

■ INDICATIONS AND   The nine causes of knee arthroplasty failure describe indications and a contraindication
CONTRAINDICATIONS   for revision knee surgery (Table 31-1).

   The indication for revision total knee arthroplasty is identifiable failure resulting from any of these nine causes except type IV. The patient presents usually with pain and sometimes with other mechanical symptoms, such as instability. The evaluations that are necessary to define the indications for revision knee surgery include a complete history, physi-

TABLE 31-1. TYPES OF KNEE ARTHROPLASTY FAILURE

Type I	Loosening and progression of arthritis in a unicompartmental replacement
Type II	Tibial/femoral instability
Type III	Malrotation and patellar instability
Type IV	Undiagnosed pain
Type V	Component breakage
Type VI	Sepsis
Type VII	Extensor mechanism rupture
Type VIII	Stiffness
Type IX	Fracture

cal examination, radiographic evaluation, aspiration of the knee, and at other times aspiration arthrograms, stress views, fluoroscopic views (5), scintigraphic studies (6), and computed tomographic scanning (7).

One of the most important factors is the time of onset of the patient's pain. The knee arthroplasty that has never provided pain relief presents a different range of problems from the one that served the patient well for a period of time and then began to develop difficulties. For example, the patient who never enjoyed pain relief after the primary arthroplasty may be experiencing referred pain from a site remote to the knee. An arthritic hip or femoral neck fracture ipsilateral to the knee arthroplasty always should be considered. Internal rotation of this hip usually reproduces the symptoms. The diagnosis should be apparent on radiographs or bone scan. Similarly, the spine can be a source of pain referred to the knee and should be evaluated thoroughly. The patient whose knee radiographs prior to the primary arthroplasty show a minimum of arthritic changes presents a significant challenge. He or she may have a low pain threshold, and the primary knee arthroplasty may have been a poor idea to begin with.

The patient who had pain prior to knee arthroplasty surgery and has a different pain afterwards may be suffering from sepsis or sympathetically mediated pain (reflex sympathetic dystrophy). Aspiration of the knee is necessary to evaluate these patients. The fluid should be sent for cell count, differential, and culture and sensitivity. Something has gone wrong with this knee, originating at the time of surgery. Pain associated with stiffness or poor motion indicates a problem with component size or position.

New onset of pain after a period of relief occurs in the patient with component loosening, progression of arthritis in the contralateral compartment of a unicompartmental replacement, late-onset sepsis, or breakage.

Some of the indications for revision knee arthroplasty surgery are mechanical. The patient with instability may suffer excessive laxity with the knee in extension varus, valgus, or both directions. In addition, instability may occur with knee flexion if the tibia dislocates anteriorly or posteriorly. Virtually all patellar complications, including fracture, loosening of the component, and breakage of the component can be related to tracking problems. These in turn usually have at their root malrotation of the femoral or tibial components. Correction of the patellar complication requires complete revision knee arthroplasty (8). Breakage of a component may present with mechanical symptoms such as grinding or instability or simply with recurrent effusions.

Extensor mechanism rupture is one of the most challenging indications for revision knee surgery. These patients present with buckling and an extensor lag. Trauma may or may not have been present. Stiffness, whether limited to a flexion contracture, poor flexion, or a combination of the two, long has been regarded as an inappropriate indication for revision surgery. As our techniques and understanding of knee arthroplasty failure have become more complete, stiffness also has become amenable to revision surgery (9). The role of sympathetically mediated pain in the stiff knee must be considered completely. This often is evaluated with therapeutic and diagnostic lumbar sympathetic blocks. Long-bone fracture, usually of the femur, is a dramatic presentation that sometimes is treated best with complete revision knee surgery, in which allograft bone often is required.

Undiagnosed pain should be regarded as a contraindication to revision knee surgery. Often these so-called mystery knees look generally good on plain radiographs, and it is difficult for the surgeon to understand precisely why the patient is suffering. This individual may indeed have referred pain from a distant source, in which case a bone scan is revealing. Many of these cases result from reflex sympathetic dystrophy, which should be diagnosed and treated. Ultimately, many knees with undiagnosed pain are suffering from malrotation of components, with a sense of painful binding as the knee moves. Accordingly, a computed tomographic scan is the best way to evaluate three-dimensional positioning of the components (Fig. 31-2).

At times, failure of solid bone ingrowth into porous coated components is at the root of undiagnosed pain. Fluoroscopic views of all interfaces of the femoral component as well as the tibia can be revealing.

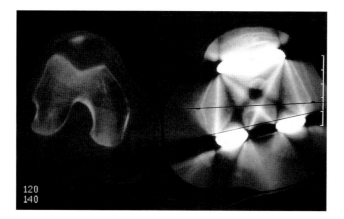

Bilateral computerized tomographic scans of the knees. The image on the *right* is the left total knee arthroplasty. One line through the transepicondylar axis shows the ideal position for the femoral component. The component, however, is rotated internally dramatically with respect to this axis. Internal rotation of the femoral component usually causes patellar tracking problems, except in cases such as this in which the patient suffers pain and stiffness as a result of the malrotation. If the knee flexes poorly, the patella does not dislocate.

Active sepsis should be regarded as a contraindication to revision knee arthroplasty. One-stage reimplantation protocols have been discussed but should not be regarded as equivalent to the gold standard, two-stage reimplantation protocol for the infected knee arthroplasty. Some dual failures, such as sepsis and extensor mechanism rupture, have been regarded as contraindications to revision. Entering this patient, however, into a two-stage protocol to eliminate infection and then reimplanting the knee with an extensor mechanism allograft improves the outcome.

■ SURGICAL
TECHNIQUES

A simple three-step revision technique may be employed, regardless of the cause of failure of a knee arthroplasty. Each of these steps represents a plateau in the progression of the revision. The basic work should be finished in one stage before ascending to the next. By the time the patient enters the operating room, there is a precise explanation for the failure and a specific mechanical plan established for the revision. The details of the mechanical plan are carried out during the three sequential steps described here. This technique has evolved over the course of more than a decade, and the preliminary results of the first 100 consecutive revision knee arthroplasties have been reported (10).

Step 1: Tibial Platform   Step 1 is reestablishment of the tibial platform. This creates a foundation on which to build the arthroplasty. The tibia is selected because it is always in contact with the femoral articular surface. By contrast, in extension it is only the distal femoral articular surface, and in flexion the posterior femur, that has a role in the arthroplasty.

It should be clear that step 1 reestablishes the bony tibial "platform" and not the articular surface. The articular polyethylene is chosen as a part of step 2. The concept of a platform can be equated to that of a "foundation" for the tibial component.

In all revision knee arthroplasties, except those in which the tibial cancellous and cortical bone is well maintained, augmented intramedullary fixation is preferred. Accordingly, the intramedullary canal of the tibia should be opened to determine the position of the intramedullary guide. It must be remembered that the position of any intramedullary stem will in turn determine the position of the implants. Unlike hip arthroplasties where a maximum fit and fill of the intramedullary canal is often desired, the surgeon risks being a "slave to the stem" by trying to completely fill the asymmetric tibial canal with an uncemented intramedullary stem. This will often result in valgus alignment or overhang of the component or both. Alignment remains the most important single factor in the reconstruction of any knee—revision or primary.

Intramedullary rods unload the proximal surface of the tibia, helping dissipate forces across the joint that would otherwise induce tilting and subsidence of the tibia (Fig. 31-3). They may prove useful for intramedullary fixation of fractures that have occurred in the tibia. Intramedullary rods are necessary to fix proximal tibial allografts, if these are necessitated by significant bone loss. Improved stem designs include offset intramedullary stems, which enhance the surgeon's ability to fill the intramedullary canal and accommodate the asymmetry in most tibias. This enables the surgeon to place the intramedullary rod in the center of the tibial canal and also have the tibial component centered on the cut bone surface proximally (Fig 31-3B).

Bone Defects   Tibial bone defects frequently are encountered in revision knee surgery. A general rule, which was established for primary knee arthroplasties, should be respected in the revision: Do not cut to the base of the defect, but preferentially reconstruct the defective bone so that the component is not seated distally on bone of smaller dimension and poor quality. Several classification systems describe bone defects in revision knee arthroplasty (11). There is a more pragmatic grading system that can be employed (Table 31-2) (12): Three types of defect are recognized, the first of which is "contained," meaning that there is a rim of bone around the defect. Small defects of this configuration sometimes can be filled with methacrylate cement. If feasible, particulate graft, whether autograft or allograft, can be compacted into these defects. This yields an excellent surface that is entirely satisfactory for cement fixation.

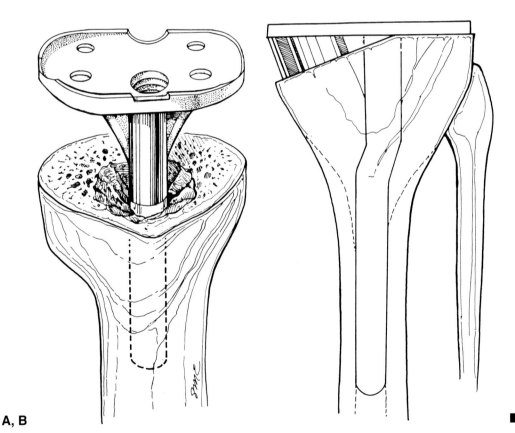

A, B   ■ FIGURE 31-3

A: Reestablishing the tibial platform provides a foundation to build the rest of the arthroplasty upon. Intramedullary stem extension often is required if bone has been compromised. These stems can alter the position of the component. Only the baseplate is required at this step. The polyethylene is chosen in step 2, stabilizing the knee in flexion. **B:** Because of the asymmetry of the tibia, offset intramedullary stems may be required to fill the diaphysis of the canal without compromising the position, size, or alignment of the prosthesis proximally. In the knee shown in this figure, a noncontained defect will be reconstituted with a modular augment.

TABLE 31-2. BONE DEFECTS

Defect	Solution
Contained	Particulate graft/methacrylate cement
Noncontained	Modular prosthetic augment
Massive	Structural allograft

A second more difficult type of defect is noncontained, which generally occurs if components have subsided and loosened or were implanted initially in malalignment. There is no peripheral rim to contain bone graft in this instance, and these are best dealt with using modular prosthetic augments of either a wedge or block shape.

The most challenging defect is the massive loss of a hemicondyle or the complete metaphysis. These require massive structural allograft. At times, surgeons have chosen to implant linked constrained devices that are cemented fully into the medullary canal femur and tibia in the face of extensive bone loss. Although these provide an easier surgical technique and a "quick fix," the results are poor with time.

With the bone defect evaluated and the intramedullary canal opened, the appropriate length and dimension as well as the offset of the intramedullary stem should be selected in accord with preoperative planning. Intramedullary "reamers" should be used to gauge the size of the canal, and not to remove bone. A trial component is attached to this intramedullary stem and implanted. The surgeon can use the component to define the defects in tibial bone and should not be concerned about reconstructing them at the present time. Alignment is more important, and a simple extramedullary device placed on the trial component reveals whether it is sitting at right angles to the long axis of the bone. For a grossly asymmetric tibia (for which an intramedullary fit cannot be achieved), full cement fixation of a smaller stem extension in the intramedullary canal may be considered.

It should be remembered that any intramedullary stem may need removal in the future, and that revision surgeries are at greater risk for infection than primaries. Accordingly, extralong intramedullary stems intended for three-point uncemented fixation should not be employed with full cement fixation. The difficulties inherent in their later removal are destructive and can jeopardize the limb.

With a trial component attached to an intramedullary stem sitting on the tibia, alignment is reconfirmed, the bone defect is noted, and a plan should be made to reconstruct it during the revision.

Step 2: Stabilize the Knee in Flexion   Most of the difficult work in the revision arthroplasty is accomplished with the knee positioned at 90 degrees. Once the knee is stabilized in flexion, with satisfactory positioning of the correct size of components, the final step is greatly facilitated.

Femoral Component Rotation   Regardless of the prerevision knee deformity or the cause of failure, it is essential to rotate the femoral component into its appropriate position with respect to the anatomy of the femur. Sadly, most of the reliable landmarks, in particular the posterior articular surfaces, that are present for primary knee arthroplasty have been destroyed at the time of revision. Two other indicators, the transepicondylar axis (13) and the palpable bone of the residual posterior femoral condyle, should be employed. The epicondyles on either side of the femur can be difficult to palpate in the primary procedure and even more difficult at the time of revision because of scarring. Only by repeated attempts at identification do these landmarks become reliably apparent (Fig. 31-4). An area that is not visible but still is reliable to assess rotational position is the palpable amount of posterior condylar bone. This should be assessed prior to removal of the failed component.

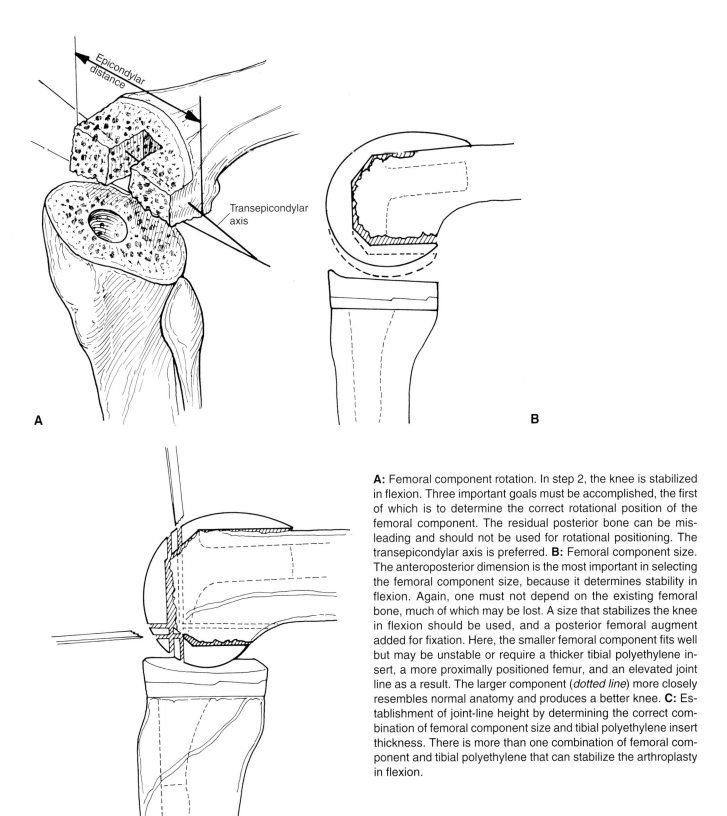

A: Femoral component rotation. In step 2, the knee is stabilized in flexion. Three important goals must be accomplished, the first of which is to determine the correct rotational position of the femoral component. The residual posterior bone can be misleading and should not be used for rotational positioning. The transepicondylar axis is preferred. **B:** Femoral component size. The anteroposterior dimension is the most important in selecting the femoral component size, because it determines stability in flexion. Again, one must not depend on the existing femoral bone, much of which may be lost. A size that stabilizes the knee in flexion should be used, and a posterior femoral augment added for fixation. Here, the smaller femoral component fits well but may be unstable or require a thicker tibial polyethylene insert, a more proximally positioned femur, and an elevated joint line as a result. The larger component (*dotted line*) more closely resembles normal anatomy and produces a better knee. **C:** Establishment of joint-line height by determining the correct combination of femoral component size and tibial polyethylene insert thickness. There is more than one combination of femoral component and tibial polyethylene that can stabilize the arthroplasty in flexion.

■   FIGURE 31-4

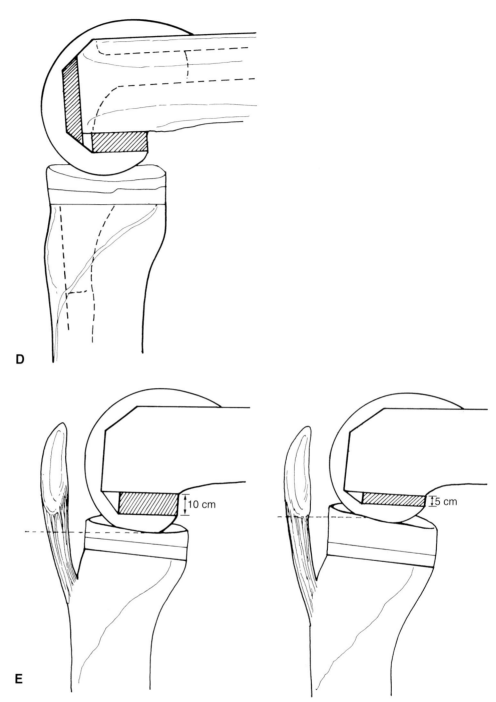

■ FIGURE 31-4
(Continued)

D: A larger femoral component and a thinner polyethylene insert not only stabilize the knee but keep the joint line in a more normal position (inferior pole of the patella is above the joint line). **E:** A smaller femoral component, which fits the remaining bone, requires a thicker polyethylene insert and a more proximal position of the femoral component. The joint line is above the inferior pole of the patella. This is less desirable.

In the situation in which a femoral component has been rotated internally, there is a greater amount of palpable bone on the medial side than the lateral. Accordingly, to correct internal malrotation of the femur at the time of reconstruction, the surgeon selects a lateral posterior femoral augment. A commitment can be made to the correct femoral rotational early in step 2 by cutting bone for the intercondylar box if a posterior stabilized or constrained condylar type implant is to be employed (Fig. 31-4A).

Femoral Component Sizing   One of the most common errors in revision knee arthroplasty surgery is to select the anteroposterior dimension of the new femoral component based exclusively on the size of the residual bone on the femur. The femur may be reduced in size tremendously because of bone loss resulting from the failure. The anteroposterior dimension of the revision femoral component should be selected as a function of what is required to stabilize the soft tissues (collateral ligaments) in the flexed position. This frequently leaves a gap between the posterior condylar bone and the component. This gap is filled with a posterior femoral condylar augment (Fig. 31-4B).

The intramedullary canal of the femur must be opened if intramedullary stems are required for enhanced fixation. The intramedullary stem on the femoral component determines its anteroposterior position and influences its varus and valgus alignment. The surgeon can assess stability in flexion by positioning the knee at 90 degrees with trial components in place and then grasping the ankle with one hand and lifting the posterior thigh with the other. The bones are distracted at the knee, and the dimensions of the flexion gap can be assessed. If there is significant asymmetry resulting from collateral ligament incompetence or contracture, a release of the tight side may become necessary. This usually is possible only if no releases were performed at the time of the primary arthroplasty and also if a similar asymmetry exists in extension. One or more femoral component sizes may be considered at this point. The final selection is made in the next part of step 2.

Reestablishment of Joint Line Height   The revision knee can be stabilized in flexion using more than one size of femoral component. For example, a femoral component with a smaller anteroposterior dimension can be coupled with a thicker articular tibial polyethylene to fill the flexion gap. This produces a higher joint line in flexion. Conversely, a larger femoral component may be coupled with a thinner articular polyethylene and also stabilize the joint. This produces a lower joint line. The medial–lateral dimension of the bone ultimately limits the femoral component size (Fig. 31-4E).

Deciding on the perfect joint-line height in revision knee arthroplasty surgery can be difficult, especially for the more challenging cases such as reimplantation after infection or the multiply revised or unstable knee. Poilvache and colleagues (14) developed a quantitative method for determining the normal joint-line height as a function of the transepicondylar axis distance. For many revision knee arthroplasties, however, it is satisfactory to establish the joint-line height within 1 cm above the inferior pole of the patella. This frequently results in excellent stability and flexion. In knees in which the patellar tendon is scarred and short or stretched and long, this is not appropriate. At this point, in step 3, the decision is made as to which combination of femoral component and tibial articular polyethylene is selected. These trial components are positioned in the knee, and stability is examined at 90 degrees of flexion.

Step 3: Extension   Most of the difficult work in the reconstruction has been accomplished. As the knee is extended fully, the posterior soft tissue tightens. To go beyond this point either because of too thin a tibial polyethylene or because of loss of distal femoral bone would produce recurvatum and an unstable knee. The position of the femoral component relative to the distal femur is noted with the knee at full extension without recurvatum. The trial femoral component is secured in this position (Fig. 31-5). Instruments are available that enable the surgeon to make bone cuts through the trial component, removing the small amounts of irregular bone so that distal femoral augments fit perfectly on the distal femur (Fig. 31-4C, D).

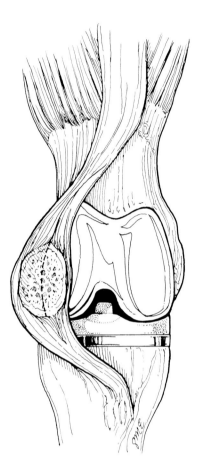

Step 3: The femur is stabilized in extension by seating the femoral component in the position that creates an extension gap equal to the thickness of the flexion gap. Cutting slots in the femoral trial component enable the surgeon to trim off excess irregular bone, which can be reconstructed with augments.

■ FIGURE 31-5

Three conditions must be satisfied at this stage:

1. Full extension of the knee without recurvatum (posterior soft tissues under tension).
2. Restoration of neutral mechanical axis (straight line from center of femoral head through center of knee and center of ankle).
3. Satisfactory varus–valgus stability.

The knee that has failed because of component loosening or catastrophic wear often has varus malalignment. Usually, the required conventional medial releases have not been performed previously and should be performed at this time. If extensive soft-tissue releases are performed, the surgeon needs to reevaluate stability in flexion, perhaps selecting a thicker tibial polyethylene insert, and then reevaluate the proximal–distal position of the femoral component with the new insert. For the majority of revision arthroplasties at this point, the knee is stable in flexion and extension, with good alignment and motion.

If nonconstrained implants have been selected, methacrylate cement can be restricted to the cut bone surfaces, and the intramedullary rods can be inserted as a "press-fit" without cement. In situations in which the bone quality is poor or a constrained articular polyethylene has been selected, some patients may benefit from full cementation of the intramedullary rods, with much the same technique as in a cemented total hip arthroplasty. This carries risk if the components ever need to be removed.

Patella   Preparation of the patella almost represents a fourth step in the reconstruction. A well-fixed, well-positioned, all-polyethylene patellar component should be left in place if it is compatible with the revision implant. Tolerating small amounts of incompatibility may prove to be a better option than removal of the component, with attendant bone loss.

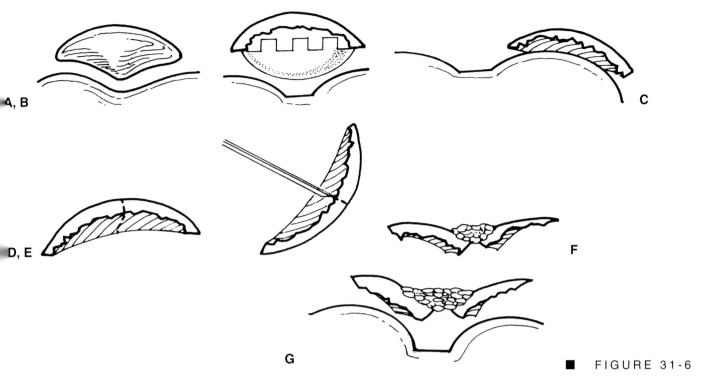

A, B

C

D, E

F

G

A "gull-wing" patellar osteotomy may be useful if the residual patella bone is too small or thin to accept a new prosthetic surface, and if it has a scaphoid shape that hugs the lateral femoral condyle, risking lateral subluxation. **A:** The normal patella tracks centrally and has a shape that matches the intercondylar groove on the femur. **B:** A well positioned, resurfaced patella in a primary arthroplasty similarly tracks centrally. **C:** The problem arises with the scaphoid-shaped patella at revision in which there is inadequate bone for resurfacing. **D:** Sagittal osteotomy. The residual patella is split from top to bottom with the saw. **E:** The patella is everted in preparation for the osteotomy. **F:** The medial and lateral halves are cracked upwards, still intact, with the patellar tendon distal and the quadriceps tendon proximal. Lateral soft tissues still are attached to the lateral half of the bone. **G:** Small pieces of bone graft can be placed on the osteotomy site. This consolidates well and is shaped to track well in the trochlear groove.

Metal-backed components should be removed and replaced if possible (15). The knee with stiffness may have an inordinately thick patellar construct. In this case, the prosthesis should be removed, the patella bone resected to a more desirable thickness, and a new surface placed (Fig. 31-5).

If patellar components have loosened and there is adequate bone available, another cemented all-polyethylene component should be used. Loosening of the patellar components, however, sometimes precludes revision, because of poor quality or inadequate amounts of bone. Patellectomy is undesirable, because it weakens the extensor mechanism and may result in rupture. A patellaplasty can be performed, in which the shape of the residual bone is enhanced to track centrally on the femoral component. Still more demanding situations occur if a scaphoid shell of bone is left on the patella. This bone, shaped much like a bottle cap, has a tendency to hug the lateral femoral condyle and to sublux laterally. This can be improved by a sagittal osteotomy, performed from the inside of the patella. The bowl or scaphoid shape of this residual bone then opens like a pair of wings (Fig. 31-6). The deep central part of the patella is then free to ride between the condyles. A small particulate bone graft may be applied to the osteotomy. The sagittal cut in the bone does not threaten the extensor mechanism, and rehabilitation can proceed normally (Fig. 31-5).

There are few alternatives to a well-performed revision total knee arthroplasty if the primary arthroplasty has failed. Limited revisions, in which only one component is changed, have been considered. In general, these are less good and paradoxically take a greater

■ TECHNICAL
ALTERNATIVES AND
PITFALLS

length of time. By removing all failed components, the surgeon is free to select components of a more modern design and to manipulate all of the variables in the reconstruction of the knee to better improve the patient's comfort and function. The few situations in which limited revision might be appropriate include the stiff knee that flexes and extends poorly because of an overly tight arthroplasty. If such a knee has been reconstructed with an unacceptably thick articular polyethylene, it is reasonable to exchange the polyethylene component. Stiffness is a multifaceted problem, however, and usually is associated with malrotation of the components, oversizing of the femoral component, and an unacceptably thick patellar construct. Sympathetically mediated pain also may contribute. Only if the surgeon can be certain that these problems do not pertain should a limited revision be performed. Arthrodesis is more difficult to achieve than revision, and the results are difficult to live with. Resection arthroplasty sometimes results if a patient simply cannot have a reimplantation after infection. The results are miserable, and this should not be considered an alternative to revision arthroplasty—only what is left if nothing more is possible. Amputation, by definition above the knee, may be necessary in rare cases of uncontrollable infection.

An experimental alternative to conventional revision arthroplasty surgery with cement fixation is the uncemented revision. Contrary to the experience with total hip arthroplasty, in which uncemented revisions sometimes proved superior to cemented ones, this has not been the case in the knee. There are a few proponents of uncemented revision knee arthroplasty (16,17), but more information has been published on cement fixation. Some problems inherent in the knee arthroplasty that could be remedied with revision may be helped by bracing. A patient with an unstable knee arthroplasty who is a poor candidate for further surgery may benefit from a long leg brace. This is generally an unappealing alternative. Any residual instability further threatens catastrophic wear or breakage of the component.

There are many pitfalls in revision arthroplasty surgery; most result from failure to diagnose the cause of failure. The worst situation is a revision with no diagnosis whatsoever. This patient is unlikely to benefit from revision surgery.

A common error in revision knee surgery is the surgeon's reflex if faced with dramatic radiographic evidence of failure to assume that a constrained implant is required. The specific indications for constraint include varus—valgus instability secondary to a failed medial collateral ligament, in cases in which ligament reconstruction or allograft substitution are not feasible. The second indication for constraint is a flexion gap sufficiently large that it cannot be balanced by increasing the size of the femoral component. This also usually is related to failure of collateral ligaments, and advancement of the ligament can be an alternative to constraint.

An easy way out of many failed knee arthroplasties, but a poor choice for longevity of the component, is a linked, hinged arthroplasty. This very rarely if ever is required in revision surgery. The problems that result from their implantation several years after revision surgery often are monumental and far more difficult to correct than the challenges presented at the time of the first revision.

Two relatively common diagnoses that remain occult are infection and reflex sympathetic dystrophy. Every knee should be aspirated prior to revision surgery to ensure that infection is not present. If the complaints of pain exceed the objective findings, reflex sympathetic dystrophy should be considered. These patients may present with skin hypersensitivity, although it is unusual to see the full-blown clinical scenario, including waxy pallor of the skin.

The diagnosis of reflex sympathetic dystrophy is facilitated with diagnostic lumbar sympathetic blocks. A series of these blocks is often beneficial for treatment. If revision is still necessary for mechanical reasons, it is best performed under an indwelling epidural catheter, which remains in place for 3 days postsurgery. The involvement of a pain-management expert benefits the patient and the revision surgeon alike.

Another problem in revision surgery results from recreating the environment of failure in the primary knee arthroplasty. Accordingly, treating a loose patellar button that resulted from malrotation of the components probably will result in further patellar problems. A simple exchange of modular articular polyethylene inserts in treating catastrophic wear is likely to recreate the environment of failure with another thin, and perhaps flat, insert.

The surgeon should strive to create a revision knee arthroplasty sufficiently stable and mobile so that these patients can enjoy aggressive rehabilitation identical to the protocol offered to patients undergoing primary knee arthroplasty. Exceptions would include reconstruction of collateral ligaments that require functional bracing and limited motion for several months following surgery. Extensor mechanism allografts similarly require a phase of incorporation before full active motion and unlimited weight bearing are permitted. The extensor mechanism allograft benefits from a hinged knee brace that is limited to between 60 and 90 degrees of flexion depending on what was achieved at surgery. This prevents the patient from stumbling, hyperflexing the knee under load, and disrupting the allograft completely. Some surgeons, after revising the knee with extensive amounts of bone graft, require prolonged periods of protected weight bearing. It is clear, however, from the biology of bone allografting that the graft does not strengthen, but rather weakens with time. Accordingly, it has been our practice to encourage full weight bearing in all of these patients as soon as comfort permits.

■ REHABILITATION

The outcomes of revision knee arthroplasty are difficult to assess, given the wide variety of causes of failure that has been reported. Three studies of a contemporary prosthesis were presented recently. It is very important in future research that the causes of failure be defined and the results depicted according to the cause of failure (2,10,18). Superior understanding of bone-grafting techniques and biology will go a long way toward enhancing the ability to reconstruct the knee. Further development of techniques for soft- tissue reconstruction, including allograft ligament reconstruction, will enable surgeons to avoid constrained components and the high loosening rates that have accompanied them. Bone-graft substitutes will prove very useful in the reconstruction of bone defects.

■ OUTCOMES AND FUTURE DIRECTIONS

References

1. Jacobs MA, Hungerford DS, Krackow KA, et al. Revision of septic total knee arthroplasty. *Clin Orthop* 1989; 238:159–166.
2. Vince KG, Long W. Revision knee arthroplasty: The limits of press fit medullary fixation. *Clin Orthop* 1995; 317:172–177.
3. Gustke K. Planning and techniques for unconstrained revision total knee replacement. In: Fu C, Vince K, eds. *Knee surgery.* Baltimore: Williams & Wilkins, 1994:1553–1562.
4. Vince K. Revision total knee arthroplasty. In: Chapman M, ed. *Operative orthopedics.* Philadelphia: JB Lippincott Co, 1993, pp. 1981–2010.
5. Fehring TK, McAvoy G. Fluoroscopic evaluation of the painful total knee arthroplasty. *Clin Orthop* 1996; 331:226–233.
6. Henderson JJ, Bamford DJ, Noble J, et al. The value of skeletal scintigraphy in predicting the need for revision surgery in total knee replacement. *Orthopedics* 1996; 19:295–299.
7. Kharrazi FD, Spitzer AI, Vince KG. Evaluation of femoral component rotation in failed total knee arthroplasty using computerized tomography. Presented at the meeting of the Societé Internationale de Chirurgie Orthopedique et Traumatologique (SICOT). Sydney, Australia, January, 1999.
8. Briard JL, Hungerford DS. Patellofemoral instability in total knee arthroplasty. *J Arthroplasty* 1989; 4(suppl):87–97.
9. Vince KG. Stiff total knee arthroplasty. In: Fu C, Vince K, eds. *Knee surgery.* Baltimore: Williams & Wilkins, 1994, pp. 1529–1538.
10. Vince KM, Mark, Kharrazi D, et al. Revision total knee arthroplasty with a modular prosthesis and a three step reconstruction technique: 2 to 10 year follow up. Presented at the *10th meeting of the Combined Orthopedic Associations of the English Speaking World,* Auckland, New Zealand, 1998.

11. Engh GA, Ammeen DJ. Classification and preoperative radiographic evaluation: Knee. *Orthop Clin North Am* 1998; 29:205–217.
12. Ortaaslan SVK. Reconstruction of bone defects in knee arthroplasty. In: Vince K, ed. *Waverly atlas of knee surgery.* Baltimore: Williams & Wilkins, in press.
13. Berger RA, Rubash HE, Steel MJ, et al. Determining the rotational alignment of the femoral component in total knee arthroplasty using the epicondylar axis. *Clin Orthop* 1993; 286:40–47.
14. Poilvache PL, Insall JN, Scuderi GR, et al. Rotational landmarks and sizing of the distal femur in total knee arthroplasty. *Clin Orthop* 1996; 331:35–46.
15. Dennis D. Removal of metal backed patellar button. In: Vince K, ed. *Waverly atlas of knee surgery.* Baltimore: Williams & Wilkins, in press.
16. Whiteside LA. Cementless revision total knee arthroplasty. *Clin Orthop* 1993; 286:160–167.
17. Mow CS, Wiedel JD. Noncemented revision total knee arthroplasty. *Clin Orthop* 1994; 309:110–115.
18. Peters CL, Hennessey R, Barden RM, et al. Revision total knee arthroplasty with a cemented posterior-stabilized or constrained condylar prosthesis: A minimum 3-year and average 5-year follow-up study. *J Arthroplasty* 1997; 12:896–903.

SUBJECT INDEX

Note: Page numbers followed by f refer to figures; page numbers followed by t refer to tables.

A

Abrasion arthroplasty, for chondral defects, 27, 37, 146
Achilles tendon allograft
  for arthroscopy-assisted PCL reconstruction, 83–93
    with ACL reconstruction, 90
    anatomic factors in, 84, 84f
    debridement in, 86, 87f
    femoral tunnel in, 87–89, 89f
    future directions for, 93
    graft insertion and fixation in, 89–90, 90f
    graft preparation for, 85–86, 86f
    guide wire placement in, 86–87, 88f
    history of, 83
    indications and contraindications for, 83–84
    instrumentation for, 84, 85f
    outcomes of, 92
    pitfalls of, 91–92
    preparation for, 85
    rehabilitation after, 92
    surgical techniques for, 84–90
    technical alternatives in, 90–91
    tibial tunnel in, 87, 88f, 89f
  for dislocation with lateral ligament injury, 111, 114f, 115
  for popliteus reconstruction, 101, 102
ACL. *See* Anterior cruciate ligament (ACL)
Albee procedure, 136
Allograft
  Achilles tendon. *See* Achilles tendon allograft
  lateral tibial plateau, 195f, 197, 198f
  medial femoral condylar, 194f, 197, 198f
  meniscal, 10–22
    ACL reconstruction with, 10, 19–20
    alternative techniques for, 17–18
    bed preparation for, 12
    closure and dressing for, 14
    diagnostic arthroscopy prior to, 12
    future of, 21–22
    graft fixation in, 14, 17–18
    graft insertion in, 14, 15f, 17
    graft selection, sizing, and preparation for, 12, 16
    history of, 10
    immunologic considerations in, 16–17
    indications for, 10–11
    osseous tunnel placement in, 12–14, 13f
    outcomes of, 18–21
    pitfalls of, 17–18
    positioning for, 12
    rehabilitation after, 18

    surgical techniques of, 11–14, 11f
  osteochondral, 150, 156
    for posttraumatic knee defects, 193–200
      graft procurement in, 194
      history of, 193
      indications and contraindications for, 193–194
      outcomes of, 197–200, 199t
      procedure for, 194–197, 194f–196f, 198f
      rehabilitation after, 197
    for tibial defect reconstruction, 247, 252–253, 253f
Anderson classification, for bone defects, 245, 246t
Anesthesia
  for arthroscopic meniscal repair, 3
  for multiple ligament reconstruction, 109
Anterior cruciate ligament (ACL), in arthroscopic meniscal repair, 2
Anterior cruciate ligament (ACL) reconstruction
  for dislocation with lateral ligament injury, 110–113, 110f, 112f, 116
  with double looped hamstring tendon graft, 57–71
    diagnostic arthroscopy in, 59
    graft harvest in, 59–60, 60f–62f
    graft insertion and fixation in, 64–70, 68f, 69f
    graft preparation in, 60–63
    history of, 57–58
    indications for, 58
    outcomes of, 71
    positioning and preparation for, 58
    rehabilitation after, 70
    surgical techniques for, 58–70
    technical alternatives in, 70
    tunnel placement and creation in, 63–64, 65f–67f
  with meniscal allograft reconstruction, 10, 19–20
  with miniarthrotomy, 73–81
    bone plugs in, 78
    bone tunnels in, 76–77, 76f–78f
    diagnostic arthroscopy in, 73–74
    graft harvesting and preparation in, 77–78
    history of, 73
    indications for, 73
    lateral oblique incision in, 74
    ligament-fixation buttons in, 78–79, 79f
    medial, 74
    notchplasty in, 74–75, 75f
    outcomes of, 81

Anterior cruciate ligament reconstruction (*continued*)
  pitfalls of, 81
  postoperative management of, 79–81
  preparation for, 73–74
  rehabilitation after, 80–81
  with patellar tendon substitution, 41–55
    diagnostic arthroscopy in, 44
    femoral tunnel preparation in, 47–51,
      48f–52f
    graft harvest in, 42, 43f
    graft passage in, 51–54, 52f, 53f
    graft preparation in, 43–44, 43f
    history of, 41–42
    indications for, 42
    notch preparation and notchplasty in,
      44–46, 45f
    outcomes of, 55
    pitfalls of, 54–55
    positioning for, 42
    rehabilitation after, 55
    surgical techniques for, 42–54
    tibial tunnel preparation in, 46–47, 46f, 48f
  with PCL reconstruction, 90
Anteromedial tibial tubercle transfer
  indications for, 123
  rehabilitation after, 128
  technique of, 124–128, 125f–128f
Arcuate-complex advancement, 105
Arcuate ligament, 96
Arthroplasty
  abrasion, for chondral defects, 27, 37, 146
  patellofemoral, 202–207
    history of, 202
    indications and contraindications for,
      202–203, 203f
    outcomes of, 207
    rehabilitation after, 207
    surgical techniques for, 203–206, 204f–206f
    technical alternatives and pitfalls of, 207
  total knee. *See* Total knee arthroplasty (TKA)
Arthroscopic biopsy, for articular autologous
      chondrocyte transplantation, 32–33
Arthroscopic meniscal repair, 1–8
  all-inside technique of, 7
  anesthesia for, 3
  complications of, 7
  contraindications to, 2–3
  fibrin clot in, 7
  history of, 1
  indications for, 1–2
  inside-out technique of, 5–7, 6f
  meniscal zones and, 1, 2f
  open technique of, 7
  outcomes of, 7–9, 8f
  outside-in technique of, 3–5, 4f
  positioning for, 3
  preoperative evaluation for, 1–2
  rehabilitation after, 7
  skin incisions for, 3
  surface anatomy in, 3

timing of, 2
vascular access channels in, 7
Arthroscopic reduction and internal fixation,
      for chondral and osteochondral
      lesions, 146–149, 147f–153f, 153–154
Arthroscopic treatment, of degenerative joint
      disease, 159–163
  history of, 159
  indications and contraindications for, 159
  outcomes and future directions of, 163
  rehabilitation after, 162
  surgical techniques for, 159–160, 160f–163f
  technical alternatives and pitfalls of, 161
Arthroscopy, diagnostic
  in ACL reconstruction
    with hamstring tendon graft, 59
    with miniarthrotomy, 73–74
    with patellar tendon substitution, 44
  of dislocation with lateral ligament injury,
      110–111, 110f
  in meniscal allograft reconstruction, 12
Arthroscopy-assisted ACL reconstruction, with
      patellar tendon substitution, 41
Arthroscopy-assisted meniscal allograft
      reconstruction, 10–22
  ACL reconstruction with, 10, 19–20
  alternative techniques for, 17–18
  bed preparation for, 12
  closure and dressing for, 14
  diagnostic arthroscopy prior to, 12
  future of, 21–22
  graft fixation in, 14, 17–18
  graft insertion in, 14, 15f, 17
  graft selection, sizing, and preparation for, 12,
      16
  history of, 10
  immunologic considerations in, 16–17
  indications for, 10–11
  osseous tunnel placement in, 12–14, 13f
  outcomes of, 18–21
  pitfalls of, 17–18
  positioning for, 12
  rehabilitation after, 18
  surgical techniques of, 11–14, 11f
Arthroscopy-assisted PCL reconstruction, 83–93
  with ACL reconstruction, 90
  anatomic factors in, 84, 84f
  debridement in, 86, 87f
  femoral tunnel in, 87–89, 89f
  future directions for, 93
  graft insertion and fixation in, 89–90, 90f
  graft preparation for, 85–86, 86f
  guide wire placement in, 86–87, 88f
  history of, 83
  indications and contraindications for, 83–84
  instrumentation for, 84, 85f
  outcomes of, 92
  pitfalls of, 91–92
  preparation for, 85
  rehabilitation after, 92

surgical techniques for, 84–90
technical alternatives in, 90–91
tibial tunnel in, 87, 88f, 89f
Arthrotomy
    mini-, for ACL reconstruction, 73–81
        bone plugs in, 78
        bone tunnels in, 76–77, 76f–78f
        diagnostic arthroscopy in, 73–74
        graft harvesting and preparation in, 77–78
        history of, 73
        indications for, 73
        lateral oblique incision in, 74
        ligament-fixation buttons in, 78–79, 79f
        medial, 74
        notchplasty in, 74–75, 75f
        outcomes of, 81
        pitfalls of, 81
        postoperative management of, 79–81
        preparation for, 73–74
        rehabilitation after, 80–81
    subvastus, for total knee arthroplasty,
            165–170
        future directions for, 170
        history of, 165
        indications and contraindications for, 165
        rehabilitation after, 169–170
        surgical techniques for, 166–168, 166f, 167f,
            169f
        technical alternatives and pitfalls of, 169
Articular autologous chondrocyte
            transplantation, 27, 32–39
    alternatives to, 36–38
    arthroscopic biopsy in, 32–33
    cell culture and expansion in, 33
    future directions in, 39
    history of, 32
    indications and contraindications for, 32
    outcomes of, 39
    rehabilitation after, 39
    surgical techniques for, 32–36, 33f–36f
Articular cartilage
    artificial, 156
    defined, 140
    structure of, 140
Articular cartilage defects
    abrasion arthroplasty for, 27, 37, 146
    autologous chondrocyte transplantation for,
            32–39
        arthroscopic biopsy in, 32–33
        cell culture and expansion in, 33
        future directions in, 39
        history of, 32
        indications and contraindications for, 32
        outcomes of, 39
        rehabilitation after, 39
        surgical techniques for, 32–36, 33f–36f, 146
        technical alternatives and pitfalls of, 36–38,
            152
    basic science of, 140–141
    classification of, 141

debridement for, 37, 144, 144f
microfracture procedure for, 23–31, 37–38
    alternatives to, 27
    contraindications to, 24
    future considerations for, 29–30
    history of, 23
    indications for, 23
    outcomes of, 28–29, 29f
    pitfalls of, 26, 29, 151
    rehabilitation after, 27–28, 27f
    surgical technique of, 24–26, 24f–26f, 144,
            144f, 145f, 146
nonoperative treatment of, 36–37
osteochondral transplantation for, 38–39,
            149–150, 154f, 155f, 156
perichondral transplantation for, 38, 146
periosteal transplantation for, 38, 146,
            151–152, 156
reduction and internal fixation for, 146–149,
            147f–153f, 153–154
repair vs. regeneration of, 141
subchondral drilling for, 37–38, 146, 151
surgical management of, 140–157
    biologic resurfacing technique for, 146
    choice of technique in, 142, 142f
    history of, 140
    indications for, 141–142
    marrow-stimulating technique for, 146
    osteochondral transplantation for, 149–150,
            154f, 155f
    outcomes of, 155–157
    reduction and internal fixation for, 146–149,
            147f–153f
    rehabilitation after, 155
    technical alternatives and pitfalls in,
            151–155
Autograft, for tibial defect reconstruction,
            246–252, 249f–251f
Autograft osteochondral transplantation, 38–39,
            149–150, 154f, 155f, 156
Autologous chondrocyte transplantation, 27,
            32–39
    arthroscopic biopsy in, 32–33
    cell culture and expansion in, 33
    future directions in, 39
    history of, 32
    indications and contraindications for, 32
    outcomes of, 39
    rehabilitation after, 39
    surgical techniques for, 32–36, 33f–36f, 146
    technical alternatives and pitfalls of, 36–38,
            152

B
Biceps tendon
    LCL augmentation with, 100, 100f, 103
    popliteus augmentation with, 99
Biceps tenodesis, 105
Biologic resurfacing techniques, for chondral
            and osteochondral lesions, 146

Bone defects
    classification of, 245, 246t
    management of, 245, 246t
    reconstruction of, 245, 246t. *See also* Tibial
        defect reconstruction
    in revision total knee arthroplasty, 295–296,
        296t
Bone-patellar tendon-bone (BPTB) autograft. *See
    also* Patellar tendon graft
    for ACL reconstruction, 57
Bone-tendon-bone graft
    for LCL reconstruction, 103, 104f
    for popliteus reconstruction, 101–102, 102f

C
Cartilage
    artificial, 156
    structure of, 140
Cartilage defects
    abrasion arthroplasty for, 27, 37, 146
    autologous chondrocyte transplantation for,
        32–39
        arthroscopic biopsy in, 32–33
        cell culture and expansion in, 33
        future directions in, 39
        history of, 32
        indications and contraindications for, 32
        outcomes of, 39
        rehabilitation after, 39
        surgical techniques for, 32–36, 33f–36f, 146
        technical alternatives and pitfalls of, 36–38,
            152
    basic science of, 140–141
    biologic resurfacing technique for, 146
    classification of, 141
    debridement for, 37, 144, 144f
    marrow-stimulating technique for, 146
    microfracture procedure for, 23–31, 37–38
        alternatives to, 27
        contraindications to, 24
        future considerations for, 29–30
        history of, 23
        indications for, 23
        outcomes of, 28–29, 29f
        pitfalls of, 26, 29, 151
        rehabilitation after, 27–28, 27f
        surgical technique of, 24–26, 24f–26f, 144,
            144f, 145f, 146
    nonoperative treatment of, 36–37
    osteochondral transplantation for, 38–39,
        149–150, 154f, 155f, 156
    perichondral transplantation for, 38, 146
    periosteal transplantation for, 38, 146,
        151–152, 156
    reduction and internal fixation for, 146–149,
        147f–153f, 153–154
    repair *vs.* regeneration of, 141
    subchondral drilling for, 37–38, 146, 151
    surgical management of, 140–157
        choice of technique in, 142, 142f

history of, 140
    indications for, 141–142
    outcomes of, 155–157
    rehabilitation after, 155
    technical alternatives and pitfalls in, 151–155
Chondral defects. *See* Cartilage defects
Chondral fracture, microfracture technique for,
    144, 144f, 145f
Chondral loose bodies, 144, 149, 149f–153f
Chondrocyte transplantation, autologous, 27,
    32–39
    alternatives to, 36–38
    arthroscopic biopsy in, 32–33
    cell culture and expansion in, 33
    future directions in, 39
    history of, 32
    indications and contraindications for, 32
    outcomes of, 39
    rehabilitation after, 39
    surgical techniques for, 32–36, 33f–36f, 146
Coblation, 163
Collateral ligaments. *See* Lateral collateral
        ligament (LCL); Medial collateral
        ligament (MCL)
Constrained implants, for valgus knee, 236
Coronary ligament, 96
Cruciate ligament
    anterior. *See* Anterior cruciate ligament (ACL)
    posterior. *See* Posterior cruciate ligament
        (PCL)

D
Debridement
    for chondral defects, 37, 144, 144f
    for PCL reconstruction, 86, 87f
Degenerative joint disease, arthroscopic
        treatment of, 159–163
    history of, 159
    indications and contraindications for, 159
    outcomes and future directions of, 163
    rehabilitation after, 162
    surgical techniques for, 159–160, 160f–163f
    technical alternatives and pitfalls of, 161
Dislocation(s)
    evaluation of, 108–109
    nonoperative treatment of, 120
    open, 109
    peroneal nerve injuries with, 109
Dislocation repair, 108–121
    anesthesia for, 109
    history of, 108
    indications and contraindications for, 108–109
    with lateral ligament injury, 110–116
        arthroscopy of, 110–111, 110f
        closure in, 116
        cruciate and lateral graft tensioning and
            fixation in, 116
        cruciate femoral tunnel placement for,
            112–113
        cruciate graft passage for, 113

cruciate graft preparation for, 111
cruciate tibial tunnel placement for,
    111–112, 112f
LCL reconstruction in, 114f, 115
popliteus reconstruction in, 115–116, 115f
postoperative radiographs of, 116, 117f
surgical approach for, 113–116
with medial ligament injury, 117–119, 118f
outcomes of, 121
pitfalls of, 120
rehabilitation after, 121
surgical approach and conditioning for,
    109–110
technical alternatives in, 119–121
Distal femoral osteotomy, 186–191
for combined deformities, 191
history of, 186
indications and contraindications for, 186,
    187f
with lateral plate fixation, 189–191, 190f
lateral tibial plateau allograft and, 195f, 197,
    198f
with medial plate fixation, 187–189, 188f
outcomes of, 191
rehabilitation after, 191
surgical techniques for, 186–191, 196f
Distal tibial tubercle medial transfer, in patellar
    instability repair, 133–135, 134f
Double looped hamstring tendon graft, ACL
    reconstruction with, 57–71
diagnostic arthroscopy in, 59
graft harvest in, 59–60, 60f–62f
graft insertion and fixation in, 64–70, 68f, 69f
graft preparation in, 60–63
history of, 57–58
indications for, 58
outcomes of, 71
positioning and preparation for, 58
rehabilitation after, 70
surgical techniques for, 58–70
technical alternatives in, 70
tunnel placement and creation in, 63–64,
    65f–67f
Duocondylar prosthesis, 209
Duopatellar prosthesis, 209

E
Elmslie-Trillat procedure, 130
modified, 130–139
closure in, 135
complications of, 136–137, 137f
contraindications for, 131
distal tibial tubercle medial transfer in,
    133–135, 134f
future directions in, 139
history of, 130
indications for, 130–131
lateral release in, 132
medial reefing in, 135, 135f

outcomes of, 138–139
pitfalls of, 136–137, 137f
postoperative management of, 136
preoperative preparation for, 131–132
rehabilitation after, 137–138
surgical techniques for, 131–136, 133f–135f
technical alternatives in, 136
vertical incision in, 132, 133f
EndoButton
in ACL reconstruction, with hamstring
    tendon graft, 64–69, 65f–68f
in popliteofibular ligament reconstruction,
    115–116, 115f
Endoscopic ACL reconstruction
with double looped hamstring tendon graft,
    57–71
diagnostic arthroscopy in, 59
graft harvest in, 59–60, 60f–62f
graft insertion and fixation in, 64–70, 68f,
    69f
graft preparation in, 60–63
history of, 57–58
indications for, 58
outcomes of, 71
positioning and preparation for, 58
rehabilitation after, 70
surgical techniques for, 58–70
technical alternatives in, 70
tunnel placement and creation in, 63–64,
    65f–67f
with patellar tendon substitution, 41–55
diagnostic arthroscopy in, 44
femoral tunnel preparation in, 47–51,
    48f–52f
graft harvest in, 42, 43f
graft passage in, 51–54, 52f, 53f
graft preparation in, 43–44, 43f
history of, 41–42
indications for, 42
notch preparation and notchplasty in,
    44–46, 45f
outcomes of, 55
pitfalls of, 54–55
positioning for, 42
rehabilitation after, 55
surgical techniques for, 42–54
tibial tunnel preparation in, 46–47, 46f, 48f
Epicondylar line, 227
Epicondyles, with meniscal bearing knee,
    227–228
Extensor mechanism reconstruction, with
    semitendinosus graft, 274–279
history of, 274
indications and contraindications for, 274–275
outcomes of, 278–279
rehabilitation after, 278
surgical techniques for, 275–276, 276f
technical alternatives and pitfalls of, 276–278,
    277f
External rotation recurvatum test, 95

F
Fabellofibular ligament, 96
Femoral component rotation, in revision total
          knee arthroplasty, 296, 299, 297f–298f,
          300f
Femoral component sizing, in revision total
          knee arthroplasty, 297
Femoral guide wires, for PCL reconstruction,
          87, 88f
Femoral osteotomy, distal, 186–191
    for combined deformities, 191
    history of, 186
    indications and contraindications for, 186, 187f
    with lateral plate fixation, 189–191, 190f
    lateral tibial plateau allograft and, 195f, 197,
          198f
    with medial plate fixation, 187–189, 188f
    outcomes of, 191
    rehabilitation after, 191
    surgical techniques for, 186–191, 196f
Femoral tunnel
    for ACL reconstruction
        with hamstring tendon graft, 63–64, 65f–67f
        with miniarthrotomy, 76–77, 78f
        with patellar tendon substitution, 47–51,
          48f–52f
    for dislocation with lateral ligament injury,
          112–113
    for PCL reconstruction, 87–89, 89f
    for popliteus reconstruction, 101–102
Femorotibial angle, 186, 187f
Fibrin clot, in arthroscopic meniscal repair, 7
Fibular origin, of popliteus muscle, 98, 98f
Fixed flexion contracture correction, 257–263
    history of, 257
    indications for, 257, 258f
    outcomes of, 263
    pitfalls of, 263
    rehabilitation after, 263
    surgical techniques for, 257–263, 258f–262f
Free flaps, after total knee replacement,
          280–281, 286–289, 286f–289f
Freeman-Swanson prosthesis, 209
Free-tissue transfers, after total knee
          replacement, 281
Fresh osteochondral allografts, for
          posttraumatic knee defects, 193–200
    graft procurement in, 194
    history of, 193
    indications and contraindications for, 193–194
    outcomes of, 197–200, 199t
    procedure for, 194–197, 194f–196f, 198f
    rehabilitation after, 197
Fulkerson procedure, 130, 131, 136

G
Gastrocnemius muscle transposition flap, after
          total knee replacement
    lateral, 285–286, 285f
    medial, 282–285, 282f–284f

Genu valgum. See Valgus knee
Gracilis muscle flap, after total knee
          replacement, 280–281
Gracilis tendon, in ACL reconstruction with
          hamstring tendon graft, 63, 70
Graft. See Allograft; Autograft; Hamstring
          tendon graft; Patellar tendon graft

H
Hamstring tendon graft
    ACL reconstruction with, 57–71
        diagnostic arthroscopy in, 59
        graft harvest in, 59–60, 60f–62f
        graft insertion and fixation in, 64–70, 68f, 69f
        graft preparation in, 60–63
        history of, 57–58
        indications for, 58
        outcomes of, 71
        positioning and preparation for, 58
        rehabilitation after, 70
        surgical techniques for, 58–70
        technical alternatives in, 70
        tunnel placement and creation in, 63–64,
          65f–67f
    PCL reconstruction with, 91
High tibial osteotomy (HTO), 178–185
    history of, 178
    indications and contraindications for, 178
    medial femoral condylar allograft and, 194f,
          197, 198f
    outcomes of, 185
    preoperative planning for, 178–180, 179f, 180f
    preparation for, 180
    procedure for, 181–184, 181f–184f
    rehabilitation after, 185
    technical alternatives and pitfalls of, 184–185
Hyaline cartilage, defined, 140

I
Iliotibial band, popliteus augmentation with, 99,
          99f
Iliotibial band release, for valgus knee, 231, 233,
          235
Immunologic considerations, in meniscal
          allograft reconstruction, 16–17
Impaction grafting, for tibial defect
          reconstruction, 253
Insall-Burstein total knee replacement, 223–224
Insall "dovetail" technique, for tibial defect
          reconstruction, 246–247, 249, 249f

J
Joint-line height, in revision total knee
          arthroplasty, 299–300
J sign, in patellar instability, 131

K
Kinematic conflict, 216

L

Laminar spreaders, for valgus knee, 235, 235f

Laskin technique, for tibial defect
        reconstruction, 247, 251–252, 251f

Lateral collateral ligament (LCL) augmentation,
        100, 100f, 103

Lateral collateral ligament (LCL) release, for
        valgus knee, 233–234

Lateral collateral ligament (LCL) repair, 95–106
    for acute injuries, 100, 100f
    anatomical basis for, 96–98, 97f, 98f
    for chronic injuries, 102–103, 104f
    with cruciate ligament repair, 105–106
    for dislocation, 114f, 115
    history of, 95
    outcomes of, 106
    with popliteus repair, 101, 103–104, 104f
    rehabilitation after, 106
    technical alternatives in, 105–106

Lateral corner repair, 95–106
    for acute injuries, 98–101, 99f, 100f
    anatomical basis for, 96–98, 97f, 98f
    for chronic injuries, 101–104, 102f–104f
    for combined injuries, 101, 103–104, 104f
    with cruciate ligament repair, 105–106
    for dislocation, 113–116, 114f, 115f, 117f
    history of, 95
    indications for, 95–96
    for LCL injuries, 100, 100f, 102–103, 104f
    outcomes of, 106
    for popliteal injuries, 98–99, 99f, 101–102,
        102f, 103f
    rehabilitation after, 106
    technical alternatives in, 105–106

Lateral femoral condyle, in valgus knee, 231,
        232f, 234

Lateral gastrocnemius muscle transposition
        flap, after total knee replacement, 280,
        285–286, 285f

Lateral ligament injury, dislocation repair with,
        110–116
    arthroscopy of, 110–111, 110f
    closure in, 116
    cruciate and lateral graft tensioning and
        fixation in, 116
    cruciate femoral tunnel placement for,
        112–113
    cruciate graft passage for, 113
    cruciate graft preparation for, 111
    cruciate tibial tunnel placement for, 111–112,
        112f
    LCL reconstruction in, 114f, 115
    popliteus reconstruction in, 115–116, 115f
    postoperative radiographs of, 116, 117f
    surgical approach for, 113–116

Lateral plate fixation, for valgus knee, 189–191,
        190f

Lateral release
    history of, 123
    indications for, 123

outcomes of, 128–129
    in patellar instability repair, 132
    pitfalls of, 128
    rehabilitation after, 128
    technique of, 123–124

Lateral tibial plateau allograft, 195f, 197, 198f

Latissimus dorsi muscle flap, after total knee
        replacement, 281

LCL. See Lateral collateral ligament (LCL)

Ligament-fixation buttons, in ACL
        reconstruction with miniarthrotomy,
        78–79, 79f

M

Marrow-stimulating techniques, for chondral
        and osteochondral lesions, 146

Medial collateral ligament (MCL) injury,
        dislocation with, 117–119, 118f, 119f

Medial collateral ligament (MCL) release, for
        varus knee, 240, 243

Medial compartment arthritis, high tibial
        osteotomy for, 178–185
    history of, 178
    indications and contraindications for, 178
    outcomes of, 185
    preoperative planning for, 178–180, 179f, 180f
    preparation for, 180
    procedure for, 181–184, 181f–184f
    rehabilitation after, 185
    technical alternatives and pitfalls of, 184–185

Medial femoral condylar allograft, 194f, 197,
        198f

Medial gastrocnemius muscle transposition
        flap, after total knee replacement, 280,
        282–285, 282f–284f

Medial plate fixation, for valgus knee, 187–189,
        188f

Medial reefing, in patellar instability repair, 135,
        135f

Medial retinaculum transfer, in patellar
        instability repair, 135, 135f

Meniscal allograft reconstruction, 10–22
    ACL reconstruction with, 10, 19–20
    alternative techniques for, 17–18
    bed preparation for, 12
    closure and dressing for, 14
    diagnostic arthroscopy prior to, 12
    future of, 21–22
    graft fixation in, 14, 17–18
    graft insertion in, 14, 15f, 17
    graft selection, sizing, and preparation for, 12,
        16
    history of, 10
    immunologic considerations in, 16–17
    indications for, 10–11
    osseous tunnel placement in, 12–14, 13f
    outcomes of, 18–21
    pitfalls of, 17–18
    positioning for, 12
    rehabilitation after, 18

Meniscal allograft reconstruction (*continued*)
  surgical techniques of, 11–14, 11f
Meniscal bearing knee, 221–229
  contact areas of, 222
  design of, 221–222
  femoral component of, 221, 222f, 227
  history of, 221–222
  indications and contraindications for,
      222–224, 223f
  outcomes of, 228–229, 229f
  posterior cruciate ligament with, 222,
      223–224, 226, 226f
  rehabilitation after, 228
  surgical techniques for, 224–227, 225f, 226f
  technical alternatives and pitfalls of, 227–228
  tibial component of, 222, 222f
Meniscal repair, arthroscopic, 1–8
  all-inside technique of, 7
  anesthesia for, 3
  complications of, 7
  contraindications to, 2–3
  fibrin clot in, 7
  history of, 1
  indications for, 1–2
  inside-out technique of, 5–7, 6f
  meniscal zones and, 1, 2f
  open technique of, 7
  outcomes of, 7–9, 8f
  outside-in technique of, 3–5, 4f
  positioning for, 3
  preoperative evaluation for, 1–2
  rehabilitation after, 7
  skin incisions for, 3
  surface anatomy in, 3
  timing of, 2
  vascular access channels in, 7
Meniscal zones, 1, 2f
Menisci, functions of, 1, 10
Mercer-Merchant patellar view, 131, 131f
Metal-backed patellar button, removal of,
      268–271, 269f–272f
Microfracture procedure, for chondral defects,
      23–31
  alternatives to, 27
  contraindications to, 24
  future considerations for, 29–30
  history of, 23
  indications for, 23
  outcomes for, 28–29
  pitfalls of, 26, 29, 151
  rehabilitation after, 27–28, 27f
  surgical technique of, 24–26, 24f–26f, 144,
      144f, 145f, 146
Miniarthrotomy, for ACL reconstruction, 73–81
  bone plugs in, 78
  bone tunnels in, 76–77, 76f–78f
  diagnostic arthroscopy in, 73–74
  graft harvesting and preparation in, 77–78
  history of, 73
  indications for, 73

  lateral oblique incision in, 74
  ligament-fixation buttons in, 78–79, 79f
  medial, 74
  notchplasty in, 74–75, 75f
  outcomes of, 81
  pitfalls of, 81
  postoperative management of, 79–81
  preparation for, 73–74
  rehabilitation after, 80–81
Mobile bearing knee. *See* Meniscal bearing knee
Modular implants, for tibial defect
      reconstruction, 247, 252
Mosaic plasty, osteochondral autograft
      transplantation and, for chondral
      defects, 38–39
Multiple ligament reconstruction, 108–121
  anesthesia for, 109
  for dislocation with lateral ligament injury,
      110–116
    arthroscopy of, 110–111, 110f
    closure in, 116
    cruciate and lateral graft tensioning and
        fixation in, 116
    cruciate femoral tunnel placement for,
        112–113
    cruciate graft passage for, 113
    cruciate graft preparation for, 111
    cruciate tibial tunnel placement for,
        111–112, 112f
    LCL reconstruction in, 114f, 115
    popliteus reconstruction in, 115–116, 115f
    postoperative radiographs of, 116, 117f
    surgical approach for, 113–116
  for dislocation with medial ligament injury,
      117–119, 118f
  history of, 108
  indications and contraindications for, 108–109
  outcomes of, 121
  pitfalls of, 120
  rehabilitation after, 121
  surgical approach and conditioning for,
      109–110
  technical alternatives in, 119–121
Muscle flaps, after total knee replacement
  gracilis, 280–281
  lateral gastrocnemius, 280, 285–286, 285f
  latissimus dorsi, 281
  medial gastrocnemius, 280, 282–285,
      282f–284f
  rectus abdominis, 286–289, 286f–289f

N

Notchplasty, in ACL reconstruction
  with miniarthrotomy, 74–75, 75f
  with patellar tendon substitution, 44–46, 45f
"No thumb" test, 226–227

O

OCD. *See* Osteochondritis dissecans (OCD)

Open reduction and internal fixation, for
        chondral and osteochondral lesions,
        146–149, 147f–153f, 153–154
Osteochondral allograft transplantation, 150,
        156
    for posttraumatic knee defects, 193–200
        graft procurement in, 194
        history of, 193
        indications and contraindications for,
                193–194
        outcomes of, 197–200, 199t
        procedure for, 194–197, 194f–196f, 198f
        rehabilitation after, 197
Osteochondral autograft transplantation,
        149–150, 154f, 155f, 156
    and mosaic plasty, 38–39
Osteochondral defects
    abrasion arthroplasty for, 146
    autologous chondrocyte transplantation for,
        146
    basic science of, 140–141
    biologic resurfacing technique for, 146
    classification of, 141
    fresh osteochondral allografts for, 193–200
        graft procurement in, 194
        history of, 193
        indications and contraindications for,
                193–194
        outcomes of, 197–200, 199t
        procedure for, 194–197, 194f–196f, 198f
        rehabilitation after, 197
    marrow-stimulating technique for, 146
    microfracture procedure for, 144, 144f, 145f,
        146
    osteochondral transplantation for, 149–150,
        154f, 155f
    periosteal transplantation for, 146
    reduction and internal fixation for, 146–149,
        147f–153f
    subchondral drilling for, 146
    surgical management of, 140–157
        choice of technique in, 142–144, 143f
        history of, 140
        indications for, 141–142
        outcomes of, 155–157
        rehabilitation after, 155
        technical alternatives and pitfalls in,
                151–155
Osteochondral fracture fragments, 144, 149,
        149f–153f
Osteochondral loose bodies, 144, 149, 149f–153f
Osteochondritis dissecans (OCD), surgical
        repair of
    biologic resurfacing techniques for, 146
    choice of technique for, 142–144, 143f
    indications for, 141, 142
    reduction and internal fixation for, 147–149,
        147f, 148f
Osteotomy
    distal femoral, 186–191

for combined deformities, 191
    history of, 186
    indications and contraindications for, 186,
        187f
    with lateral plate fixation, 189–191, 190f
    with medial plate fixation, 187–189, 188f
    outcomes of, 191
    rehabilitation after, 191
    surgical techniques for, 186–191
high tibial, 178–185
    history of, 178
    indications and contraindications for, 178
    outcomes of, 185
    preoperative planning for, 178–180, 179f,
        180f
    preparation for, 180
    procedure for, 181–184, 181f–184f
    rehabilitation after, 185
    technical alternatives and pitfalls of,
        184–185
Outerbridge classification, for articular cartilage
        lesions, 141

P
Pain, after total knee arthroplasty, 293
Particular bone graft, for tibial defect
        reconstruction, 247, 248f
Patella
    proximal shift of, 175, 176f
    in revision total knee arthroplasty, 300, 301f
Patella alta, 274
Patellar button, removal of metal-backed,
        268–271, 269f–272f
Patellar instability, modified Elmslie-Trillat
        procedure for, 130–139
    closure in, 135
    complications of, 136–137, 137f
    contraindications for, 131
    distal tibial tubercle medial transfer in,
        133–135, 134f
    future directions in, 139
    history of, 130
    indications for, 130–131
    lateral release in, 132
    medial reefing in, 135, 135f
    outcomes of, 138–139
    pitfalls of, 136–137, 137f
    postoperative management of, 136
    preoperative preparation for, 131–132
    rehabilitation after, 137–138
    surgical techniques for, 131–136, 133f–135f
    technical alternatives in, 136
    vertical incision in, 132, 133f
Patellar tendon graft
    for ACL reconstruction
        endoscopic, 41–55
            diagnostic arthroscopy in, 44
            femoral tunnel preparation in, 47–51,
                48f–52f
            graft harvest in, 42, 43f

Patellar tendon graft (*continued*)
  graft passage in, 51–54, 52f, 53f
  graft preparation in, 43–44, 43f
  history of, 41–42
  indications for, 42
  notch preparation and notchplasty in,
    44–46, 45f
  outcomes of, 55
  pitfalls of, 54–55
  positioning for, 42
  rehabilitation after, 55
  surgical techniques for, 42–54
  tibial tunnel preparation in, 46–47, 46f,
    48f
  with miniarthrotomy, 73–81
    bone plugs in, 78
    bone tunnels in, 76–77, 76f–78f
    diagnostic arthroscopy in, 73–74
    graft harvesting and preparation in,
      77–78
    history of, 73
    indications for, 73
    lateral oblique incision in, 74
    ligament-fixation buttons in, 78–79, 79f
    medial, 74
    notchplasty in, 74–75, 75f
    outcomes of, 81
    pitfalls of, 81
    postoperative management of, 79–81
    preparation for, 73–74
    rehabilitation after, 80–81
  for dislocation with lateral ligament injury,
    111
  for PCL reconstruction, 91
  for popliteus reconstruction, 102, 103f
Patellar tendon rupture, semitendinosus graft
    for, 274–279
  history of, 274
  indications and contraindications for, 274–275
  outcomes of, 278–279
  rehabilitation after, 278
  surgical techniques for, 275–276, 276f
  technical alternatives and pitfalls of, 276–278,
    277f
Patellofemoral replacement, 202–207
  history of, 202
  indications and contraindications for,
    202–203, 203f
  outcomes of, 207
  rehabilitation after, 207
  surgical techniques for, 203–206, 204f–206f
  technical alternatives and pitfalls of, 207
PCL. *See* Posterior cruciate ligament (PCL)
Perichondral transplantation, for chondral
    defects, 38, 146
Periosteal patch, for articular autologous
    chondrocyte transplantation, 34–36,
    35f, 36f
Periosteal transplantation, for chondral defects,
    38, 146, 151–152, 156

Peroneal nerve injuries, with dislocations, 109
Pes planus, from valgus knee alignment, 236
PLRI (posterolateral rotatory instability), 95
Polymethylmethacrylate (PMMA), for tibial
    defect reconstruction, 245–246, 247,
    248f, 251, 252, 253
Popliteofibular fascicle, 98, 98f
Popliteofibular ligament, 98, 98f
Popliteofibular ligament reconstruction, 102,
    103f
  after dislocation, 115–116, 115f
Popliteus augmentation, 99, 99f
Popliteus bypass procedure, 105
Popliteus muscle, fibular origin of, 98, 98f
Popliteus repair, 95–106
  for acute injuries, 98–99, 99f
  anatomical basis for, 96–98, 97f, 98f
  for chronic injuries, 101–102, 102f, 103f
  with cruciate ligament repair, 105–106
  for dislocation, 115–116, 115f
  history of, 95
  with LCL repair, 101, 103–104, 104f
  outcomes of, 106
  rehabilitation after, 106
  technical alternatives in, 105–106
Popliteus tendon recession, 105
Posterior cruciate ligament (PCL)
  in fixed flexion contracture correction,
    260–262, 261f, 262f
  normal anatomy of, 84, 84f
Posterior cruciate ligament (PCL) recession,
    215–216, 215f
  with meniscal bearing knee, 226, 226f
Posterior cruciate ligament (PCL) reconstruction
  arthroscopy-assisted, 83–93
    with ACL reconstruction, 90
    anatomic factors in, 84, 84f
    debridement in, 86, 87f
    femoral tunnel in, 87–89, 89f
    future directions for, 93
    graft insertion and fixation in, 89–90, 90f
    graft preparation for, 85–86, 86f
    guide wire placement in, 86–87, 88f
    history of, 83
    indications and contraindications for, 83–84
    instrumentation for, 84, 85f
    outcomes of, 92
    pitfalls of, 91–92
    preparation for, 85
    rehabilitation after, 92
    surgical techniques for, 84–90
    technical alternatives in, 90–91
    tibial tunnel in, 87, 88f, 89f
  for dislocation with lateral ligament injury,
    110–113, 110f, 112f, 116
Posterior cruciate ligament (PCL)-retaining
    arthroplasty, 209, 210–215, 211f–215f,
    217
Posterior cruciate ligament (PCL)-substituting
    arthroplasty, 209, 216–217, 216f

with meniscal bearing knee, 223–224
Posterior stabilized arthroplasty, 209, 216–217,
          216f
    with meniscal bearing knee, 223–224
Posterolateral corner repair, 95–106
    for acute injuries, 98–101, 99f, 100f
    anatomical basis for, 96–98, 97f, 98f
    for chronic injuries, 101–104, 102f–104f
    for combined injuries, 101, 103–104, 104f
    with cruciate ligament repair, 105–106
    for dislocation, 113–116, 114f, 115f, 117f
    history of, 95
    indications for, 95–96
    for LCL injuries, 100, 100f, 102–103, 104f
    outcomes of, 106
    for popliteal injuries, 98–99, 99f, 101–102,
          102f, 103f
    rehabilitation after, 106
    technical alternatives in, 105–106
Posterolateral drawer test, 95
Posterolateral rotatory instability (PLRI), 95
Posttraumatic knee defects, fresh osteochondral
          allografts for, 193–200
    graft procurement in, 194
    history of, 193
    indications and contraindications for, 193–194
    outcomes of, 197–200, 199t
    procedure for, 194–197, 194f–196f, 198f
    rehabilitation after, 197

Q
Q angle, in patellar instability repair, 130, 133

R
Rectus abdominis muscle transfer flap, after
          total knee replacement, 286–288,
          286f–289f
Reduction and internal fixation, for chondral
          and osteochondral lesions, 146–149,
          147f–153f, 153–154
Rehabilitation
    after ACL reconstruction
        with hamstring tendon graft, 70
        with miniarthrotomy, 80–81
        with patellar tendon substitution, 55
    after allograft for posttraumatic knee defect,
          197
    after arthroscopic meniscal repair, 7
    after arthroscopic treatment of degenerative
          joint disease, 162
    after articular autologous chondrocyte
          transplantation, 39
    after distal femoral osteotomy, 191
    after extensor mechanism reconstruction, 278
    after fixed flexion contracture correction, 263
    after high tibial osteotomy, 185
    after meniscal allograft reconstruction, 18
    with meniscal bearing knee, 228
    after microfracture procedure for chondral
          defects, 27–28, 27f

after modified Elmslie-Trillat procedure,
          137–138
    after multiple ligament reconstruction, 121
    after osteochondral transplantation, 155
    after patellofemoral replacement, 207
    after PCL reconstruction, 92
    after posterolateral corner repair, 106
    after resurfacing techniques, 155
    after soft tissue releases
        for valgus knee, 236–237
        for varus knee, 244
    after subvastus arthrotomy, 169–170
    after supracondylar fracture repair, 266
    after tibial defect reconstruction, 254
    after tibial tuberosity elevation, 176
    after total knee arthroplasty, 217–218
        revision, 302
        with subvastus arthrotomy, 169–170
    after wound problem repair, 290
Resurfacing technique, for chondral and
          osteochondral lesions, 146
Retinacular release
    history of, 123
    indications for, 123
    outcomes of, 128–129
    pitfalls of, 128
    rehabilitation after, 128
    technique of, 123–124
Revision total knee arthroplasty, 291–303
    bone defects in, 295–296, 296t
    extension in, 292f, 299–300
    femoral component rotation in, 296–299,
          297f–298f, 300f
    femoral component sizing in, 299
    history of, 291
    indications and contraindications for,
          292–294, 292t, 294f
    outcomes of, 303
    patella in, 300–301, 301f
    reestablishment of joint-line height in,
          299–300
    rehabilitation after, 303
    stabilization of knee in flexion in, 292f,
          296–300
    surgical techniques for, 292f, 294–300
    technical alternatives and pitfalls of, 301–302
    tibial platform in, 292f, 294–295, 295f
Roux-Goldthwait procedure, 130, 136
Rush rods, for supracondylar fracture repair,
          264–267, 265f–267f

S
Sculco technique, for tibial defect
          reconstruction, 246–247, 249–251, 250f
Semitendinosus graft
    ACL reconstruction with, 57–71
        diagnostic arthroscopy in, 59
        graft harvest in, 59–60, 60f–62f
        graft insertion and fixation in, 64–70, 68f,
          69f

Semitendinosus graft (*continued*)
  graft preparation in, 60–63
  history of, 57–58
  indications for, 58
  outcomes of, 71
  positioning and preparation for, 58
  rehabilitation after, 70
  surgical techniques for, 58–70
  technical alternatives in, 70
  tunnel placement and creation in, 63–64,
    65f–67f
  extensor mechanism reconstruction with,
    274–279
  history of, 274
  indications and contraindications for,
    274–275
  outcomes of, 278–279
  rehabilitation after, 278
  surgical techniques for, 275–276, 276f
  technical alternatives and pitfalls of,
    276–278, 277f
Short lateral ligament, 96
Soft-tissue expanders, after total knee
    replacement, 281
Soft tissue releases
  for valgus knee, 231–237
    history of, 231
    indications and contraindications for,
      231–233, 232f
    outcomes of, 237
    rehabilitation after, 236–237
    surgical techniques for, 233–235, 235f
    technical alternatives and pitfalls of, 236
  for varus knee, 239–244
    history of, 239
    indications and contraindications for,
      239–240
    outcomes and future directions for, 244
    rehabilitation after, 244
    surgical techniques for, 240–243, 242f
    technical alternatives and pitfalls of,
      243–244
Static alignment, 234–235
Subchondral drilling, for chondral defects,
    37–38, 146, 151
Subvastus arthrotomy, for total knee
    arthroplasty, 165–170
  future directions for, 170
  history of, 165
  indications and contraindications for, 165
  rehabilitation after, 169–170
  surgical techniques for, 166–168, 166f, 167f,
    169f
  technical alternatives and pitfalls of, 169
Supracondylar fractures, after total knee
    replacement, 264–267, 265f–267f

T
Tibial defect reconstruction, 245–255
  allograft for, 247, 252–253, 253f

autograft for, 246–252, 249f–251f
cement and particulate bone graft for, 247,
    248f
future directions in, 254–255
history of, 245
impaction grafting for, 253
indications and contraindications for,
    245–247, 246t
Insall "dovetail" technique for, 246–247, 249,
    249f
Laskin technique for, 247, 251–252, 251f
modular and special implants for, 247, 252
rehabilitation after, 254
in revision total knee arthroplasty, 295–296,
    296t
Sculco technique for, 246–247, 249–251, 250f
technical alternatives and pitfalls of, 253–254
Tibial guide wires, for PCL reconstruction,
    86–87, 88f
Tibial osteotomy, high, 178–185
  history of, 178
  indications and contraindications for, 178
  medial femoral condylar allograft and, 194f,
    197, 198f
  outcomes of, 185
  preoperative planning for, 178–180, 179f, 180f
  preparation for, 180
  procedure for, 181–184, 181f–184f
  rehabilitation after, 185
  technical alternatives and pitfalls of, 184–185
Tibial platform, in revision total knee
    arthroplasty, 292f, 294–295, 295f
Tibial tuberosity elevation, 171–177
  discussion of, 176–177
  history of, 171
  indications for, 171
  rehabilitation after, 176
  surgical techniques for, 172–176, 172f–176f
  technical alternatives and pitfalls of, 176
Tibial tunnel
  for ACL reconstruction
    with hamstring tendon graft, 63–64
    with miniarthrotomy, 76, 76f, 77f
    with patellar tendon substitution, 46–47,
      46f
  for dislocation with lateral ligament injury,
    111–112, 112f
  for PCL reconstruction, 87, 88f, 89f
  for popliteus reconstruction, 101, 102f
Toradol, after ACL reconstruction with
    miniarthrotomy, 80
Total knee arthroplasty (TKA), 209–218
  classic alignment in, 210–211, 211f, 234
  evaluation with trial components in, 213–215,
    213f, 214f
  femoral component rotation in, 211
  fixed flexion contracture correction in,
    257–263
    history of, 257
    indications for, 257, 258f

outcomes of, 263
pitfalls of, 263
rehabilitation after, 263
surgical techniques for, 257–263, 258f–262f
history of, 209
indications and contraindications for, 210
Insall-Burstein replacement in, 223–224
instrumentation for, 210
meniscal bearing knee in, 221–229
    contact areas of, 222
    design of, 221–222
    femoral component of, 221, 222f, 227
    history of, 221–222
    indications and contraindications for,
        222–224, 223f
    outcomes of, 228–229, 229f
    posterior cruciate ligament with, 222,
        223–224, 226, 226f
    rehabilitation after, 228
    surgical techniques for, 224–227, 225f, 226f
    technical alternatives and pitfalls of,
        227–228
    tibial component of, 222, 222f
outcomes of, 218
pain after, 293
PCL recession in, 215–216, 215f
PCL-retaining, 209, 210–215, 211f–215f, 217
PCL-substituting, 209, 216–217, 216f
posterior stabilized, 209, 216–217, 216f
proximal shift of patella prior to, 175, 176f
reconstruction of patellar tendon rupture
        after, 274–279
    history of, 274
    indications and contraindications for,
        274–275
    outcomes of, 278–279
    rehabilitation after, 278
    surgical techniques for, 275–276, 276f
    technical alternatives and pitfalls of,
        276–278, 277f
rehabilitation after, 217–218
removal of metal-backed patellar button
        after, 268–271, 269f–272f
revision, 291–303
    bone defects in, 295–296, 296t
    extension in, 292f, 299–300
    femoral component rotation in, 296, 299,
        297f–298f, 300f
    femoral component sizing in, 299
    history of, 291
    indications and contraindications for,
        292–294, 292t, 294f
    outcomes of, 303
    patella in, 300–301, 301f
    reestablishment of joint-line height in, 299
    rehabilitation after, 303
    stabilization of knee in flexion in, 292f,
        296–300
    surgical techniques for, 292f, 294–300
    technical alternatives and pitfalls of, 301–302

tibial platform in, 292f, 294–295, 295f
spacer blocks in, 213, 234–235
subvastus arthrotomy for, 165–170
    future directions for, 170
    history of, 165
    indications and contraindications for, 165
    rehabilitation after, 169–170
    surgical techniques for, 166–168, 166f, 167f,
        169f
    technical alternatives and pitfalls of, 169
supracondylar fractures after, 264–267,
        265f–267f
surgical techniques for, 210–217, 211f–216f
technical alternatives and pitfalls of, 217
tibial defect reconstruction in, 245–255
    allograft for, 247, 252–253, 253f
    autograft for, 246–252, 249f–251f
    cement and particulate bone graft for, 247,
        248f
    future directions in, 254–255
    history of, 245
    impaction grafting for, 253
    indications and contraindications for,
        245–247, 246t
    Insall "dovetail" technique for, 246–247,
        249, 249f
    Laskin technique for, 247, 251–252, 251f
    modular and special implants for, 247, 252
    rehabilitation after, 254
    Sculco technique for, 247–248, 249–251, 250f
    technical alternatives and pitfalls of,
        253–254
tibial tuberosity elevation prior to, 171–177
    discussion of, 176–177
    history of, 171
    indications for, 171
    rehabilitation after, 176
    surgical techniques for, 172–176, 172f–176f
    technical alternatives and pitfalls of, 176
wound coverage after, 280–289
    free flaps for, 280–281, 286–289, 286f–289f
    free-tissue transfers for, 281
    gracilis muscle flap for, 280–281
    history of, 280
    indications and contraindications for,
        280–281, 281f
    lateral gastrocnemius muscle transposition
        flap for, 280, 285–286, 285f
    latissimus dorsi muscle flap for, 281
    medial gastrocnemius muscle transposition
        flap for, 280, 282–285, 282f–284f
    outcomes of, 290
    pitfalls of, 289–290
    rectus abdominis muscle transfer for,
        286–289, 286f–289f
    rehabilitation after, 289
    soft-tissue expanders for, 281
Traumatic knee defects, fresh osteochondral
        allografts for, 150, 156
    for posttraumatic knee defects, 193–200

Traumatic knee defects (*continued*)
    graft procurement in, 194
    history of, 193
    indications and contraindications for,
        193–194
    outcomes of, 197–200, 199t
    procedure for, 194–197, 194f–196f, 198f
    rehabilitation after, 197

U
Unicompartmental replacement, 217

V
Valgus knee
    distal femoral osteotomy for, 186–191
        for combined deformities, 191
        history of, 186
        indications and contraindications for, 186,
            187f
        with lateral plate fixation, 189–191, 190f
        with medial plate fixation, 187–189, 188f
        outcomes of, 191
        rehabilitation after, 191
        surgical techniques for, 186–191
    soft tissue releases for, 231–237
        history of, 231
        indications and contraindications for,
            231–233, 232f
        outcomes of, 237
        rehabilitation after, 236–237
        surgical techniques for, 233–235, 235f
        technical alternatives and pitfalls of, 236
Varus knee, soft tissue releases for, 239–244
    history of, 239

indications and contraindications for,
        239–240
    outcomes and future directions for, 244
    rehabilitation after, 244
    surgical techniques for, 240–243, 242f
    technical alternatives and pitfalls of, 243–244
Varus-valgus constraint, 217
Vascular access channels, in arthroscopic
        meniscal repair, 7
Vastus medialis oblique (VMO) muscle transfer,
        in patellar instability repair, 135, 135f

W
Whiteside's line, 227
Wound coverage, after total knee replacement,
        280–290
    free flaps for, 280–281, 286–289, 286f–289f
    free-tissue transfers for, 281
    gracilis muscle flap for, 280–281
    history of, 280
    indications and contraindications for,
        280–281, 281f
    lateral gastrocnemius muscle transposition
        flap for, 280, 285–286, 285f
    latissimus dorsi muscle flap for, 281
    medial gastrocnemius muscle transposition
        flap for, 280, 282–285, 282f–284f
    outcomes of, 289
    pitfalls of, 289
    rectus abdominis muscle transfer for,
        286–288, 286f–289f
    rehabilitation after, 289
    soft-tissue expanders for, 281